Zoo and Wild Mammal Formulary

Zoo and Wild Mammal Formulary

Alicia Hahn, DVM, DACZM
Pittsburgh Zoo & PPG Aquarium, Pittsburgh, Pennsylvania, USA

WILEY Blackwell

This edition first published 2019

Registered Office
John Wiley & Sons, Inc., 111 River Street, Hoboken, NJ 07030, USA

Editorial Office
111 River Street, Hoboken, NJ 07030, USA

For details of our global editorial offices, customer services, and more information about Wiley products visit us at www.wiley.com.

Wiley also publishes its books in a variety of electronic formats and by print-on-demand. Some content that appears in standard print versions of this book may not be available in other formats.

Library of Congress Cataloging-in-Publication Data

Names: Hahn, Alicia, author.
Title: Zoo and wild mammal formulary / Alicia Hahn.
Description: Hoboken, NJ : Wiley-Blackwell, 2019. | Includes bibliographical references and index. |
Identifiers: LCCN 2019011595 (print) | LCCN 2019012922 (ebook) | ISBN 9781119514893 (Adobe PDF) | ISBN 9781119515081 (ePub) | ISBN 9781119515050 (paperback)
Subjects: | MESH: Veterinary Drugs | Mammals | Animals, Zoo | Animals, Wild | Drug Therapy–veterinary | Formulary
Classification: LCC SF916.5 (ebook) | LCC SF916.5 .H34 2019 (print) | NLM SF 916.5 | DDC 636.089/51–dc23
LC record available at https://lccn.loc.gov/2019011595

Cover Design: Wiley
Cover Image: © Paul A. Selvaggio

Set in 10/12pt Warnock by SPi Global, Pondicherry, India
Printed and bound in Singapore by Markono Print Media Pte Ltd

10 9 8 7 6 5 4 3 2 1

Contents

Preface

This book was born out of a clinical need voiced by myself and my many colleagues in Zoo, Exotic, and Wildlife medicine. For a number of years, I have been needing a resource similar to the *Exotic Animal Formulary* by Dr Carpenter, but for Zoo and Wild mammals. I hoped "someone" would write such a book, but eventually out of frustration elected to pursue it myself. In all honesty this was a naïve undertaking, as I had no idea how many hundreds of hours would be required to compile all this data. However, it has all been worth it, since it has already come in handy for treating many of my own institution's cases.

I find as a busy zoo clinician that I often don't have the time or access to find drug doses used in every species or track down the original paper citing such a dose. As such, like many of you, I have to extrapolate from domestic animals.

To answer this need, I compiled data from textbooks, peer-reviewed literature, relevant proceedings and personal communications. Wherever able I indicated how many animals and in what capacity the drug was used. I wanted to provide you as a clinician with as much confidence as possible when treating your cases. This is with the acknowledgement, however, that the literature available for some species is limited to n = 1 case reports. In addition, I prevailed upon the generosity of my esteemed colleagues for editing data and contributing doses that have been successful for them. Average weights for relevant species are also listed at the end of each chapter.

I included images of White-bellied tree pangolins on the cover of this formulary. This was an effort to highlight that pangolins are the most trafficked species in the world. Over one million have been killed in recent years for their scales and meat, and they are thus critically endangered. I am thankful to be a part of the US Pangolin Consortium and for the opportunity to work with this amazing species. I hope that increased awareness of their plight and the hard work of many people with in-situ research and rehabilitation, combined with research and support in captive collections, will help this imperiled animal.

I hope to continue with further editions of this formulary and welcome any constructive criticism for improvement or ideas for including additional data in the future.

In the end, I hope this formulary will be helpful for you and your patients!

Acknowledgments

This book would not have been possible without the support of my husband, family, friends and colleagues. Jennifer Hicks, you are a creative genius, and I so appreciate all of your help and ideas! I want to thank Paul Selvaggio for the use of his amazing pangolin photographs. Also, thank you very much to my co-editors and contributors. I really appreciate you devoting your precious time to these chapters! And finally, thank you to Wiley-Blackwell and my publishing team for your support and having faith in me and my idea.

List of Reviewers

Elizabeth Arnett-Chin, DVM
Staff Veterinarian
Naples Zoo at Caribbean Gardens, Naples, FL, USA

Anne Burgdorf-Moisuk, DVM, DACZM
Director of Animal Health
Great Plains Zoo and Delbridge Museum of Natural History, Sioux Falls, SD, USA

A. Margarita Woc Colburn, DVM
Associate Veterinarian
Nashville Zoo at Grassmere, Nashville, TN, USA

Gretchen A. Cole, DVM, DACZM, ECZM (ZHM)
Associate Veterinarian
Oklahoma City Zoo and Botanical Garden, Oklahoma City, OK, USA

Shannon Cerveny, DVM, DACZM
Staff Veterinarian
St. Louis Zoo, St Louis, MO, USA

Jennifer D'Agostino, DVM, DACZM
Director of Veterinary Services
Oklahoma City Zoo and Botanical Garden, Oklahoma City, OK, USA

Michelle Davis, DVM, DACZM, DECZM (ZHM)
Senior Veterinarian & Clinical Residency Coordinator
Georgia Aquarium, Atlanta, GA, USA

Gabriella L. Flacke, DVM, MVSc, PhD
Associate Veterinarian
Zoo Miami, Department of Animal Health, Miami, FL, USA

Amanda Guthrie, DVM, DACZM, DECZM
Senior Veterinary Officer
ZSL London Zoo, London, UK

Elizabeth E. Hammond, DVM, DACZM, DECZM (ZHM)
Senior Veterinarian
Lion Country Safari, Loxahatchee, FL, USA

James G. Johnson III, DVM, MS, CertAqV, DACZM
Associate Veterinarian
Zoo Miami, Miami, FL, USA

Jennifer Kilburn, DVM
Associate Veterinarian
Tulsa Zoo, Tulsa, OK, USA

R. Scott Larsen, DVM, MS, DACZM
Vice President of Veterinary Medicine
Denver Zoo, Denver, CO, USA

Michele A. Miller, DVM, MPH, PhD, DECZM (ZHM)
National Research Foundation South African Research Chair in Animal TB, Cape Town, South Africa
DST/NRF Centre of Excellence for Biomedical Tuberculosis Research, Cape Town, South Africa
SAMRC Centre for Molecular and Cellular Biology, Division of Molecular Biology and Human Genetics, Cape Town, South Africa
Faculty of Medicine and Health Sciences, Stellenbosch University, Cape Town, South Africa

Adrian Mutlow, MA, VetMB, MSc, MRCVS
Clinical Veterinarian
San Francisco Zoological Society, San Francisco, CA, USA

Hendrik Nollens, DVM, MSc, PhD
Vice President of Animal Health
SeaWorld Parks, Orlando, FL, USA

Luis R. Padilla, DVM, DACZM
Director of Animal Health
St. Louis Zoo, St Louis, MO, USA

Kristen Phair, DVM, DACZM
Associate Veterinarian
Phoenix Zoo, Phoenix, AZ, USA

Kimberly L. Rainwater, DVM
Associate Veterinarian
Fort Worth Zoo, Fort Worth, TX, USA

Rodney Schnellbacher, DVM, DACZM
Staff Veterinarian, Animal Health
Dickerson Park Zoo, Springfield, MO, USA

Ginger Sturgeon, DVM
Director of Animal Health
Pittsburgh Zoo & PPG Aquarium, Pittsburgh, PA, USA

Julie Swenson, DVM, DACZM
Associate Veterinarian
Fossil Rim Wildlife Center, Glen Rose, TX, USA

Allison D. Tuttle, DVM, DACZM
Vice President of Biological Programs
Mystic Aquarium, Mystic, CT, USA

Trevor T. Zachariah, DVM, MS, DACZM
Director of Veterinary Programs
Brevard Zoo Sea Turtle Healing Center, Melbourne, FL, USA

List of Abbreviations

BID	twice daily or every 12 hours
EOD	every other day or every 48 hours
d	days, i.e. 8d is 8 days
IC	intracoelomic
IM	intramuscular
IV	intravenous
PO	per os or by mouth
q	every, i.e. q8d is every 8 days
QID	four times daily or every six hours
SID	once daily
TID	three times daily, or every eight hours
TO	topical administration

1

Platypus and Echidnas

Drug name	Drug dose	Species	Comments
Antimicrobials and Antifungals			
Amoxicillin/clavulanic acid	20 mg/kg IM SID or PO BID [1]	Echidnas	
	12.5 mg/kg IM SID [2]	Platypus	
Amphotericin B	0.5 mg/kg injected intralesionally twice weekly [3]	Platypus	For ulcerative mycosis of *Mucor amphibiorum*.
Ceftazidime	65 mg/kg IM SID [1]	Echidnas	
Doxycycline	5 mg/kg PO SID [1]	Echidnas	
Enrofloxacin	5 mg/kg SC or PO SID [1]	Echidnas	
	5 mg/kg IM SID [1]	Platypus	
Itraconazole	5 mg/kg PO SID [1]	Echidnas	
Metronidazole	20 mg/kg IV SC PO SID [1]	Echidnas	
Nystatin	10 000 IU/kg BID [1]	Echidnas	
	Ointment applied topically [1]	Echidnas	
Oxytetracycline	20 mg/kg IM SID [1]	Echidnas	
Penicillin with benzathine	10 mg/kg IM SC SID [1]	Echidnas	
Procaine penicillin	15 mg/kg IM, SC SID [1]	Echidnas	
Trimethoprim sulfadiazine	5 mg/kg IM SID [1, 2]	Echidnas and Platypus	
Analgesic			
Buprenorphine	1 mg/kg IV IM SID [1]	Echidnas	Analgesia
Butorphanol	0.1 mg/kg IV IM BID [1]	Echidnas	
Flunixin meglumine	0.5 mg/kg IM SC IV SID [1]	Echidnas	
Ketoprofen	1 mg/kg IV IM SC SID [1]	Echidnas	
Meloxicam	0.2 mg/kg SC or PO SID [1]	Echidnas	
	0.5 IV mg/kg SC SID [1]	Echidnas	

(*Continued*)

Zoo and Wild Mammal Formulary, First Edition. Alicia Hahn.

Drug name	Drug dose	Species	Comments
Anesthetic			
Atipamezole HCl	0.5 mg/kg IM [1]	Echidnas	
Diazepam	1–5 mg/kg IM [1]	Echidnas	Sedation
	0.5–1.0 mg/kg IM [2]	Platypus	Sedation for minor procedures.
Ether	Mask induction [4]	Platypus	n = 2 wild caught animals briefly anesthetized for transponder placement and blood draw to analyze blood sample appeared to induce leukocytosis.
Isoflurane	Mask induction [2]	Platypus	Rarely have injectables been used, rather induction with a face mask via isoflurane is usually employed.
Ketamine + medetomidine	K: 5 mg/kg + M: 0.5 mg/kg IM, antagonize with 2.5 mg/kg atipamezole [1, 3, 5]	Echidnas	
	K: 5 mg/kg + M: 0.3 mg/kg IM [1]	Echidnas	
Ketamine + xylazine	K: 5–10 mg/kg + X: 1–2 mg/kg IM, antagonize with 0.1 mg/kg yohimbine IV [1, 3, 5]	Echidnas	
Pentobarbitol	200 mg/kg IV [6]	Echidnas	Euthanasia.
Telazol	3–10 mg/kg IM [1]	Echidnas	
Antiparasitic			
Fipronil	10 mg/kg Topical, once [1]	Echidnas	
Ivermectin	0.2 mg/kg SC [1, 2]	Echidnas and Platypus	To treat acariasis.
Moxidectin	0.2 mg/kg IM SC q7d[1]	Echidnas	
Praziquantel	5 mg/kg IM PO once [1]	Echidnas	
Selamectin	Topical application [3]	Echidnas	To treat acariasis.
Toltrazuril	20 mg/kg PO SID × 2d [1, 3]	Echidnas	To treat coccidiosis.
Other			
Bromhexine HCl	1 mg/kg PO TID [1]	Echidnas	To use as a mucolytic.
Dexamethasone	0.2 mg/kg IM SC SID [1]	Echidnas	
Formic acid	2% in food at 2% [1]	Echidnas	
Phytomenadione	0.1 mg/kg PO [1]	Echidnas	

Species	Weights
Echidna *(Tachyglosss aculeatus)*	2.5–6 kg
Duck-billed platypus *(Orinthorynchus anatinus)*	0.2–2 kg

References

1 Vogelnest, L. and Woods, R. (2008). Echidna. In: *Medicine of Australian Mammals* (ed. L. Vogelnest and R. Woods), 77–102. Victoria, Australia: Csiro Publishing.
2 Vogelnest, L. and Woods, R. (2008). Platypus. In: *Medicine of Australian Mammals* (ed. L. Vogelnest and R. Woods), 77–102. Victoria, Australia: Csiro Publishing.
3 Holz, P. (2015). Monotremata (Echidna, Platypus). In: *Fowler's Zoo and Wild Animal Medicine*, vol. 8 (ed. R.E. Miller and M. Fowler), 247–254. St. Louis, MO: Elsevier Saunders.
4 Whittington, R.J. and Grant, T.R. (1995). Hencalotopic changes in the platypus (*Orinthorynchus anatinus*) following capture. *Journal of Wildlife Diseases* 31 (3): 386–390.
5 Holz, P. (2014). Monotremes (Echidna and Platypus). In: *Zoo Animal and Wild Immobilization and Anesthesia* (ed. G. West, D. Heard and N. Caulkett), 517–520. Ames, IA: Wiley Blackwell.
6 Whittington, R., Middleton, D., Spratt, D.M. et al. (1992). Spayenosis in the montremes *Tachyglosss aculeatus* and *Orinthorynchus anatinus* in Australia. *Journal of Wildlife Diseases* 28 (4): 636–640.

2

Marsupials

Drug name	Drug dose	Species	Comments
Antimicrobials and Antifungals			
Macropods			In macropods dysbiosis has been reported after oral administration of antibiotics, particularly penicillins [1].
Amoxicillin (long-acting)	20 mg/kg IM q48 hrs [2]	Macropods	Intractable animals with severe dental disease.
Amoxicillin trihydrate	10 mg/kg IM [3]	Tammar wallabies	n = 5 pharmacokinetic evaluation showed minimum inhibitory concentration breakpoint (0.25 μg/ml) for *Staph* and *Strep* species for 8 hr and only exceeded 2 μg/ml for 2 hr, but the MIC breakpoint for *Enterobacteria* and *Enterococci* was not reached.
Azithromycin	15 mg/kg PO SID × 10d [4]	Eastern gray kangaroos	Oral necrobacillosis treatment.
Atovaquone	100 mg/kg PO SID [2]	Macropods	For treatment of toxoplasmosis, combine with canola oil to enhance absorption.
Ceftiofur	2 mg/kg IM SID 7–10d [2]	Macropods	For the empiric treatment/ suspicion of salmonellosis if susceptibility results are not available.
Ceftiofur sodium	1–2 mg/kg IM or IV SID [2]	Macropods	To treat bacterial pneumonia of susceptible infections.
Ceftiofur crystalline free acid (Excede)	4.3 mg/kg IV intraoperatively, IV BID postoperatively [5]	Bennett's wallabies	n = 1. 4 yr old male wallaby who suffered traumatic cervical spinal fracture and received intraoperative antibiotics.

(*Continued*)

Zoo and Wild Mammal Formulary, First Edition. Alicia Hahn.

Drug name	Drug dose	Species	Comments
Clindamycin	11 mg/kg PO BID [2]	Macropods	Necrobacillosis, toxoplasmosis, and for severe periodontal disease, alone or in combination with metronidazole 20 mg/kg PO BID or oxytetracycline 40 mg/kg IM q48 hr, continued until complete resolution of lesions. Up to 30 days treatment for toxoplasmosis. May result in a dysbiosis (author's experience in one animal).
	17–21 mg/kg IV BID for 40–55d [6]	Red-necked wallabies	n = 1 captive-born Red-necked wallaby, treated with clindamycin and benzathine penicillin G long term for mandibular osteomyelitis.
Enilconazole	Weekly topical baths [2]	Macropods, tractable or readily anesthetized	For the treatment of dermatophytosis.
Enrofloxacin	5 mg/kg SC or PO SID [2]	Macropods	For susceptible infections.
Fluconazole	10–20 mg/kg PO BID [2]	Macropods	For the treatment of cryptococcosis until serum testing is negative.
Gentamicin + amoxicillin	G: 4–7 mg/kg IM BID + A: 10 mg/kg IM TID [2]	Macropods	For severe cases of pneumonia in pouch young.
Griseofulvin	5–10 mg/kg PO BID administered until 2 wks after the cessation of clinical signs [2]	Macropods	For the treatment of dermatophytosis. At the higher end of dosing, diarrhea, and neurological signs have been seen after only 1 wk of treatment.
Itraconazole	5 mg/kg PO SID administered until 2 wks after resolution of signs [2]	Macropods	For the treatment of dermatophytosis and candidiasis in pouch young. Pulse therapy of 5 mg/kg PO SID for 1 wk then off for 2 wks for a total of 12 weeks has also been successful.
	20–40 mg/kg PO SID [2]	Macropods	For the treatment of cryptococcosis until serum testing is negative.
Metronidazole	20 mg/kg PO BID [2]	Wallaroos, Macropods	For the treatment/suspicion of gastric amoebiasis. Also for anaerobic infections. Often unpalatable.
Miconazole	Topical SID to BID [2]	Macropods	For the treatment of dermatophytosis.
Nystatin cream	Topical [2]	Macropods	For the treatment of candidiasis.

Drug name	Drug dose	Species	Comments
Nystatin	5000–5010 000 IU/kg PO TID for 3–5d [2]	Hand reared Macropods	For the treatment of candidiasis in milk for oral cavity, esophageal and gastric lesions. Higher doses may result in diarrhea. itraconazole 5 mg/kg PO SID × 5d has also been used.
Oxytetracycline	40 mg/kg IM, IV q48 h [2, 7, 8]	Macropods	For susceptible infections. Pharmacokinetic parameters in Tammar wallabies comparable to those reported for eutherians of equivalent size; allometric scaling for marsupials may not be valid. In Red-necked wallabies (n = 3), elimination half-life is 11.4 h.
Oxytetracycline (long-acting, LA 200)	20 mg/kg IM, IV q72 hrs for 7–21d [2, 8]	Macropods	For the treatment of dermatophilosis. Topical povidone iodine solution is an alternative. Also helpful with intractable animals with severe periodontal disease. Pharmacokinetic parameters of oxytetracycline in Tammar wallabies comparable to those reported for eutherians of equivalent size; allometric scaling for marsupials may not be valid; questionable therapeutic efficacy based on plasma concentrations.
Procaine penicillin/ Benzathine penicillin G	25–30 mg/kg IM q48 hrs [2, 8]	Macropods	For bacterial infections. Also for the treatment of tetanus in addition to boostering tetanus toxoid.
Procaine penicillin/ Benzathine penicillin	80 000 U/kg SC BID × 150d [6]	Red-necked wallabies	n = 1 captive born Red-necked wallaby, Treated with clindamycin and benzathine penicillin G long term for mandibular osteomyelitis.
Penicillin G procaine	20 000 U/kg SC SID [9]	Red kangaroos	n = 1 case of an 8 yr old male red kangaroo with 2 wk history of vomiting, mesenteric volvulus diagnosis.
Sodium penicillin G	30 mg/kg IV [8]	Tammar wallabies	Pharmacokinetic parameters in Tammar wallabies comparable to those reported for eutherians of equivalent size; allometric scaling for marsupials may not be valid.
Terbinafine	Topical SID to BID [2]	Macropods	For the treatment of dermatophytosis.

(*Continued*)

Drug name	Drug dose	Species	Comments
Tulathromycin	2.5 mg/kg SC, IM q7d [2]	Macropods	Registered for respiratory infections in pigs and cattle. Has been used in macropods without adverse effects.
Koalas and Wombats			Parenteral oxytetracycline and oral erythromycin have resulted in wasting and death within 2–6 weeks in Koalas. Nystatin may induce diarrhea at higher doses [1].
Amoxicillin	10 mg/kg PO, SC, IM BID [2]	Koalas	For susceptible infections.
Amoxicillin/ clavulanic acid (Clavamox)	12.5 mg/kg PO, SC, IM BID [2]	Koalas	Some clinicians avoid PO route.
Amphotericin B + an oral triazole	A: 0.5 mg/kg in 300 ml 2.5% dextrose and 0.45% NaCl, given SC twice weekly + itraconazole 100 mg/ day PO or fluconazole 50–100 mg PO BID [2]	Koalas	Treatment of cryptococcal lesions (nasal, lower respiratory, and central nervous system disease).
Ampicillin	5–10 mg/kg IV TID-QID [2]	Koalas	For the treatment of septicemia in combination with gentamicin.
Ceftazidime	15 mg/kg SC IM BID [2]	Koalas	Bacterial infections, particularly useful for *Pseudomonas aeruginosa*.
Chloramine 0.3–0.6%	Daily topical application [2]	Koalas	For treatment of dermatophytosis.
Chloramphenicol	30 mg/kg SC BID × 10–14d beyond resolution of clinical signs [2]	Koalas	For treatment of chlamydiosis.
	60 mg/kg SC SID [2, 10, 11]	Koalas	For anti-chlamydial therapy, for 45 days. In study with 9 koalas, controlled mild chlamydial infection and prevented shedding, but severe urogenital disease did not respond to this chloramphenicol regimen [11]. In study of 19 koalas, pharmacokinetics data do not support current dosing regimen for chlamydiosis [10].
Chloramphenicol 10 mg/g with Hydrocortisone acetate 5 mg/g	topical ocular instillation [2]	Koalas	For chlamydial keratoconjunctivitis.

Drug name	Drug dose	Species	Comments
Ciprofloxacin	10 mg/kg PO BID [2]	Koalas	For anti-chlamydial therapy.
Enrofloxacin	6 mg/kg IV SID-BID [2]	Koalas	For susceptible infections. Increased frequency of dosing for serious infections. Can be given in combination with metronidazole and cephalosporin for broad antibacterial coverage.
	5–10 mg/kg PO or SC SID [2, 12]	Koalas	For anti-chlamydial therapy. A pharmacokinetics study (n = 43) indicates that Enrofloxacin doses of 10 mg/kg SC, 5 mg/kg SC, or 20 mg/kg PO and marbofloxacin doses 1–3.3 mg/kg PO, 10 mg/kg PO, or 5 mg/kg SC are unlikely to inhibit growth of chlamydial pathogens *in vivo*.
Fluconazole	6 mg/kg loading dose then 3 mg/kg PO SID × 14d [2]	Koalas	n = 1 with diarrhea due to *Candida* infection, treated for 14 days and resolved.
Fluconazole	50–100 mg per koala PO BID [2]	Koalas	Nasopharyngeal cryptococcosis.
Gentamicin sulfate + ampicillin	2–4 mg/kg IV + A: 5–10 mg/kg IV [2]	Koalas	After this initial dose gentamicin at 2–4 mg/kg IM or SC q8 hr, and ampicillin at 5–10 mg/kg IV q6 hr. Stagger IV administration of the two drugs.
Gentamicin sulfate	2 mg/kg to 2–3 ml saline nebulization [2]	Koalas	Respiratory tract infection treatment.
Griseofulvin	100 mg PO SID for 4 months [2]	Koalas	n = 1 animal with a fungal paronychial infection that resolved.
Hexamine (methenamine) hippurate	250 mg/koala PO SID [2]	Adult Queensland koalas	For the treatment of cystitis.
Itraconazole (10 mg/ml oral solution)	Pulse therapy of 5 mg/kg PO SID for 1 wk, stop for 2 weeks then repeat for 12 weeks [2]	Koalas	For treatment of dermatophytosis.
	100 mg/koala PO SID [2]	Koalas	Cryptococcosis.
Ketoconazole	10 mg/kg PO × 7d [2]	Koalas	Antifungal.
Metronidazole	20–25 mg/kg IV slowly BID [2]	Koalas	Anaerobic infections.
Nystatin	5000–10 000 IU/kg PO TID [2]	Koalas	Oral candidiasis.

(*Continued*)

Drug name	Drug dose	Species	Comments
	10 000–20 000 IU/kg PO TID × 7d [2]	Koalas	To treat mycotic diarrhea.
Ofloxacin (3 mg/ml)	Topical ocular instillation [2]	Koalas	Chlamydial conjunctivitis.
Oxytetracycline HCl 18.5 mg/ml + oleandomycin phosphate 10 mg/ml + neomycin sulfate 10 mg/ml	Topical ocular instillation [2]	Koalas	Chlamydial conjunctivitis.
Oxytetracycline 5 mg/g + polymixin B 10000 U/g	Topical ocular instillation [2]	Koalas	Chlamydial conjunctivitis.
Procaine penicillin/ Benzathine penicillin G	26.5 mg/kg SC IM q72 hrs [2]	Koalas	Bacterial infections.
Terbinafine cream	Topically on lesion SID [2]	Koalas	Dermatophytosis.
Ticarcillin sodium	45–50 mg/kg IV q4–6 hr [2]	Koalas	Serious infection.
Trimethoprim sulfadiazine	30 mg/kg PO BID [2]	Koalas	
Trimethoprim sulfamethoxazole	15 mg/kg PO BID [2]	Koalas	
Dasyurids and Numbats			
Amikacin	3 mg/kg BID [2]	Dasyurids	For treatment of granulomatous dermatitis.
	7.5 mg/kg IM BID × 6d, then 7.5 mg/kg IM BID × 10d, 6 wks later [2]	Numbats	Bacterial dermatitis.
Amoxicillin/ clavulanic acid (Clavamox)	12.5 mg/kg PO BID added to food, 8.75 mg/kg SC SID for 3–5d [2]	Numbats	Salmonella enteritis treatment.
Azithromycin	20 mg/kg SID [2]	Dasyurids	Mycobacteriosis; treatment is difficult, prolonged, and usually unsuccessful.
Enrofloxacin	2.5 mg/kg BID [2]	Dasyurids	For treatment of granulomatous dermatitis.
Ethambutol	20 mg/kg SID [2]	Dasyurids	Mycobacteriosis; treatment is difficult, prolonged, and usually unsuccessful.
Myambutol	20 mg/kg SID [2]	Dasyurids	Mycobacteriosis; treatment is difficult, prolonged, and usually unsuccessful.
Rifabutin	20 mg/kg SID [2]	Dasyurids	For treatment of granulomatous dermatitis.

Drug name	Drug dose	Species	Comments
Trimethoprim sulfamethoxazole	10 mg/kg of trimethoprim PO BID × 14d [2]	Numbats	Salmonella enteritis treatment.
Possums, Gliders, and American opossums			Subadult Ringtail possums *(Pseuocheirus peregrinus)* appear to be particularly sensitive to antibiotics, with dysbiosis, wasting and death seen [1, 2].
Amoxicillin/ clavulanic acid	20 mg/kg SC, IM SID to BID up to 4 weeks [2]	Possums, Common brushtails	Exudative dermatitis.
	12.5–20 mg/kg SC BID for 3–5d [2]	Common ringtails and Common brushtails	
Clindamycin	11 mg/kg BID for 2–3 wks [2]	Possums	Treating dental disease.
	10–15 mg/kg PO BID up to 4 weeks [2]	Possums	Toxoplasmosis.
	10 mg/kg PO BID for 7–10d [2]	Yellow-bellied gliders	
Doxycycline	5 mg/kg initially then 2.5 mg/kg PO SID for 3–5d [2]	Common ringtails	
Enrofloxacin	5 mg/kg SC SID × 5d [2]	Common ringtails	
Nystatin	5000–10 000 U/kg TID × 5d [2]		To prevent secondary fungal or yeast overgrowth during antibiotic therapy.
	10 000 U/kg PO TID × 7d [2]		To treat oral candidiasis.
Procaine penicillin with benzathine penicillin	Procaine 150 mg/ml and benzathene 112.5 mg/ml used a 1 ml/10 kg q48 hr repeated 2–3 times [2]	Common brushtails	
Bandicoots and Bilbies			
Amoxicillin	20 mg/kg IM or SC SID or PO BID [2]		Rarely used since amoxicillin/ clavulanic acid is available.
Amoxicillin/ clavulanic acid (Clavamox)	12.5 mg/kg SC SID or PO BID [2]		Commonly used as first choice for minor wounds.
Ceftazidime	15 mg/kg IM BID [2]	Bandicoots	Used for complicated toe infections.
Cephalexin	20–30 mg/kg PO BID [2]		
Clindamycin	11 mg/kg PO BID [2]		Periodontal disease and toe infections.

(*Continued*)

Drug name	Drug dose	Species	Comments
Doxycycline	5 mg/kg PO loading dose, 2.5 mg/kg PO BID × 2 doses, then SID [2]		Likely to be useful.
Enrofloxacin	5 mg/kg PO or IM BID [2]		
Metronidazole	50 mg/kg PO SID [2]		
Trimethoprim/ sulfamethoxazole	15 mg/kg PO BID [2]		
Analgesia			
Macropods			
Buprenorphine	0.01–0.05 mg/kg SC or IM TID [2]	Macropods	
Butorphanol	0.4 mg/kg SC or IM [2]	Macropods	
Carprofen	2–4 mg/kg SC SID [2]	Macropods	
Flunixin meglumine	0.5–1 mg/kg IM or IV SID × 3d [2, 9]	Macropods	
Ketoprofen	2 mg/kg SC SID [2]	Macropods	
Meloxicam	0.2 mg/kg SC or PO SID [2]	Macropods	
Tolfenamic acid	4 mg/kg SC q48 hrs [2]	Macropods	Good for intractable animals due to dosing interval.
Koalas and Wombats			Avoid rump for IM injections in wombats due to sacral plate [1]
Buprenorphine hydrochloride	0.01 mg/kg SC or IM BID [2, 13]	Koalas	n = 5 institutions responding to a survey about analgesics used in koalas in Australia (dosage range 0.01–0.05 mg/kg with 0.01 mg/kg the most common dosage).
Acetaminophen (paracetamol) ± codeine	15 mg/kg PO SID to BID [2, 13]	Koalas	n = 4 institutions responding to a survey about analgesics used in koalas in Australia (dosage range reported 10–15 mg/kg acetaminophen) to provide interim analgesia in washout period between different NSAIDS or when switching between corticosteroid and NSAID.
Butorphanol tartrate	0.2 mg/kg IM, SC, IV [2, 13]	Koalas	n = 3 institutions responding to a survey about analgesics used in koalas in Australia. Dosage range reported as 0.1–0.4 mg/kg.
Carprofen	4 mg/kg PO SID to BID for 24 hr then 2 mg/kg PO SID after [2, 13]	Koalas	Some advise maximum 4d duration to reduce risk of gastrointestinal tract ulceration. Do not give with corticosteroids.

Drug name	Drug dose	Species	Comments
Fentanyl	5ug/kg IV bolus then 3ug/kg/hr IV infusion [2, 13]	Koalas	Intraoperative and postoperative pain management. n = 1 institution responding to a survey about analgesics used in koalas in Australia.
Flunixin meglumine	1 mg/kg SC IM IV SID for 1–3d [2]	Koalas	
Lidocaine	<1 mg/kg as regional infusion [13]	Koalas	Local anesthetic. n = 2 institutions responding to a survey about analgesics used in koalas in Australia. Variable efficacy reported.
Meloxicam	0.1–0.2 mg/kg PO, SC, IV SID [2, 14]	Koalas	Oral bioavailability is negligible. Parenteral route recommended. Pharmacokinetics study indicates SID dosing may be insufficient, but this requires further investigation regarding safety.
	0.075–0.4 mg/kg (suggested 0.1–0.2 mg/kg IM SC PO) [13, 14]	Koalas	n = 11 institutions responding to a survey about analgesics used in koalas in Australia. Oral bioavailability is negligible. Parenteral route recommended. Higher end of dosage range may be more effective.
Meperidine	1 mg/kg q4–8 h IM [13]	Koalas	n = 1 institution responding to a survey about analgesics used in koalas in Australia. Less potent than morphine, but faster onset. Give IM as SC route can cause local tissue irritation/pain. IV route can cause histamine release.
Methadone	0.25–0.5 mg/kg SC or IM q4–6 hrs [2, 13]	Koalas	n = 5 institutions responding to a survey about analgesics used in koalas in Australia. Moderate to severe pain. Titrate dose according to response.
Pethidine (aka meperidine)	1 mg/kg SC IM or IV q4–8 hrs [2, 13]	Koalas	Mild to moderate pain.
Tramadol	0.2–4 mg/kg PO [13]	Koala	n = 3 institutions responding to a survey about analgesics used in koalas in Australia.
Dasyurids, Possums, Gliders, and American opossums			
Buprenorphine	0.005–0.01 mg/kg SC or IV BID [2]	Possums and Gliders	

(*Continued*)

Drug name	Drug dose	Species	Comments
	0.01 mg/kg SC once [15]	Opossums	n = 1 North American opossum undergoing scrotal ablation given as premedication with midazolam 10 minutes prior to chamber induction with isoflurane.
Butorphanol	0.4 mg/kg SC or IM [2]	Possums and Gliders	
Butorphanol tartrate	0.5 mg/kg IM once [15]	Sugar gliders	n = 5 sugar gliders undergoing scrotal ablation. Dose given 5–10 minutes prior to chamber induction with isoflurane.
Carprofen	4 mg/kg SC once [2]	Possums and Gliders	
	3 mg/kg SC SID × 3d [2]	Numbats	
Ketoprofen	1 mg/kg SC SID × 5d [2]	Numbats	
Meloxicam	0.2 mg/kg PO or SC followed by 0.1 mg/kg PO SID × 5d [2]	Possums and Gliders	
	0.2 mg/kg SC once, then 0.1–0.2 mg/kg PO SID × 6d [2]	Numbats	
	0.2 mg/kg SC once, then PO × 3d [15]	Sugar gliders, Opossums	n = 5 sugar gliders and n = 1 opossum undergoing scrotal ablation treated for postoperative pain.
Tolfenamic acid	4 mg/kg SC SID × 5d [2]	Possums and Gliders	
Bandicoots and Bilbies			
Buprenorphine	0.01 mg/kg SC or IM BID [2]	Bandicoots and Bilbies	Has been used intra-and postoperatively.
Carprofen	2 mg/kg SC/PO BID [2]	Bandicoots and Bilbies	
Meloxicam	0.3 mg/kg PO followed by 0.1 mg/kg PO SID × 5d [2]	Bandicoots and Bilbies	
Anesthesia and Sedation			
Macropods			
Alfaxalone (alphaxalone)	5–8 mg/kg IM or 1.5–3 mg/kg IV [1, 2, 16]	Macropods	Sedation, very short duration of action. Useful for induction prior to inhalant anesthetic use. Better in tame animals.

Drug name	Drug dose	Species	Comments
Alphaxalone + alphadolone combo solution (Althesin)	(In solution: ALX: 9 mg/ml and ALD: 3 mg/ml) Give 0.25 ml-0.5 ml/kg IV to effect [17]	Macropods and phalangers	Short duration, can top up, recover fast.
Alfaxalone + medetomidine	A: 4 mg/kg + M: 0.1 mg/kg; antagonized with atipamezole 0.5 mg/kg half IV and half IM if necessary [16, 18]	Semi-free-ranging Bennett's wallabies	n = 26 adult animals split into two groups receiving AM or 0.1 mg/kg medetomidine + 5 mg/kg ketamine IM in a 3 ml dart. Induction and maintenance satisfactory for both, no significant differences, both had bradycardia, and mean cloacal temperature was lower in the AM group.
Azaperone	1–2 mg/kg IM [1, 2, 16]	Macropods	Sedation, onset in 15–20 min duration of 3–8 hours.
	2–4 mg/kg IM [17]	Large macropods	Tranquilization.
Diazepam	0.1–2 mg/kg IM or 0.1–1 mg/kg IV [1, 2, 16]	Macropods	Sedation, duration of 1–2 hours. If necessary can antagonize with flumazenil 1 mg per 25 mg benzodiazepine. As little as 0.1 mg/kg in wild brush-tailed rock wallaby *(Petrogale penicillata).* Better to overdose than underdose. Oral administration very unreliable and not recommended.
Diazepam	2–4 mg/kg IM or IV [17]	All Marsupials	Tranquilization or anticonvulsant.
Fluphenazine decanoate	2.5 mg/kg IM [1, 2]	Macropods	Sedation, duration of 10 days.
Haloperidol decanoate	4–6 mg/kg IM [1, 2]	Macropods	Sedation, duration unknown, possibly up to 30 days.
Isoflurane		Macropods	Immobilization, induction, maintenance, or both [1].
Ketamine	K: 5–25 mg/kg IM [2]	Macropods	Inferior quality of immobilization compared to Telazol.
	K: 5 mg/kg IM [19]	Matschie's tree kangaroos *(Dendrolagus matschiei)*	
	K: 9 mg/kg IM [19]	Eastern gray kangaroos	
Ketamine + dexmedetomidine	K: 5 mg/kg + D: 0.05 mg/kg IM [16]	Bennett's wallabies	

(*Continued*)

Drug name	Drug dose	Species	Comments
Ketamine + medetomidine	K: 5 mg/kg + M: 0.1 mg/kg [16]	Macropods (docile Red kangaroos, Western gray kangaroos, Bennett's wallabies). Did not work for Eastern gray kangaroos, pademelons, or Parma wallabies.	KM combo provides superior relaxation compared to Telazol, but longer induction times,.
	K: 5 mg/kg + M: 0.1 mg/kg IM. Antagonize with atipamezole 4–5 × the medetomidine dose [1, 2]	Macropods	Immobilization, use higher doses in nervous or excited animals. Less salivation than Telazol combinations. Recovery to standing 30 minutes after antagonist administration [2].
	K: 4 mg/kg + M: 0.04 mg/kg IM. Antagonize with atipamezole 0.2 mg/kg IM [2]	Eastern gray kangaroos	Provided safe and reliable anesthesia. Atipamezole administration at least 30 minutes after ketamine injection to improve recovery quality [2].
	K: 5 mg/kg + M: 0.05 mg/kg IM. Antagonize with atipamezole 0.2 mg/kg [19]	Eastern gray kangaroos	Supplement with ketamine 2–5 mg/kg as needed. Give atipamezole >30 minutes after last ketamine dose.
	K: 4–7 mg/kg + M: 0.04–0.07 mg/kg IM; antagonize with atipamezole at 5 × the medetomidine dose in mg [17]	Most kangaroo species	
	K: 4.3–6.6 mg/kg + M: 0.036–0.064 mg/kg IM. Antagonized with atipamezole 0.21–0.33 mg/kg IM [20]	Bennett's wallabies	n = 14 animals divided into two groups-group one received a combination of BAM, and group two KM. The former group did not provide sufficient sedation in all animals and may not be suitable. KM worked well but did require supplemental gas anesthesia.
	K: 5 mg/kg + M: 0.1 mg/kg IM in a 3 ml dart. Antagonized with atipamezole 0.5 mg/kg half IV and half IM if necessary [18]	Semi-free-ranging Bennett's wallabies	n = 26 adult animals split into two groups receiving KM or 0.1 mg/kg medetomidine + 4 mg/kg Alfaxalone IM in a 5 ml dart. Induction and maintenance satisfactory for both, no significant differences, both had bradycardia, and mean cloacal temperature was lower in the AM group.

Drug name	Drug dose	Species	Comments
Ketamine + medetomidine	K: 4.4–5.1 mg/kg + M: 0.078–0.09 mg/kg IM. Antagonized with atipamezole 0.29–0.37 mg/kg IM [21]	Bridled nailtail wallabies	n = 301 wallabies anesthetized with combination listed to the left (protocol 1) or with K: 4.8–5.6 mg/kg M: 0.096–0.112 mg/kg (protocol 2). In protocol 2, 5 animals died during induction. No animals died during induction with protocol 1.
	K: 4 mg/kg + M: 0.015 mg/kg [22]	Matschie's tree kangaroos	Chemical restraint.
Ketamine + medetomidine + midazolam	K: 3–4 mg/kg + M: 0.05 mg/kg + Mid: 0.02–0.1 mg/kg IM. Antagonize with atipamezole 0.25 mg/kg IM [1]	Macropods	Immobilization.
Ketamine + xylazine	K: 5 mg/kg + X: 2 mg/kg IM via dart [17]	Macropods	Immobilization.
	K: 8 mg/kg + X: 8 mg/kg IM [19]	Red kangaroos	
	K: 10–25 mg/kg + X: 2–5 mg/kg; start w/5 mg/kg each drug [2, 16]	Macropods	Quality of restraint inferior to Telazol.
	K: 15 mg/kg + X: 2 mg/kg IM [16]	Bennett's wallabies	
Midazolam	0.3 mg/kg IM or 0.2 mg/kg IV [1]	Macropods	Sedation
	0.3–0.4 mg/kg IM or IV [16]	Macropods	Sedation, shorter acting than diazepam; antagonize with 1 mg flumazenil per 25 mg benzodiazepine.
Telazol	T: 2–8 mg/kg IM [17]	Macropods	Supplement with ketamine 1–2 mg/kg IV to prolong anesthesia. Instead could use propofol 6–8 mg/kg IV to effect to achieve additional anesthesia.
	4–5 mg/kg IM for tractable animals, and 7–10 mg/kg IM non-tractable or 1–3 mg/kg IV [1, 2, 16]	Macropods	Immobilization, lower doses can be used for tractable animals, higher doses for excited animals and Western gray kangaroos. Recoveries in general can be prolonged at 1–5 hrs.
	4.7–4.9 mg/kg [16]	Wild Eastern gray kangaroos	Induction in 7–10 min, recovery time of 116–130 min.

(*Continued*)

Drug name	Drug dose	Species	Comments
	5–7 mg/kg IM [2]	Macropods	Can use 4 mg/kg in tractable animals. Rapid and smooth induction and good relaxation, appears to be quite safe in macropods, adverse reactions are rare. Excess salivation can be controlled with atropine 0.3–0.6 mg IV or IM total.
	5 mg/kg IM [19]	Bennett's tree kangaroos *(Dendrolagus bennettianus)*, Matschie's tree kangaroos *(Dendrolagus matschiei)*	Supplement with ketamine 2.5 mg/kg as needed.
Telazol	5–7 mg/kg IM [19]	Eastern, Western gray and Red kangaroos	Supplement in Red kangaroos with ketamine 2.5–3.5 mg/kg as needed.
	T: 10 mg/kg [19]	Brush-tailed bettongs *(Bettongia penicillata)*	Supplement with ketamine 10 mg/kg IM as needed.
Telazol + acepromazine	T: 3–4 mg/kg + A: 0.3 mg/kg IM [1]	Macropods	Immobilization.
Telazol + dexmedetomidine	T: 0.5–1 mg/kg + D: 0.03–0.04 mg/kg IM [16]	Red kangaroos	For remote injection of captive animals, immobilization.
Telazol + medetomidine	T: 2–3 mg/kg IM + M: 0.04 mg/kg IM; antagonize with atipamezole at 4 × the medetomidine dose [1, 2]	Macropods (specifically Red kangaroos in the reference)	Immobilization.
	T: 0.5–1 mg/kg + M: 0.03–0.04 mg/kg IM [16]	Red kangaroos	For remote injection of captive animals, immobilization.
Telazol + xylazine	T: 3–5 mg/kg + X: 0.5–2 mg/kg IM; antagonize with yohimbine 0.2 mg/kg IV or atipamezole 0.05–0.4 mg/kg IV [2]	Macropods	
Thiopental	T: 28 mg/kg IV [17]	Small kangaroos: Tammar wallabies and Quokkas	Can be induced, intubated, and maintained on inhalant anesthesia. Rat kangaroos aka Potoroo have lower tolerance to Thiopental and pentobarbital than other kangaroo species.

Drug name	Drug dose	Species	Comments
Thiopentone	15–20 mg/kg IV. Give 2/3 of dose as a bolus then titrate to effect with the rest [2]	Macropods	
Zuclopenthixol acetate	4–10 mg/kg IM [1, 2, 16]	Macropods	Sedation, duration of 48–72 hrs.
Zuclopenthixol decanoate and Pipothiazine palmitate	10 mg/kg of each drug IM [2, 16]	Red-necked wallabies	Lower doses proved ineffective, onset within 24 h [2], duration for approximately 10 days.
Koalas and Wombats			
Alfaxalone	3 mg/kg IM or 1.5 mg/kg IV [1, 2, 16]	Koalas	Immobilization, provides approximately 10 min of anesthesia IV.
	3–5 mg/kg IM [1, 16]	Wombats	Immobilization, effect is dose dependent. Adults may require 10 or more milliliters.
Alphaxalone + alphadolone combo solution (Althesin)	A:3–6 mg/kg IM or 1–2 mg/kg IV [17]	Koalas	Safe and rapid immobilization.
Diazepam	0.5–1 mg/kg IM or 0.5 mg/kg IV [1, 2]	Koalas	Sedation
	0.5–1 mg/kg IM [1, 16]	Wombats	Sedation for several hours.
Fluphenazine	Not recommended [16]	Wombats	2 mg/kg resulted in 4 weeks of sedation and anorexia in both Common, Southern and Northern hairy-nosed wombats.
Isoflurane	Via facemask, 3.5–5% [1, 2, 16]	Koalas and Wombats	Immobilization induction, maintenance or both. Juvenile wombats can be induced and maintained on isoflurane.
Ketamine	10–15 mg/kg IM [2]	Koalas	Anesthetic induction resulting in light anesthesia with muscle hypertonicity. Addition of alpha 2 agonist is advisable.
Ketamine + medetomidine	K: 2 mg/kg + M: 0.125 mg/kg IM; antagonize with atipamezole at 4 × medetomidine dose IM [1, 16]	Wombats	Immobilization.
Ketamine + xylazine	K: 20 mg/kg + X: 4 mg/kg [16]	Wombats	Immobilization.
	K: 5 mg/kg + X: 5 mg/kg IM. Antagonize with yohimbine 0.2 mg/kg IV [2]	Koalas	Deep sedation.

(*Continued*)

Drug name	Drug dose	Species	Comments
	K: 15 mg/kg + X: 5 mg/kg IM [2, 16, 19]	Koalas	Immobilization, surgical level of anesthesia.
Midazolam	0.5 mg/kg IM [1]	Wombats	Sedation
Propofol	2.5–3 mg/kg IV bolus, 4–5 mg boluses for maintenance [1, 2]	Koalas	Immobilization, short duration of action.
	2.5–3 mg/kg IV bolus [2]	Koalas	Recumbency and light anesthesia in tame, captive animals.
	6–8 mg/kg IV [2, 16]	Koalas	Used for very short procedures.
Telazol	2–9 mg/kg (2 mg/kg heavy sedation, 3–5 mg/kg light anesthesia) [1, 16]	Wombats	Effect and duration are dose-dependent. More agitated animals may require higher doses (up to 15 mg/kg has been used safely). Combination of choice for wombats with rapid induction and good relaxation. Recoveries can take several hours.
	4–10 mg/kg [16]	Koalas	7 m/kg IM alone can be used for minor surgical procedures, relaxation is variable, and moderate salivation can occur, with 3–4 hr recoveries.
	5–10 mg/kg IM or 2.5 mg/kg IV [1, 2]	Koalas	Immobilization.
	7 mg/kg IM [19]	Koalas	Supplement with ketamine 3.5 mg/kg.
Telazol + medetomidine	T: 3.5 mg/kg + M: 0.055 mg/kg IM; antagonize with atipamezole 2 mg IV [1, 2]	Victorian koalas	Immobilization, in a study of 19 animals, 50% were light to surgical anesthesia and 50% were heavily sedated with this protocol.
	T: 3 mg/kg + M: 0.04 mg/kg IM; antagonize with atipamezole 5 × medetomidine dose IM [1]	Wombats	Immobilization.
Dasyurids (Tasmanian devils, Numbats, Quolls, etc.)			
Alfaxalone	2–3 mg/kg IM [16]		Immobilization.
Diazepam	1–2 mg/kg IM [1, 2]		Sedation
Isoflurane	via facemask [1, 2]		Immobilization induction, maintenance or both. 5% induction, 2% maintenance.
Ketamine + xylazine	K: 20 mg/kg + X: 4 mg/kg IM [2, 16]	Tasmanian devils, Dasyurids	Immobilization.
Telazol	7–10 mg/kg IM [1, 2, 16]		Immobilization. Can result in prolonged recoveries.

Drug name	Drug dose	Species	Comments
Telazol	T: 5.5 mg/kg IM [19]	Tasmanian devils	Supplement with ketamine 4 mg/kg as needed. Relaxation is variable with hypersalivation and constant jaw and limb movement and recoveries can be prolonged >6 hr.
Possums, Gliders, and North American Opossums			
Alfaxalone	5–8 mg/kg IM or 5 mg/kg IV [1, 2, 16]	Common brushtails and Common ringtail possums	Rapid, short-acting anesthesia.
Butorphanol tartrate	0.4–1 mg/kg SC or IM [1, 2]	Possums and Gliders	Sedation
Diazepam	0.5–2 mg/kg IM, PO or IV [1]	Opossums	Sedation
	0.5–1 mg/kg IM [1, 2]	Possums and Gliders	Sedation
Isoflurane	via facemask [1, 2]	Possums, Gliders, and Opossums	Immobilization induction, maintenance or both.
Ketamine	10–30 mg/kg IM [2]	Common ringtail and Brushtail possums	Immobilization.
	30–50 mg IM [1]	Opossums	Immobilization.
Ketamine + fentanyl-droperidol	K: 20–25 mg/kg + FD:0.75–1 ml/kg IM [17]	Opossums	Immobilization.
Ketamine + medetomidine	K: 1–3 mg/kg + M: 0.02–0.1 mg/kg IM; antagonize with atipamezole 0.05–0.4 mg/kg IV [1, 2, 16]	Possums and Gliders	Immobilization.
	K: 2–3 mg/kg + M: 0.05–0.1 mg/kg IM; antagonize with atipamezole 0.05–0.4 mg/kg IV [1, 16]	Opossums	Immobilization.
Ketamine + medetomidine + butorphanol	K: 10 mg/kg + M: 0.07–0.1 mg/kg + B: 0.2–0.5 mg/kg IM [1, 16]	Opossums	Immobilization.
Ketamine + xylazine	K: 2–3 mg/kg + X: 2–5 mg/kg IM; antagonize with yohimbine 0.2 mg/kg IM [2]	Brushtail possums	
	K: 10 mg/kg + X: 5 mg/kg [16]	Opossums	

(*Continued*)

Drug name	Drug dose	Species	Comments
	K: 20–30 mg/kg + X: 5 mg/kg IM [17]	Possums	Surgical anesthesia.
	K: 30 mg/kg + X: 6 mg/kg [2, 16]	Possums and Gliders	
Midazolam	0.1 mg/kg SC [15]	Opossum	n = 1 North American opossum undergoing scrotal ablation given as premedication with midazolam 10 minutes prior to chamber induction with isoflurane.
Propofol	6 mg/kg IV [2]	Possums	
Telazol	1–3 mg/kg IV [2]	Possums	
Telazol	4–10 mg/kg IM or 1–3 mg/kg IV [2, 16, 17]	Possums and Gliders	Relaxation was variable and deaths occurred when used in Squirrel gliders. Can be combined with medetomidine at 0.05–0.4 mg/kg IV or IM.
	15 mg/kg IM [1, 16]	Opossums	Immobilization.
Bandicoots and Bilbies			
Diazepam	0.5–1 mg/kg IM; antagonize with flumazenil at 0.05–0.1 mg per mg of benzodiazepine IM or IV [1, 2]		Sedation
Isoflurane	via facemask [1]	Bandicoots	Immobilization induction, maintenance or both.
Ketamine + xylazine	K: 30 mg/kg + X: 10 mg/kg IM [16]		Immobilization.
Midazolam	0.1–0.2 mg/kg IM, antagonize with flumazenil at 0.05–0.1 mg per mg of benzodiazepine IM or IV [1, 2]		Sedation
Telazol	T: 0.005 mg/g [19]	Long-nosed bandicoots	Supplement with ketamine 0.005 mg/g.
	T: 10 mg/kg IM [19]	Short-nosed bandicoots	Supplement with ketamine 10 mg/kg IM as needed.
Antiparasitic			
Macropods			
Albendazole	3.8 mg/kg PO once [23]	Eastern gray kangaroos	n = 12 animals wild caught and treated then fecal egg counts monitored.

Drug name	Drug dose	Species	Comments
Atovaquone	100 mg/kg PO SID [2]	Macropods	For treatment of toxoplasmosis, combine with canola oil to enhance absorption.
Fenbendazole	25 mg/kg PO SID × 5d [2]	Macropods	For the treatment of verminous bronchitis and pneumonia.
Fipronil	Topical application (Domestic animal dose) [2]	Macropods	For the treatment of ticks and fleas.
Imidacloprid	10 mg/kg topical [2]	Macropods	For the treatment of lice or flea infestations.
Ivermectin	0.2–0.4 mg/kg topically applied, PO or SC [2]	Macropods	Topical for the treatment of lice infestation, all three methods of application for ticks, once weekly for 4 treatments for mites. Also effective for strongyloides infestation given topically.
Levamisole	10 mg/kg PO [2]	Macropods	For the treatment of strongyloides infestation. Also may be useful for other helminths.
Mebendazole	Do not use at high doses [24]	Red-legged pademelons; Macropods	n = 5 treated with mebendazole at 50 mg/kg SID × 5–6d developed bone marrow aplasia and subsequent septicemia.
Moxidectin	0.5 mg/kg topically applied, PO or SC [2]	Macropods	Topical for the treatment of lice infestation, all three methods of application for ticks, once weekly for 4 treatments for mites. Also effective for strongyloides infestation given topically.
Selamectin	Topical application (domestic animal dose) [2]	Agile Wallabies	To treat sarcoptic mange.
Thiabendazole	44 mg/kg PO [2]	Macropods	For the treatment of strongyloides infestation.
Toltrazuril	25 mg/kg PO SID × 3d [2]	Macropods	To treat coccidiosis. Consider adding fluids and enrofloxacin 5 mg/kg IM or SC SID × 5d to treat secondary bacterial infections in hand reared kangaroos with a suspicion of disease. Homologous plasma transfusions from healthy adults, 10 ml/kg IV, may be useful. If hemorrhagic enteritis is seen, adding Phytomenadione, 2.5 mg/kg IM or SC SID × 5 day, may be beneficial.

(*Continued*)

Drug name	Drug dose	Species	Comments
Koalas and Wombats			
Amitraz (50 g/l acaricidal dog wash solution)	0.025% topical application [2]	Koalas, Wombats	Thoroughly wet all fur, for treatment of sarcoptic mange or for nymphal tick infestation.
Fipronil	Topical spray [2]	Koalas	To treat for ticks.
Ivermectin	0.2–0.3 mg/kg PO SC 3 treatments 10 days apart, repeat with a second course after 2 weeks to totally eradicate mites [2]	Wombats	Treatment of sarcoptic mange. Another option is to treat at weekly intervals until 2 weeks past negative skin scrapes.
	0.3 mg/kg SC q10d for 3 treatments [2]	Wombats, Koalas	For treatment of sarcoptic mange.
	0.6 mg/kg PO SID [2]	Koalas	To treat refractory demodicosis treated daily for up to 6 wks after negative scrapes obtained.
Malathion	0.2% solution immersion for topical administration q10d × 3 treatments [2]	Koalas	n = 1 hand-reared individual with sarcoptic mange, treated 3 times at 10 day intervals.
Moxidectin	0.2–0.3 mg/kg PO SC 3 treatments 10 days apart, repeat with a 2nd course after 2 weeks to totally eradicate mites [2, 25]	Wombats	Treatment of sarcoptic mange. Another option is to treat at weekly intervals until 2 weeks past negative skin scrapes [25].
Praziquantel	5 mg/kg PO once [2]	Koalas	To treat Anoplocephalid cestode Bertiella obesa.
Pyrimethamine + Sulfadiazine	P: 0.5 mg/kg SID PO + S: 20 mg/kg PO TID [2]	Wombats	Treatment for toxoplasmosis based on treatment of choice in humans. Supplement with folinic acid 1 mg/kg PO SID.
Toltrazuril	25 mg/kg PO SID × 3d [2]	Southern hairy-nosed wombats	For treatment of coccidiosis. Anecdotal reports of adverse reactions including deaths in a small number of Common wombats.
Trimethoprim sulfonamide	15 mg/kg PO BID for at least 4 weeks [2]	Wombats	Treatment for toxoplasmosis.
Dasyurids, Numbats, Possums, Gliders, and North American Opossums			
Albendazole	23.75 mg/kg PO, twice 7 days apart [2]	Possums	
Doramectin	0.8 mg/kg PO [2]	Possums	For treatment of nematodes.
Eprinomectin	7.5 mg/kg PO [2]	Possums	For treatment of nematodes.
Fenbendazole	20–50 mg/kg PO SID × 3d [2]	Possums and Gliders	

Drug name	Drug dose	Species	Comments
Imidacloprid	10–11.3 mg/kg topically [2, 26]	Yellow-bellied gliders, Eastern barred bandicoots, Eastern quells, Fat-tailed dunnarts, Lead beaters possums, and Ring-tailed possums	Cleared a flea infestation by applying to the gliders and nests, and no live fleas were seen for 27 d.
Ivermectin	0.2 mg/kg PO or SC [2]	Possums, Dasyurids, Numbats	
Levamisole	37.5 mg/kg [2]	Possums	
Moxidectin	0.2 mg/kg SQ [2]	Dasyurids	
Oxfendazole	5 mg/kg PO once [2]	Possums and Gliders	
Selamectin	6 mg/kg topically once per month [2]	Possums	For treating Trichosurolaelaps crassipes infestations in Common brushtails.
Toltrazuril	25 mg/kg PO SID × 3d, in combination with enrofloxacin 5 mg/kg IM SID × 5d [2]	Brushtail possums	Coccidiosis.
Bandicoots and Bilbies			
Fenbendazole	10–30 mg/kg PO SID for 3 days [2]	Bandicoots	For treating Physaloptera peramelis.
Fipronil	2.5 g/l sprayed lightly over coat [2]	Bandicoots	To treat flea and louse infestations.
Imidacloprid	100 mg/ml deposited as a 10 mg/kg dose percutaneously [2]	Bandicoots	To treat flea infestations.
Ivermectin	0.2 mg/kg SC, repeat in 14 days [2]	Bandicoots	For treating heavy tick or mite burdens. Light tick burdens are removed by hand.
Moxidectin	0.2–0.4 mg/kg PO or SC, repeat in 14 days [2]		May be useful for treating Phylsaloptera peramelis and Capillaria spp. infections.
Pyrimethamine + Sulfonamide and trimethoprim + folic acid	P: 0.5 mg/kg PO SID + ST: 25 mg/kg PO SID + F: 1 mg/kg PO SID [2]	Bandicoots	For the treatment of toxoplasmosis.
Pyrimethamine + Sulfadiazine + folic acid	P: 2 mg/kg PO SID + S: 20 mg/kg PO TID + F: 1 mg/kg PO SID [2]		Toxoplasmosis treatment.

(*Continued*)

Drug name	Drug dose	Species	Comments
Toltrazuril	2.5 mg/kg PO as single dose [2]		Coccidial infection treatment; limited success.
Trimethoprim/ Sulfonamide	5 mg/kg of trimethoprim component SC or PO SID [2]		Coccidial infection treatment. Local ulceration at injection site seen in an Eastern barred bandicoot.
Other			
Acetyl cystine in saline		Macropods	Nebulization for Bordetella rhinitis or pneumonia [2].
Bromhexine HCl	2 mg/kg PO BID × 5d, then 1 mg/kg PO BID afterward [2]	Koalas	Mucolytic for treating rhinitis or bronchitis.
Chlorhexidine varnish (sustained release containing chlorhexidine diacetate 1.5 g, ethyl cellulose 3.0 g, polyethylene glycol 400 0.3 g, ethanol up to 50 ml)	Topically applied [4]	Macropods	Treatment of oral necrobacillosis or lumpy jaw. Applied in 3 layers each 1–2 mm thick with long-handled standard No. 4 horsehair paintbrush. Allow time to dry between each layer. Application frequency of 10–12 days.
Cisapride	0.1–0.2 mg/kg PO TID 30–60 min prior to feeding [2]	Koalas	For treatment of delayed gastric emptying.
Crystalloid fluids	3 ml/kg/hr IV CRI [9]	Red kangaroos	n = 1 case of an 8 yr old male Red kangaroo with 2 wk. history vomiting, mesenteric volvulus diagnosis; crystalloid fluid was supplemented with 2.5% dextrose and potassium chloride 15 mEq/l.
Dantrolene sodium	1 mg/kg IV [2]	Macropods	For treatment of capture myopathy, as a muscle relaxant. Consider giving with IV fluids, prednisolone sodium succinate 5–10 mg/kg IV.
Desoxycorticosterone pivalate (DOCP)	2.4 mg/kg IM q25d [27]	Matschie's tree kangaroos	Mineralocorticoid replacement n = 1 female 20 yr old diagnosed with hypoaldosteronism; successfully managed with DOCP for 12 months.
Dexamethasone 0.1% ophthalmic suspension	1–2 drops per eye BID [2]	Koalas	For treating chlamydial keratoconjunctivitis to reduce proliferative inflammation of conjunctivae. Given concurrently with appropriate antibiotic therapy.
Dexamethasone	2 mg/kg SC SID × 3d [2]	Numbats	Anti-inflammatory for degenerative disease.
Dextrose 10%	20 ml/kg IV [2]	Hand-reared Macropods	For treatment of hypoglycemia.

Drug name	Drug dose	Species	Comments
Dextrose 50%	Dilute 1:4, give 1 ml/kg of 12.5% dextrose IV, followed by a CRI of isotonic fluids supplemented with 1.25–5% dextrose [28]	Neonatal Macropods	If glucose <3.2 mmol/l or 60 mg/dl.
Enalapril	0.5 mg/kg PO SID [22]	Matschie's tree kangaroos	n = 1 case of successful management of hypertrophic cardiomyopathy. Animal received enalapril, furosemide 2.5 mg/kg PO SID to BID, and extended release diltiazem 6 mg/kg PO BID. No progression of HCM 74+ months later.
Famotidine	0.5 mg/kg SID IV [9]	Red Kangaroo	n = 1 case of an 8 yr old male red kangaroo with 2 wk. history vomiting, mesenteric volvulus diagnosis, surgical correction- given famotidine, buprenorphine, flunixin meglumine and procaine penicillin intraoperatively.
Furosemide	5 mg/kg IV or SC [2]	Koalas	Diuretic
Human Chorionic gonadotropin	250 IU IM on day 2 of estrus [2]	Koalas	Induction of ovulation.
Iohexol	700 mg/kg IV once during CT evaluation [9]	Red kangaroo	n = 1 case of an 8 yr old male Red kangaroo with 2 wk history vomiting, mesenteric volvulus diagnosis with CT and contrast.
Mannitol	0.5–1 g/kg given slowly IV [2]	Koalas	For lowering intracranial pressure.
Methylprednisolone sodium succinate	30 mg/kg given slowly IV [2]	Koalas	For treating spinal trauma, give over 30 min, useful if given within 8 hrs of trauma.
Metoclopramide	0.5 mg/kg IV IM or SC TID [2]	Koalas	To encourage gastric emptying and accelerate intestinal transit.
	0.2 mg/kg SC BID [9]	Red Kangaroos	n = 1 case of an 8 yr old male red kangaroo with 2 wk history vomiting, mesenteric volvulus diagnosis, postoperatively had ileus, so gave metoclopramide.
Mirtazapine	0.4 mg/kg PO SID [9]	Red Kangaroos	n = 1 case of an 8 yr old male red kangaroo with 2 wk history vomiting, mesenteric volvulus diagnosis, gave mirtazapine to stimulate appetite with apparent positive effect.
Nandrolone laurate	1 mg/kg SC [2]	Koalas	Anabolic
Oxytocin	1 IU/kg IM SC [2]	Koalas	To stimulate milk let-down.
Potassium chloride	1–2 mmol PO SID-TID [2]	Koalas	Oral potassium supplement.

(*Continued*)

Drug name	Drug dose	Species	Comments
Psyllium	2 g/kg/d mixed with low lactose milk powder [2]	Koalas	n = 1 case of sand impaction to assist with passage of sand. Also hydrated well with IV SC and oral fluids. Given over a 2-month period (decreased psyllium dose to 1 g/kg/d for 2nd month).
Phytomenadione	2.5 mg/kg IM SC SID × 5d [2]	Macropods	For treatment of hemorrhagic enteritis associated with coccidiosis or anemia due to hematoazoan infections.
Prednisolone sodium succinate	5–10 mg/kg IV [2]	Macropods	For administration in capture myopathy with dantrolene and IV fluids.
Vitamin E	200–600 mg PO SID [2]	Macropods	For the treatment of nutritional myopathy or muscular dystrophy.
	40 U/kg SC once [9]	Red kangaroos	n = 1 case of an 8 yr old male red kangaroo with 2 wk history vomiting, mesenteric volvulus diagnosis. Vitamin E administered postoperatively as Capture myopathy prophylaxis.
Vitamin E (alpha-tocopherol)	25 mg PO total dose [2, 29]	Tree kangaroos	Muscular dystrophy treatment.
Vitamin K1	2.5–5 mg/kg SC or IM initially then orally [2]	Macropods	Treat until coagulation profiles return to normal, usually 7–10 d.

Species	Weight [1, 16, 19]
Bilby	0.8–2.5 kg
Brown antechinus	20–70 g
Brush-tailed phascogale	100–300 g
Brush-tail possum	1.2–4.5 kg
Common wombat	22–39 kg
Eastern quoll	0.7–2 kg
Eastern gray Kangaroo	17–85 kg
Fat-tailed dunnart	10–20 kg
Feather-tailed glider	10–15 g
Koala	4–15 kg
Kowari	70–170 g
Marsupial mole	40–70 g
Parma wallaby	3–6 kg
Tammar wallaby	4–10 kg
Tasmanian devil	7–10 kg
Tasmanian pademelon	2–12 kg
Tiger quoll	1–5 kg

Species	Weight [1, 16, 19]
Red kangaroo	17–92 kg
Red-necked wallaby	12–24 kg
Ring-tail possum	700–900 g
Southern brown bandicoot	0.4–1.8 kg
Southern hairy-nosed wombat	18–36 kg
Sugar glider	95–160 g
Swamp wallaby	10–20 kg
Western gray kangaroo	17–72 kg
Virginia opossum	2–5.5 kg

References

1 Vogelnest, L. (2015). Marsupialia (*Marsupials*). In: *Fowler's Zoo and Wild Animal Medicine*, vol. 8 (ed. R.E. Miller and M. Fowler), 255–274. St Louis, MO: Elsevier Saunders.
2 Vogelnest, L. and Woods, R. (2008). Marsupials. In: *Medicine of Australian Mammals* (ed. L. Vogelnest and R. Woods). Victoria, Australia: Csiro Publishing.
3 McLelland, D.J., Rich, B.G., and Holz, P.H. (2009). The pharmacokinetics of single dose intramuscular amoxicillin trihydrate in Tammar wallabies (*Macropus eugenii*). *Journal of Zoo and Wildlife Medicine* 40 (1): 113–116.
4 Bakal-Weiss, M., Steinberg, D., Friedman, M. et al. (2010). Use of a sustained release chlorhexidine varnish as treatment of oral necro-bacillosis in Macropus spp. *Journal of Zoo and Wildlife Medicine* 41 (2): 371–373.
5 Kragness, B.J., Graham, J.E., Bedenice, D. et al. (2016). Surgical correction of a cervical spinal fracture in a Bennett's wallaby (*Macropus rufogriseus*). *Journal of Zoo and Wildlife Medicine* 47 (1): 379–382.
6 Kane, L.P., Langan, J.N., Adkesson, M.J. et al. (2017). Treatment of mandibular osteomyelitis in two Red-necked wallabies (*Macropus rufogriseus*) by means of intensive long-term parenteral drug administration and serial computed tomographic monitoring. *Journal of the American Veterinary Medical Association* 251 (9): 1070–1077.
7 Kirkwood, J.K., Gulland, F.M., Needham, J.R. et al. (1988). Pharmacokinetics of Oxytetracycline in clinical cases in the red-necked wallaby (*Macropus rufogriseus*). *Research Veterinary Science* 44 (3): 335–337.
8 McLelland, D.J., Barker, I.K., Crawshaw, G. et al. (2011). Single-dose pharmacokinetics of Oxytetracycline and Penicillin G in Tammar wallabies (*Macropus eugenii*). *Journal of Veterinary Pharmacologic Therapy* 34 (2): 160–167.
9 Knafo, S.E., Rosenblatt, A.J., Morrisey, J.K. et al. (2014). Diagnosis and treatment of mesenteric volvulus in a Red kangaroo (*Macropus rufus*). *Journal of the American Veterinary Medical Association* 244 (7): 844–850.
10 Black, L.A., McLachlan, A.J., Griffith, J.E. et al. (2013). Pharmacokinetics of chloramphenicol following administration of intravenous and subcutaneous chloramphenicol sodium succinate, and subcutaneous chloramphenicol, to koalas (*Phasolarctos cinereus*). *Journal of Veterinary Pharmacologic Therapy* 36 (5): 478–485.
11 Govendir, M., Hnager, J., Loader, J.J. et al. (2012). Plasma concentrations of Chloramphenicol after subcutaneous administration to koalas (*Phascolarctos cinereus*) with chlamydiosis. *Journal of Veterinary Pharmacologic Therapy* 35 (2): 147–154.

12 Griffith, J.E., Higgins, D.P., Li, K.M. et al. (2010). Absorption of Enrofloxacin and Marbofloxacin after oral and subcutaneous administration in diseased koalas (*Phascolarctos cinereus*). *Journal of Veterinary Pharmacologic Therapy* 33 (6): 595–604.

13 de Kauwe, T., Kimble, B., and Govendir, M. (2014). Perceived efficacy of analgesic drug regimens used for Koalas (*Phasolarctos cinereus*) in Australia. *Journal of Zoo and Wildlife Medicine* 45 (2): 350–356.

14 Kimble, B., Black, L.A., Valtchev, P. et al. (2013). Pharmacokinetics of Meloxicam in koalas (*Phascolarctos cinereus*) after intravenous, subcutaneous, and oral administration. *Journal of Veterinary Pharmacologic Therapy* 36: 486–493.

15 Cusack, L., Cutler, D., and Mayer, J. (2017). The use of the ligasure™ device for scrotal ablation in marsupials. *Journal of Zoo and Wildlife Medicine* 48 (1): 228–231.

16 Holz, P. (2014). Marsupials. In: *Zoo Animal and Wild Immobilization and Anesthesia* (ed. G. West, D. Heard and N. Caulkett), 521–528. Ames, IA: Wiley Blackwell.

17 Carpenter, R. (2007). Exotic and zoo animal species. In: *Lumb and Jones' Veterinary Anesthesia and Analgesia* (ed. W.J. Tranquilli, J.C. Thurmon and K.A. Grimm), 788, 798–799. Ames, IA: Wiley Blackwell.

18 Bouts, T., Karunaratna, D., Berry, K. et al. (2011). Evaluation of Medetomidine-Alfaxalone and Medetomidine-Ketamine in semi-free ranging Bennett's wallabies (*Macropus rufogriseus*). *Journal of Zoo and Wildlife Medicine* 42 (4): 617–622.

19 Kreeger, T., Arnemo, J.M., and Raath, J.P. (2012). *Handbook of Wildlife Chemical Immobilization*. Fort Collins, Colorado: Wildlife Pharmaceuticals Inc.

20 Watson, M.K., Thurber, M., and Chinnadurai, S.K. (2016). Comparison of Medetomidine-Ketamine and Butorphanol-Azaperone-Medetomidine in captive Bennett's Wallabies (*Macropus rufogriseus*). *Journal of Zoo and Wildlife Medicine* 47 (4): 1019–1024.

21 Boardman, W.S., Caraguel, C.G., Gill, S. et al. (2014). Mass capture and anesthesia of Australian bridled nailtail wallabies (*Onychogalea fraenata*) with the use of medetomidine and ketamine. *Journal of Wildlife Diseases* 50 (4): 858–863.

22 Fredholm, D.V., Jones, A.E., Hall, N.H. et al. (2015). Successful management of hypertrophic cardiomyopathy in a Matschie's tree kangaroo (*Dendrolagus matshiei*). *Journal of Zoo and Wildlife Medicine* 46 (1): 95–99.

23 Cripps, J., Beveridge, I., and Coulson, G. (2013). The efficacy of anthelmintic drugs against nematodes infecting free-ranging Eastern Grey kangaroos (*Macropus giganteus*). *Journal of Wildlife Diseases* 49 (3): 535–544.

24 Speare, R., Skerratt, L.F., Berger, L. et al. (2004). Toxic effects of Mebendazole at high doses on the haematology of Red-legged pademelons (*Thylogale stigmatica*). *Australian Veterinary Journal* 82 (5): 300–303.

25 Death, C.E., Taggart, D.A., Williams, D.B. et al. (2011). Pharmacokinetics of moxidectin in the Southern hairy-nosed wombat (*Lasiorhinus latifrons*). *Journal of Wildlife Diseases* 47 (3): 643–649.

26 Baker, R.T. and Beveridge, I. (2001). Imidacloprid treatment of marsupials for fleas (*Pygiopsylla hoplia*). *Journal of Zoo and Wildlife Medicine* 32 (3): 391–392.

27 Whoriskey, S.T., Bartlett, S.L., and Baitchman, E. (2016). Hypoaldosteronism in a Matschie's tree kangaroo (*Dendrolagus matschiei*). *Journal of Zoo and Wildlife Medicine* 47 (2): 628–631.

28 Campbell-Ward, M. (2019). Macropod pediatric medicine. In: *Fowler's Zoo and Wild Animal Medicine Current Therapy*, vol. 9 (ed. R.E. Miller, N. Lamberski and P.P. Calle), 500–501. St. Louis, MO: Elsevier.

29 Portas, T.J. (2019). Medical aspects of potoroid marsupial conservation translocations. In: *Fowler's Zoo and Wild Animal Medicine Current Therapy*, vol. 9 (ed. R.E. Miller, N. Lamberski and P.P. Calle), 494–495. St. Louis, MO: Elsevier.

3

Xenarthra: Anteaters, Armadillos, and Sloths

Drug name	Drug dose	Species	Comments
Antimicrobials and Antifungals			
Amikacin	20 mg/kg IV SID [1]	Tamanduas	n = 1 case of anemia requiring blood transfusion after tail tip surgery. After blood and Oxyglobin transfusion, also given IV Amikacin and penicillin G potassium IV daily in fluids for 48 hrs.
Amoxicillin	10–11 mg/kg IM or PO SID × 5d [2]	Sloths	
	10 mg/kg PO or IM SID-TID × 5d [2]	Anteaters	First choice for respiratory infections.
Amoxicillin/clavulanic acid	10–14 mg/kg PO BID [3]	Anteaters	Used for generalized infections.
	10 mg/kg PO BID [1]	Tamanduas	n = 1 case of anemia requiring blood transfusion after tail tip surgery.
	10–14 mg/kg PO BID [3]	Tamanduas	Used in cases of inflammatory bowel disease in conjunction with prednisolone or chloramabucil.
Ampicillin	10–20 mg/kg IM TID × 5–10d [2]	Armadillos	
	10–20 mg/kg IM or IV BID for 5–8d [2]	Sloths	IV was effective in septicemia.
	10–20 mg/kg IM BID for 7–10d [2]	Anteaters	Used for dermatitis or pneumonia.
Ceftiofur sodium	2.2–4.4 mg/kg IM SID to BID × 5d [2]	Anteaters	Used for dermatitis or pneumonia.
Ceftiofur crystalline free acid (Excede)	6.6 mg/kg IM q5d [3]	Anteaters, Tamanduas	For pneumonia.

(Continued)

Zoo and Wild Mammal Formulary, First Edition. Alicia Hahn.

Drug name	Drug dose	Species	Comments
Cephalexin	15–20 mg/kg IM BID 5–10d [4]	Sloths	Dermatitis.
Ceftriaxone	20 mg/kg IM SID × 3d [4]	Sloths	Used for pneumonia.
Chloramphenicol	27–75 mg/kg IM BID × 10d [2]	Armadillos	Used for bacterial enteritis. 50–100 mg/kg used for pneumonia.
	100 mg/kg IM SID 5–10d [4]	Sloths	Used for pneumonia.
	20–100 mg/kg IM BID × 7d [2]	Anteaters	Used for dermatitis or pneumonia.
Doxycycline	5 mg/kg PO BID for 5–10d [2]	Anteaters	Broad spectrum coverage.
Enrofloxacin	1.25 mg/kg IM or PO BID × 5d [2]	Armadillos	Hypersensitivity reaction noted in Dwarf anteaters.
	2.5–5 mg/kg IM SID [2]	Armadillos	Used for generalized or systemic infections.
	10 mg/kg IM SID × 12d [2]	Armadillos	Used for *Salmonella sp.* infections.
	2.5–3.5 mg/kg IM SID [2]	Sloths	Used for respiratory and urogenital problems.
	5 mg/kg IM BID × 20d [5]	Hoffmann's two-toed sloths	n = 1 case of *Bordatella bronchiseptica* successfully treated with IM enrofloxacin, in addition to nebulization daily with albuterol and gentamicin for 14 days. SC administration painful.
Enrofloxacin	2.5 mg/kg IM or PO SID × 5d [2]	Anteaters	Broad spectrum coverage.
	2.5–5 mg/kg PO SID [3]	Tamanduas	Broad spectrum coverage.
Gentamicin	30 mg of 40 mg/ml was added to albuterol 1.25 mg and diluted in 0.9% saline [5]	Hoffmann's two-toed sloths	n = 1 case of *Bordatella bronchiseptica* successfully treated with IM enrofloxacin, in addition to nebulization daily with albuterol and gentamicin for 14 days.
	50 mg of 100 mg/ml added to 0.5 ml of acetylcysteine in 5 ml of 0.9% saline. Nebulized BID to TID for 10–15 min × 5d [3]	Anteaters, Tamanduas	Used in cases of pneumonia in neonates.
Itraconazole	5 mg/kg PO SID × 4–6 weeks [4]	Sloths	Systemic dermatophytosis. In combination with chlorhexidine shampoo baths.

Drug name	Drug dose	Species	Comments
Ketaconazole	5 mg/kg PO SID × 4–6 weeks [4]	Sloths	Systemic dermatophytosis.
Metronidazole	10–15 mg/kg PO BID × 5–7d [3]	Anteaters, Tamanduas	Used in cases of clostridial colitis.
Penicillin G	40 000 IU/kg IM SID × 5d [2]	Armadillos	
Penicillin G potassium	15 000 IU/kg IV every 6 hrs [1]	Tamanduas	n = 1 case of anemia requiring blood transfusion after tail tip surgery. After blood and Oxyglobin transfusion, also given IV Amikacin and penicillin G potassium IV daily in fluids for 48 hrs.
Penicillin G benzathine and Penicillin G procaine	50 000 IU/kg IM or SC, followed by 10 000 IU IM or SC SID for 5–10d [2]	Anteaters	Can be used as preventative treatment during bacterial culture and while awaiting sensitivity results.
Terbinafine	Topical spray BID × 3–4 weeks [4]	Sloths	Focal dermatophytosis.
Trimethoprim sulfamethoxazole	15 mg/kg IM SID × 5d [2]	Armadillos	
	15–40 mg/kg IM SID for 7–10d [2]	Sloths	Used for pneumonia.
	15 mg/kg PO BID for 3–5d [2]	Anteaters	First choice for gastrointestinal infections. Given IM resulted in bone marrow hypoplasia in a juvenile Tamandua *(Tamandua tetradactyla)*.
Analgesic			
Flunixin meglumine	2.5 mg/kg SC SID × 3d [2]	Armadillos	For analgesia.
	1 mg/kg SC SID × 3d [2]	Sloths	For analgesia, and gastrointestinal tract disorders like colic.
	1 mg/kg SC SID × 3d [2]	Anteaters	For analgesia, and gastrointestinal tract disorders like colic.
Gabapentin	3–5 mg/kg PO SID × 3d [4]	Sloths	Analgesic postop. Can cause lethargy, sedation and anorexia at higher dosages.
Ketoprofen	2 mg/kg SQ on first day, then 1 mg/kg SQ × 2d [4]	Sloths	Analgesic and anti-inflammatory therapy.

(Continued)

Drug name	Drug dose	Species	Comments
	1–2 mg/kg IM SID for 3–5d [2]	Anteaters	Anti-inflammatory therapy.
Meloxicam	0.05–0.1 mg/kg IM q48 hrs for 3–4 doses [2]	Sloths	Analgesia, anti-inflammatory therapy.
	0.1–0.15 mg/kg PO SID [3]	Anteaters, Tamanduas	Analgesia, anti-inflammatory therapy.
Tramadol	0.5 mg/kg IM SID to BID [2]	Armadillos	Analgesia, may cause anorexia or gastrointestinal tract problems.
	2–3 mg/kg IM, IV TID-QID × 3–4d [4]	Sloths	Analgesic, for postoperative or traumatic wounds.
	2–3 mg/kg PO BID [3]	Anteaters	For analgesia in severe osteoarthritis cases.
Anesthetic			It has been recommended to fast smaller xenarthrans for 4–6 hrs and larger for 12–24 hrs prior to immobilization [2]
Acepromazine + ketamine	A: 0.1 mg/kg + K: 10 mg/kg [6]	Two-toed sloths	n = 30 free-ranging adults >2 kgs, resulted in poor anesthetic level and lack of muscle relaxation.
Acepromazine + diazepam + ketamine + buprenorphine	A: 0.06 mg/kg + D: 0.3 mg/kg + K: 8.8 mg/kg + B: 5.9 microg/kg [7]	Giant anteaters	n = 5 animals evaluated for osteosynthesis, gastrostomy, or treatment of burns. Animals were maintained with isoflurane via facemask. Induction in 10–15 min, good muscle relaxation.
Fentanyl citrate/ Droperidol combo	0.11–0.25 ml/kg [2]	Armadillo	Captive
Isoflurane	4–5% induction, 2–3% maintenance [8]	Southern naked-tailed armadillos	Rapid induction and recovery, no analgesia.
Ketamine	10–15 mg/kg IM [9]	Armadillos	
	65–90 mg/kg IM [8]	Armadillos	Poor anesthetic quality.
	6 mg/kg [8]	Sloths	Poor anesthetic quality.
	9 mg/kg [8]	Anteaters	Poor anesthetic quality.
Ketamine + acepromazine	K: 25 mg/kg + A: 0.3 mg/kg IM [2]	Armadillos	Free-ranging.
	K: 10 mg/kg + A: 0.1 mg/kg IM [2, 8]	Sloths	Free-ranging, rapid induction but poor sedation and muscle relaxations.

Drug name	Drug dose	Species	Comments
	K: 1.3 mg/kg + A: 0.1 mg/kg IM [2, 8].	Sloths *(Braduypus torquatus)*	Free-ranging, Mild sedation, for exams and diagnostic sampling.
Diazepam + buprenorphine	K: 8.8 mg/kg + A: 0.06 mg/kg + Diaz: 0.3 mg/kg + Bup: 0.006 mg/kg IM [2, 8]	Giant anteaters	Associated with isoflurane for maintenance. Diazepam in separate syringe to prevent precipitation.
Ketamine + dexmedetomidine	K: 1–3 mg/kg + Dexmed: 0.006–0.018 mg/kg IM; antagonize with atipamezole 0.145 mg/kg [8]	Hoffmann's two-toed sloths, Brown-throated three-toed sloths	Short procedures in free-ranging animals, may requires supplementation.
Ketamine + dexmedetomidine	K: 4 mg/kg + Dexmed: 0.04 mg/kg IM [10]	Linnaeus's two-toed sloths	n = 7 (4.3).
Ketamine + medetomidine	K: 7.5 mg/kg + M: 0.075 mg/kg IM; antagonized with atipamezole [8, 11]	Nine-banded armadillos (NBA) and Great long-nosed armadillos (GLA)	n = 47 nine-banded (NBA) and 31 Great long-nosed (GLA) in a comparison of 3 anesthetic protocols. 1. Telazol at 8.5 mg/kg for 12 NBA and 10 GLA, 2. Ketamine 40 mg/kg + xylazine 1 mg/kg IM for 18 NBA and 9 GLA. 3. Ket + Med for 17 NBA and 12 GLA. The latter protocol resulted in better muscle relaxation and animals were standing within 16 min post atipamezole administration. The Telazol resulted in long irregular recoveries up to 3 hrs. All protocols had overall 50% hypoxemia with SpO2 < 85%. Ket+ Med produces a 30–40 min immobilization with quick recovery.
	K: 3 mg/kg + M: 0.04 mg/kg IM; antagonize with atipamezole 0.2 mg/kg [6, 8]	Two toed sloths	n = 46 animals, free-ranging >2 kg, bradypnea noted, good anesthesia with good muscle relaxation and analgesia for minor surgery for up to 40 minutes.
	K: 4–7.5 mg/kg + M: 0.075 mg/kg IM; antagonize with atipamezole 0.38 mg/kg [2, 12]	Long-nosed armadillos	Free-ranging, supplement with 5 mg/kg ketamine as needed.

(Continued)

Drug name	Drug dose	Species	Comments
	K: 5 mg/kg + M: 0.02–0.07 mg/kg IM; antagonize with 0.25 mg/kg atipamezole [12, 9]	Armadillos, Six-banded and three-banded armadillos	Supplement with 5 mg/kg ketamine as needed.
	K: 5 mg/kg + M: 0.02 mg/kg IM, antagonize with 0.1 mg/kg atipamezole [8]	Brown-throated three-toed sloths	Good muscle relaxation, rapid recovery after antagonist.
	K: 3 mg/kg + M: 0.04 mg/kg IM; antagonize with atipamezole 0.2 mg/kg [2, 8, 9, 12]	Sloths	Free-ranging, supplement with ketamine 1.5 mg/kg as needed.
	K: 2.5–3 mg/kg + M: 0.02 mg/kg IM; antagonize with atipamezole 0.1 mg/kg IM [2, 12, 13]	Two toed sloths, Three-toed sloths	n = 26 Two-toed and 15 Three-toed sloths, free-ranging, supplement with ketamine 1.5 mg/kg as needed. Able to examine within 10 minutes after drug administration. Recoveries were smooth and uneventful. All animals experienced a time-dependent decrease in heart rate and blood pressure and an increase in respiratory rate during the course of anesthesia.
Ketamine + medetomidine	K: 2–4 mg/kg + M: 0.02–0.04 mg/kg IM; antagonize with atipamezole at 5 × the M dose [2, 8, 9, 12].	Giant Anteaters, Tamanduas, Silky anteaters	Good muscle relaxation, supplement with ketamine 2 mg/kg.
Ketamine + butorphanol + dexmedetomidine	K: 2 mg/kg + B: 0.2 mg/kg + D: 0.02 mg/kg IM; antagonize with atipamezole 10 × dexmedetomidine dose [3]	Anteaters	Good analgesia and muscle relaxation.
Ketamine + butorphanol + medetomidine	K: 15 mg/kg + B: 0.1 mg/kg + M: 0.07 mg/kg IM; antagonize with atipamezole 0.35 mg/kg IM [12, 8].	Long-nosed/Nine-banded armadillos	Good analgesia and muscle relaxation.
Ketamine + butorphanol + propofol	K: 7 mg/kg + B: 0.4 mg/kg IM, then P: 5 mg/kg IV [8]	Six-banded armadillos	For semen collection by electroejaculation.

Drug name	Drug dose	Species	Comments
Ketamine + medetomidine + midazolam	K: 7 mg/kg + M: 0.08 mg/kg + Mid: 0.1 mg/kg; antagonize with atipamezole 0.4 mg/kg [8]	Andean hairy armadillos	Rapid induction and recovery.
Ketamine + midazolam	K: 8–13 mg/kg + Mid: 0.22–0.42 mg/kg IM [2]	Sloths	Captive, associated with isoflurane anesthesia for maintenance.
	K + 5–10 mg/kg + Mid: 0.2 mg/kg IM [4, 8, 9, 12]	Sloths	
	K: 5–10 mg/kg + Mid: 0.2 mg/kg IM; antagonize with flumazenil 0.01–0.02 mg/kg [2, 8, 9]	Giant anteaters, Nine-banded armadillos	For short procedures.
	K: 5 mg/kg + Mid: 0.2 mg/kg IM [9, 12]	Armadillos, Giant armadillos, Six-banded armadillos, Three-banded armadillos	
	K: 8–12 mg/kg + Mid: 0.2–0.4 mg/kg [2, 8, 12]	Silky/Pygmy anteaters	Short procedures.
Ketamine + midazolam + dexmedetomidine	K:2 mg/kg + Mid: 0.1 mg/kg + Dex: 0.012 mg/kg IM; antagonize with atipamezole 0.12 mg/kg [2, 8]	Brown-throated three-toed sloths	Rapid induction and recovery after antagonist.
	K: 2.42–2.92 mg/kg + Mid: 0.1 mg/kg + Dex: 0.008–0.016 mg/kg IM [2, 8]	Sloths	Captive
	K: 4 mg/kg + Mid: 0.1 mg/kg + Dex: 0.015 mg/kg IM; antagonize with atipamezole 0.15 mg/kg [2, 8]	Giant anteaters, Pygmy anteaters	Rapid induction and recovery after antagonist.
	K: 4–5 mg/kg + Mid: 0.1 mg/kg + Dex: 0.02 mg/kg IM; antagonize with atipamezole 0.15 mg/kg [2, 8]	Tamanduas	Rapid induction and recovery after antagonist.
	K: 4 mg/kg + Mid: 0.1 mg/kg + Dex: 0.015–0.03 mg/kg IM; antagonize with atipamezole 0.15 mg/kg [2, 8]	Silky anteaters	Rapid induction and recovery after antagonist.

(Continued)

Drug name	Drug dose	Species	Comments
	K: 5 mg/kg + Mid: 0.1 mg/kg + Dex: 0.015 mg/kg IM; antagonize with atipamezole 0.4 mg/kg [2, 8]	Nine-banded armadillos, Southern naked-tailed armadillos)	Rapid induction and recovery after antagonist.
Ketamine + midazolam + dexmedetomidine	K: 7 mg/kg + Mid: 0.1 mg/kg + Dex: 0.04 mg/kg IM; antagonize with atipamezole 0.4 mg/kg [2, 8]	Andean hairy armadillos	Captive
	K: 7 mg/kg + Mid: 0.05 mg/kg + Dex: 0.05 mg/kg IM [2, 8]	Pichi/dwarf armadillos	Captive
Ketamine + midazolam + xylazine	K: 15 mg/kg + X : 1 mg/kg + Mid: 0.04 mg/kg IM; antagonize with 0.2 mg/kg yohimbine [8, 12].	Hairy anteaters, Andean hairy armadillos	Supplement with ketamine 7.5 mg/kg IM as needed, NO regurgitation, mild salivation, rapid recovery after antagonist.
	K: 3 mg/kg + X: 1 mg/kg + Mid:0.2 mg/kg I; antagonize with 0.125 mg/kg yohimbine and flumazenil 0.005 mg/kg [8]	Linnaeus's two-toed sloths	Rapid induction and recovery, mild hypertension.
Ketamine + midazolam + xylazine + atropine	K: 30 mg/kg + Mid: 0.5 mg/kg + X: 0.5 mg/kg + A: 0.02 mg/kg IM in pelvic limbs [14]	Yellow armadillos	n = 10 animals immobilized successfully for intrabdominal radio transmitter surgical implantation. Mean surgery time was 50 min, and animals were deemed fit for release in 2–3 hrs post recovery. This dosage of ketamine is higher than used previously for restraint and exam of Hairy armadillos and Yellow armadillo semen collection, but lower than restraint for abdominal surgical implantation in Nine-banded armadillos. Atropine is recommended to prevent sialorrhea.
Ketamine + xylazine	K: 5 mg/kg + X: 3.5 mg/kg IM; antagonize with yohimbine 0.125 mg/kg IM [12]	Giant anteaters	Supplement with 5 mg/kg ketamine as needed.

Drug name	Drug dose	Species	Comments
	K: 40 mg/kg + X: 1 mg/kg IM [2, 8, 12]	Long-nosed armadillos	Free-ranging, Prolonged recoveries.
	K: 20–37 mg/kg + X : 0.6–1.25 mg/kg IM; antagonize with yohimbine 0.12–0.14 mg/kg [2, 8]	Armadillos	Free-ranging, risk of hypothermia, K: 30–32 mg/kg: no regurgitation, frequent salivation. Good muscle relaxation. Tachypnea and apnea.
	K: 10 mg/kg + X: 1 mg/kg IM [2, 6, 8, 12]	Two-toed sloths	n = 89, free-ranging, >2 kg, and was characterized by suitable anesthesia with good muscle relaxation, moderate bradycardia, recovery was smooth with being able to hang at 34 minutes.
	K: 10 mg/kg + X: 1.5 mg/kg IM [12]	Silky anteaters	
	K: 5–10 mg/kg + X: 0.5–1.5 mg/kg; antagonize with yohimbine 0.12–0.2 mg/kg [2, 8, 9]	Giant anteaters	No regurgitation.
	K: 13 mg/kg + X: 3.4 mg/kg IM; antagonize with atipamezole 0.4 mg/kg IM [15]	Giant anteaters	n = 1 animal anesthetized to treat tongue tip constriction.
Ketamine + xylazine	K: 20 mg/kg + X: 1 mg/kg [2, 8, 16]	Tamandua	n = 10 wild animals. This study evaluated ketamine alone at 9.8–12.6 mg/kg in 7 animals or Ket + Xyl in 10 animals. The latter protocol resulted in longer immobilization time (>40 min) without lengthening recovery time, and better muscle relaxation and overall is recommended.
	K: 5 mg/kg + X: 1 mg/kg IM [12, 8, 9]	Armadillos, Giant armadillos, Six-banded armadillos, Three-banded armadillos	Rapid recovery after agonist in Giant armadillo.
Ketamine + xylazine + propofol	K: 7 mg/kg + X: 1 mg/kg IM, then P: 5 mg/kg IV [8]	Six-banded armadillos	For semen collection by electroejaculation.

(Continued)

Drug name	Drug dose	Species	Comments
Medetomidine + midazolam + butorphanol	M: 0.01 mg/kg + Mid: 0.21–0.25 mg/kg + B: 0.21–0.25 mg/kg IM; antagonize with atipamezole 0.05 mg/kg [2]	Sloths	Captive
Telazol	T: 8.5 mg/kg IM [2, 8, 12]	Long-nosed/ Nine-banded armadillos	Free-ranging, Prolonged recoveries.
	T: 3.85–11.9 mg/kg [2, 8]	Three-banded armadillos	Free-ranging, Rapid induction, duration approx. 40 min, regular muscle relaxation, tachypnea and apnea.
	15 mg/kg [2, 8]	Pichi/dwarf armadillos	Captive, Prolonged recoveries.
	4.4 mg/kg [2]	Sloths	
	10 mg/kg [2, 6, 8, 12]	Two-toed sloths	n = 37 free-ranging, 2 kg, characterized by good anesthesia and muscle relaxation but irregular respiration, low SpO2, and a long irregular recovery of up to 3 hrs.
	1.9–6 mg/kg IM [2, 8]	Sloths	Captive
	6 mg/kg IM [12]	Sloths	
	15 mg/kg IM [2, 8, 12]	Tamanduas	Rapid induction and recovery after induction.
	2–8 mg/kg IM [9]	Armadillos	
	8 mg/kg IM [12]	Giant armadillos, Six-banded armadillos, Three-banded armadillos	
	2–6 mg/kg IM [9]	Sloths	
Telazol + medetomidine	T: 3 mg/kg + M: 0.06 mg/kg IM; antagonize with atipamezole 0.3 mg/kg [8]	Three-banded armadillos	Rapid induction, very prolonged recovery, used with isoflurane.
Xylazine + butorphanol + midazolam	X: 1.2 mg/kg + B: 0.4 mg/kg + Mid: 0.2 mg/kg; antagonize with yohimbine 0.125 mg/kg + naltrexone 0.25 mg/kg [8]	Giant armadillos	Maintenance with isoflurane, rapid induction and recovery after antagonists.

Drug name	Drug dose	Species	Comments
Antiparasitic			
Fenbendazole	25 mg/kg PO SID × 3d [4]	Sloths	Nematodes
	25–50 mg/kg [2]	Anteaters	
	20–25 mg/kg PO SID × 5d [3].	Tamanduas	
Imidacloprid	7.3 mg/kg Topically, divided in four places along dorsum [17]	Giant anteaters	n = 2 animals with a flea infestation *(Pulex simulans)* given medication topically and substrate removed. Within 10 days infection was cleared from animals and the building.
Ivermectin	0.14 mg/kg SC once or twice a week during a 3–4 week period [2, 4].	Sloths	For the treatment of sarcoptic mange. Toxicity seen in Bradypus (seizures, death).
	0.2 mg/kg SC, once [2]	Anteaters	
Levamisole	100 mg/kg IM q2 wks × 2 treatments [4]	Sloths	Nematodes
Menbendazole	100 mg/kg PO BID × 7d [4]	Sloths	Nematodes
Metronidazole	25 mg/kg SID × 5d [4]	Sloths	Entamoeba, Giardia.
	12–15 mg/kg PO BID × 5d [3]	Anteaters, Tamanduas	Giardia (in combination with fenbendazole).
Metronidazole + Azithromycin combo	M: 10–20 mg/kg + A: 10–12 mg/kg [2]	Anteaters	For the treatment of amoeba infections leading to diarrhea.
Praziquantel	5 mg/kg [2]	Anteaters	
	5 mg/kg PO BID-SID × 1–3d [4]	Sloths	
Pyrantel pamoate	10–20 mg/kg [2]	Anteaters, Tamanduas	
Selamectin	6 mg/kg TO q21d [4]	Sloths	Mange
	6 mg/kg TO q30d [3]	Anteaters, Tamanduas	For flea preventative. Also used to treat mites if repeated in 14 days.
Sulfadimethoxine	55 mg/kg first dose, afterwards 27.5 mg/kg [2, 18]	Anteaters	For the treatment of coccidiosis. Toxicity has been documented.
Other			
Acyclovir	20 mg/kg PO BID × 21 d+ [4]	Sloths	Antiviral for suspected Herpesvirus.
Albuterol sulfate	0.042% inhalation solution, 3 ml nebulized by facemask over 30 min [2]	Sloths	Used as decongestant or expectorant.

(*Continued*)

Drug name	Drug dose	Species	Comments
Amlodipine	0.18 mg/kg PO SID [19]	Sloths	For hypertension.
Bismuth subsalicylate	20 mg/kg PO BID × 3d [4]	Sloths	Anti-diarrheal.
Bromhexine	0.6 mg/kg PO SID for 5–7d [2]	Sloths	Used as decongestant or expectorant.
Canine distemper vaccine Recombitek C3	1 ml given on day 0 and day 21 [10]	Linnaeus's two-toed sloths	n = 7 (4.3), after day 1, one sloth had oral mucosal ulcerations. On day 21, a booster was administered. On day 49, 4 animals were sedated and blood drawn for comparison to pre-vaccination. 3/4 had a threefold increase in serum titer. This study followed an outbreak of canine distemper virus infection in 6 adult sloths and 5/6 died or were euthanized after exhibiting lethargy, anorexia, ocular and nasal discharge, oral and nasal ulcerations and diarrhea. Necropsy and histopathology diagnosed CDV infection.
Purevax ferret distemper vaccine (live Canary pox)	1 ml given at 12 weeks, booster at 16 and 20 weeks of age. Booster annually [3]	Giant anteaters, Tamanduas	No adverse effects have been noted.
Chlorambucil	0.2–0.25 mg/kg PO q72 hrs [3]	Tamanduas	n = 1, irritable bowel disease case. Monitor CBCs. Once remission occurs, the dosage is reduced or dosage interval can be extended. Can be used in conjunction with prednisolone therapy.
Corticotrophin	4-5.5 IU/Kg IM [20]	Armadillos	ACTH stimulation test.
	10 mg/kg IM [3]	Anteaters	ACTH stimulation test. Used compounded Wedgewood gel.
Cortrosyn	5 µg/kg IM [21]	Sloths	ACTH stimulation test.
Cyclosporine	Initial 5 mg/kg PO SID [3].	Anteaters	n = 1 Treatment for IBD. Once IBD is under control, can wean down to lowest possible dose that will control IBD.

Drug name	Drug dose	Species	Comments
Dexamethasone	0.4 mg/kg IM once [2]	Armadillos	For shock therapy.
	0.3–0.6 mg/kg IM SID × 4d [2].	Sloths	For respiratory problems.
	2 mg/kg IM once [2]	Anteaters	For shock therapy.
Diazepam	0.2 mg/kg PO SID × 5d [3]	Anteaters	For anti-anxiety.
Digoxin	0.007–0.01 mg/kg PO q48 hrs [19]	Sloths	Monitor levels.
Doxapram	2–4 mg/kg IM once [2]	Sloths	For apnea and other complications with gas anesthesia.
	1–4 mg/kg IM SID for 5–10d [2]	Anteaters	For apnea and other complications with gas anesthesia.
Enalapril	0.5 mg/kg PO SID [19]	Sloths	Heart failure, for hypertension.
Famotidine	0.5 mg/kg SQ, PO SID [3]	Anteaters, Tamanduas	Anorexia, GI ulcer.
Furosemide	3 mg/kg IM BID [19]	Sloths	Heart failure.
Iron dextran	5 mg/kg IM [1]	Tamanduas	n = 1 case of anemia requiring blood transfusion after tail tip surgery. After blood and Oxyglobin transfusion, also given Iron dextran, Vitamin K and prednisolone.
Maropitant Citrate(Cerenia)	1 mg/kg SQ, PO SID × 5d [3]	Anteaters, Tamanduas	Anti-nausea.
Metoclopramide	0.2 mg/kg PO SID [4]	Sloths	Give 30 minutes before feeding.
	0.3 mg/kg SQ BID-TID × 5d [3]	Anteaters, Tamandua	Anti-emetic.
	0.5 mg/kg PO BID [3]	Anteaters, Tamanduas	Anti-emetic.
Mirtazapine	0.4 mg/kg PO SID [3]	Anteaters	Appetite stimulant.
Omeprazole	0.5–1 mg/kg PO SID [3]	Anteaters, tamanduas	GI ulceration.
Oxyglobin	55 ml IV 10 ml/kg/hr [1]	Tamanduas	n = 1 case of anemia requiring blood transfusion after tail tip surgery. After a whole blood transfusion, additional Oxyglobin was administered.
Oxytocin	3 units IM SID to BID [3]	Anteaters	Can cause colic episodes at the twice a day dose.

(*Continued*)

Drug name	Drug dose	Species	Comments
Prednisone	1 mg/kg PO SID × 10d then EOD [4]	Sloths	
Prednisolone	0.5 mg/kg PO BID [3]	Tamanduas	For irritable bowel disease therapy. Once is controlled, can slowly be weaned to lowest dose possible.
Rabies vaccine (Imrab 3, killed)	1 ml given at 20 weeks, booster at 1 year, then every 3 years [3]	Giant anteaters, Tamanduas	
Simethicone suspension or tablets	50–100 mg total dose PO with food BID to TID [2]	Sloths	For treatment of bloat and overfermentation.
Simethicone suspension		Tamanduas	Bloat [3].
Sucralfate	1 g PO TID × 7d [3]	Anteaters	Give in a slurry. For GI ulceration.
Vitamin K	0.5 mg/kg IM [1]	Tamanduas	n = 1 case of anemia requiring blood transfusion after tail tip surgery. After blood and Oxyglobin transfusion, also given Iron dextran, Vitamin K and prednisolone.
	5–10 mg/kg IM SID × 7d [2]	Anteaters	For the treatment of hypovitaminosis K and coagulation disorders.
	2 mg/kg PO q2–3 times a week [3]	Anteaters, Tamanduas	Preventative, during administration of antibiotics or during illness.
West Nile Virus Vaccine (killed)	1 ml given at 12 weeks, booster at 16 and 20 weeks of age. Booster annually [3]	Giant anteaters, Tamanduas	No adverse effects have been noted.
Whole blood	65 ml in acid citrate dextrose [1]	Tamanduas	n = 1 case of anemia requiring blood transfusion after tail tip surgery. Collected via 60 ml syringe and butterfly from conspecific, transfused with a 170u filter in-line, over 90 min at a rate of 50 ml/hr IV.

Species	Weights [12, 8, 9]
Giant anteater *(Myrmecophaga tridactyla)*	18–39 kg
Lesser anteater/Tamandua *(Tamandua tetradactyla)*	2–7 kg
Silky anteater *(Cyclopes didactylus)*	0.4–0.8 kg
Giant armadillo *(Priodontes maximus)*	18–33 kg
Hairy armadillo *(Chaetophractus nationi)*	1–2 kg
Long-nosed armadillo *(Dasypus novemcinctus)*	3–10 kg
Six-banded armadillo *(Euphractus sexcinctus)*	3–6.5 kg
Three-banded armadillo *(Tolypeutes spp.)*	1–2 kg
Three-toed sloth *(Bradypus variegatus)*	2–6 kg
Two-toed sloth *(Choloepus spp.)*	4–8.5 kg

References

1 Raines, J.A. and Storms, T. (2015). A successful transfusion in a tamandua (*Tamandua tetradactyla*) using both whole blood and blood replacement products. *Journal of Zoo and Wildlife Medicine* 46 (1): 161–163.

2 Aguilar, R.F. and Superina, M. (2015). Xenarthra. In: *Fowler's Zoo and Wild Animal Medicine*, vol. 8 (ed. R.E. Miller and M. Fowler), 355–368. St Louis, MO: Elsevier Saunders.

3 Margarita Woc Colburn, A., DVM (2018). Personal communication.

4 Dinner, C.O. and Pastor, G.N. (2017). *Manual de manejo, medicina y rehabilitaciŮn de perezosos*. Chile: Fundación Hualamo.

5 Hammond, E.E., Sosa, D., Beckerman, R. et al. (2009). Respiratory disease associated with *Bordetella bronchiseptica* in a Hoffmann's two-toed sloth (*Choloepus hoffmanni*). *Journal of Zoo and Wildlife Medicine* 40 (2): 369–362.

6 Vogel, I., de Thoisy, B., and ViÈ, J.C. (1998). Comparison of injectable anesthetic combinations in free-ranging two-toed sloths in French Guiana. *Journal of Wildlife Diseases* 34 (3): 555–556.

7 Carregaro, A.B., Gerardi, P.M., and Honsho, D.K. (2009). Allometric scaling of chemical restraint associated with inhalant anesthesia in giant anteaters. *Journal of Wildlife Diseases* 45 (2): 547–551.

8 Moreno, G.R. (2019). Xenarthra immobilization and restraint. In: *Fowler's Zoo and Wild Animal Medicine Current Therapy*, vol. 9 (ed. R.E. Miller, N. Lamberski and P.P. Calle), 527–535. St Louis, MO: Elsevier Saunders.

9 West, G., Carter, T., and Shaw, J. (2014). Edentata. In: *Zoo Animal and Wild Immobilization and Anesthesia* (ed. G. West, D. Heard and N. Caulkett), 533–542. Ames, IA: Wiley Blackwell.

10 Sheldon, J.D., Cushing, A.C., Wilkes, R.P. et al. (2017). Serologic response to canine distemper vaccination in captive Linnaeus's two-toed sloths (*Choloepus didactylus*) after a fatal canine distemper virus outbreak. *Journal of Zoo and Wildlife Medicine* 48 (4): 1250–1253.

11 Fournier-Chambrillon, C., Vogel, I., Fournier, P. et al. (2000). Immobilization of free-ranging nine-banded and great long-nosed armadillos with three anesthetic combinations. *Journal of Wildlife Diseases* 36 (1): 131–140.

12 Kreeger, T.J., Arnemo, J.M., and Raath, J.P. (2002). *Handbook of Wildlife Chemical Immobilization*. Fort Collins, Colorado: Wildlife Pharmaceuticals Inc.

13 Hanley, C.S., Siudak-Campfield, J., Paul-Murphy, J. et al. (2008). Immobilization of free-ranging Hoffmann's two-toed and brown-throated three-toed sloths using Ketamine and Medetomidine: a comparison of physiologic parameters. *Journal of Wildlife Diseases* 44 (4): 938–945.

14 de Oliveira Gasparotto, V.P., Attias, N., Miranda, F.R. et al. (2017). Chemical immobilization of free-ranging yellow Armadillos (*Euphractus sexcinctus*) for implantation of intra-abdominal transmitters. *Journal of Wildlife Diseases* 53 (4): 896–900.

15 Steinmetz, H.W., Clauss, M., Feige, K. et al. (2007). Recurrent tongue tip constriction in a captive giant anteater (*Myrmecophaga tridactyla*). *Journal of Zoo and Wildlife Medicine* 38 (1): 146–149.

16 Fournier-Chambrillon, C., Fournier, P., and ViÈ, J.C. (1997). Immobilization of wild collared anteaters with ketamine- and xylazine-hydrochloride. *Journal of Wildlife Diseases* 33 (4): 795–800.

17 Mutlow, A.G., Dryden, M.W., and Payne, P.A. (2006). Flea (*Pulex simulans*) infestation in captive giant anteaters (*Myrmecophaga tridactyla*). *Journal of Zoo and Wildlife Medicine* 37 (3): 427–429.

18 Hatt, J., Wenker, C., Isenbuegel, E. et al. (1998). Suspected sulfadimethoxine intoxication in a captive Giant Anteater (*Myrmecophaga tridactyla*). *Annual Proceeding of the American Association of Zoo Veterinarians*. 188–192.

19 Rosenburg, S.R. and Snyder, P.S. (2000). Myocardial failure in a two-toed sloth (*Choloepus didactylus*). *Annual Proceedings of the International Association of Aquatic Animal Medicine*. 4.

20 Howell-Stephens, J.A., Brown, J.S., Bernier, D. et al. (2012). Characterizing adrenocortical activity in zoo-housed southern three-banded armadillos (*Tolypeutes matacus*). *General and Comparative Endocrinology* 178: 64–74.

21 Kline, S., Rooker, L., Nobrega-Lee, M. et al. (2015). Hypoadrenocorticism (Addison's disease) in a Hoffmann's two-toed sloth (*Choloepus hoffmanni*). *Journal of Zoo and Wildlife Medicine* 46 (1): 171–174.

4

Pangolins

Drug name	Drug dose	Species	Comments
Antimicrobials and Antifungals			**A group of 45 White-bellied pangolins *(Manis tricuspis)* are held in North American zoos as part of the US Pangolin Consortium. They have been treated anecdotally for a variety of conditions. However, pharmacokinetic data is not available.**
Amikacin sulfate	4.4 mg/kg loading dose, then 2.2 mg/kg SQ BID [1]	White-bellied pangolins	
Amoxicillin/clavulanic acid (Clavamox)	10 mg/kg PO BID [1]	White-bellied pangolins	
Ampicillin	20–40 mg/kg IV TID-QID [1]	White-bellied pangolins	
Cephalexin (Ceff DT 250)	50 mg PO SID × 5d [2]	Indian pangolins	n = 1 hand-reared neonate. For treatment of a swelling in neck region resulting in protrusion of tongue.
Ceftazidime	20 mg/kg IM SID to BID [1]	White-bellied pangolins	
Ceftiofur crystalline free acid (Excede)	6 mg/kg SQ q3d [1]	White-bellied pangolins	
Ciprofloxacin	15 mg/kg PO BID [1]	White-bellied pangolins	
Clindamycin phosphate	20 mg/kg SQ BID [1]	White-bellied pangolins	

(*Continued*)

Drug name	Drug dose	Species	Comments
Doxycycline	9 mg/kg PO SID [1]	White-bellied pangolins	n = 1 animal treated for 8 weeks after atypical mycobacterium (sensitive to doxycycline) was cultured from gastric wash. No apparent ill effects. Initially after administration salivation and signs of bitter taste were seen.
Enrofloxacin	10–15 mg/kg PO SID to BID or 2.5–5 mg/kg IV or IO [1]	White-bellied pangolins	
Marbofloxacin	8 mg/kg PO SID [1]	White-bellied pangolins	
Metronidazole	13 mg/kg PO BID [1]	White-bellied pangolins	
	15–17 mg/kg PO SID [1]	White-bellied pangolins	
Trimethoprim sulfadimethoxine	30 mg/kg PO SID to BID [1]	White-bellied pangolins	
Analgesia			
Buprenorphine	0.01 mg/kg IM q8 hrs OR 0.2 mg/kg SQ SID [1]	White-bellied pangolins	
Meloxicam	0.1–0.3 mg/kg SQ SID [1]	White-bellied pangolins	
Anesthesia and Sedation			
Isoflurane	Chamber induction [1, 3]	White-bellied pangolins	Induction in small chamber, then use facemask for maintenance. Recovery may be longer than expected but similar to other burrowing species.
Ketamine	10–20 mg/kg IM [4]	Pangolins	
Ketamine	22 mg/kg IM [5]	Long tailed pangolins	Supplement with 11 mg/kg ketamine, as needed.
	16–25 mg/kg IM [3]	Long tailed and Chinese pangolins	At higher doses uncoiling is possible, but some muscle tone and salivation persists. Lasts for 10–20 min.
Midazolam	0.2 mg/kg IM 20 min prior to tube feeding/medicating [1]	White-bellied pangolins	n = 1 captive animal post abdominal surgery that required tube feeding. Midazolam resulted in sedation that allowed easy uncoiling of animal to allow medicating. Did not reverse, lasted <8 hrs. Gave SID for 10 days with no ill effects.

Drug name	Drug dose	Species	Comments
Telazol	3–5 mg/kg IM [4]	Pangolins	
Antiparasitic			
Albendazole	10 mg PO [2]	Indian pangolins *(Manis crassicaudata)*	n = 1 hand-reared juvenile, for treatment of *strongyloides* eggs in feces
Doramectin	0.2 mg/kg SC [4]	Pangolins	For the treatment of nematodes
Fenbendazole	25–50 mg/kg PO SID × 3d [1]	White-bellied pangolins	n = 3 captive animals, treated for relevant parasites, CBC after both dose levels did not indicate toxicity.
Ivermectin	0.2 mg/kg SC or PO [1]	Pangolins	For the treatment of nematodes
Lindane dust 0.5%	Topical dusting [4]	Pangolins	For the treatment of ticks
Niclosamide (Yomesan)	157 mg/kg PO [4]	Pangolins	For the treatment of platyhelminths such as tapeworms
Praziquantel	8 mg/kg PO [1]	White-bellied pangolins	
Pyrantel pamoate	10 mg/kg PO once, repeat in 7 days [1]	White-bellied pangolins	n = 3 captive animals treated for relevant parasites without clinical adverse effects.
Thiabendazole	55–110 mg/kg PO once [4]	Pangolins	For the treatment of nematodes. No side effects were noted.
Other			
Aluspray aerosol bandage	Topical as needed for dermatitis [1]	White-bellied pangolins	
Ascorbic acid (vitamin C)	22 mg/kg PO BID [1]	White-bellied pangolins	
Bismuth subsalicylate	8.7 mg/kg PO TID [1]	White-bellied pangolins	
Capromorelin	2.88 mg/kg PO SID [1]	White-bellied pangolins	
Cerenia (maropitant)	1–2 mg/kg PO or SQ, or 0.3 mg/kg SQ SID [1]	White-bellied pangolins	
Cimetidine	5–10 mg/kg PO BID × 14d [4]	Pangolins	Hemorrhagic gastric ulcers with enteritis have been commonly reported as a cause of death in rescued animals. Treatment may control early-stage gastric ulcers for 2 weeks.

(*Continued*)

Drug name	Drug dose	Species	Comments
Cyanocobalamin	500 μg SQ [1]	White-bellied pangolins	
Distemper vaccine (Purevax Canary pox vectored)	1 ml SQ [1]	White-bellied pangolins	n = 1 captive animal, vaccinated animal was lame and hyporexic for 3 days afterward.
Famotidine	0.15–0.25 mg/kg SQ SID [1]	White-bellied pangolins	
Ferric hydroxide	10 mg/kg IM once [1]	White-bellied pangolins	
Iron dextran	15 mg/kg IM once [1]	White-bellied pangolins	n = 1 captive animal, anemia of chronic disease at 15% HCT with hypochromic red cells, 30 days after injection 31% HCT with normal RBCs. A second animal required 2 injections for full recovery over 2 months.
Lactated Ringer's solution	60–120 ml SQ/ pangolin; IV or IO fluid rates 1–3 × maintenance [1]	White-bellied pangolins	
Metoclopramide	0.2–0.6 mg/kg PO SID to BID [1]	White-bellied pangolins	n = 2 captive animals during periods of ileus. Once defecating again weaned slowly from BID to SID for 14 days then EOD for 7 days.
Mineral oil	1 ml/pangolin PO SID × 7d [1]	White-bellied pangolins	n = 2 captive animals during periods of ileus/ constipation.
Mineral oil + KY lubricant	5 ml of each given as an enema with a lubricated red rubber tube [1]	White-bellied pangolins	n = 2 captive animals during periods of constipation.
Omeprazole	2 mg/kg PO [1]	White-bellied pangolins	
Ondansetron	1 mg/kg PO BID [1]	White-bellied pangolins	
Phytonadione	1.5 mg/kg IM SID or 3.21 mg/kg PO SID [1]	White-bellied pangolins	
Poly-Vi-Sol (Vitamin complex drops)	0.45 ml/kg PO SID × 7d [1]	White-bellied pangolins	
Ranitidine	2–3 mg/kg PO BID × 14d [4]	Pangolins	Hemorrhagic gastric ulcers with enteritis have been commonly reported as a cause of death in rescued animals. Treatment may control early stage gastric ulcers for 2 weeks.
SamE	17.5 mg/kg PO [1]	White-bellied pangolins	

Drug name	Drug dose	Species	Comments
Sensorcaine (95% lidocaine 20 mg/ml + 5% epinephrine 1 mg/ml)	0.15 ml given SQ as a local block prior to abdominal incision [1]	White-bellied pangolins	n = 1 captive animal with abdominal surgery to relieve obstipation.
Sucralfate	5–100 mg/kg PO [1]	Pangolins	Administered to assist in treatment of gastric ulcers with antacid medications 1 hour prior to feeding on an empty stomach, for best results in severe cases.
Vitamin B complex	0.09 ml/kg in SQ fluids [1]	White-bellied pangolins	n = 3 captive animals upon arrival into quarantine

Species	Weight [4, 5]
Chinese Pangolin *(Manis pentadactyla)*	Male up to 9 kg, female 6–7 kg
Giant Pangolin *(Manis gigantea)*	up to 33 kg
Ground Pangolin *(Manis temminckii)*	2–4 kg
Indian Pangolin *(Manis crassicaudata)*	5–35 kg
Indian Pangolin *(Manis crassicaudata)*	5–35 kg
Long tailed Pangolin *(Manis tetradactyla)*	2–3 kg
Sundra Pangolin *(Manis javanica)*	up to 10 kg
White-bellied or Tree Pangolin *(Manis tricuspis)*	1–2 kg

References

1 US Pangolin Consortium (2018). Personal communication.
2 Mohaptra, R.K., Panda, S., Sahu, S.K. et al. (2013). Hand-rearing of rescued Indian pangolin (*Manis crassicaudata*) at Nandankanan Zoological Park, Odisha. *Indian Zoo Yearbook* 5: 17–25.
3 Langan, J. (2014). Tubulidentata and Pholidota. In: *Zoo Animal and Wild Immobilization and Anesthesia* (ed. G. West, D. Heard and N. Caulkett), 539–542. Ames, IA: Wiley Blackwell.
4 Shih-Chien, J. and Hsienshao Tsao, E. (2015). Pholidota. In: *Fowler's Zoo and Wild Animal Medicine*, vol. 8 (ed. R.E. Miller and M. Fowler), 369–374. St Louis, MO: Elsevier Saunders.
5 Kreeger, T.J., Arnemo, J.M., and Raath, J.P. (2002). *Handbook of Wildlife Chemical Immobilization*. Fort Collins, Colorado: Wildlife Pharmaceuticals Inc.

5

Aardvarks

Drug name	Drug dose	Species	Comments
Antimicrobials and Antifungals			
Amikacin	15.24 mg/kg SC SID × 26d [1]	Aardvarks	n = 1, 17 yr old male with intervertebral disc disease that underwent hemilaminectomy, drug given postoperatively for urinary tract infection.
Ceftiofur HCl	3.8 mg/kg IM [2]	Aardvarks	n = 1, 5 yr old captive animal undergoing Caesarian section, given perioperatively.
Clavamox	14 mg/kg PO BID × 14d [2]	Aardvarks	n = 1, 5 yr old captive animal undergoing Caesarian section, given postoperatively.
	12.5 mg/kg PO BID × days [3]	Aardvarks	n = 1, 23 yr old male underwent eyelid surgery, given postoperatively.
Clindamycin	5 mg/kg IM then 12 mg/kg IV BID × 27d [1]	Aardvarks	n = 1, 17 yr old male with intervertebral disc disease that underwent hemilaminectomy, drug given perioperatively and postoperatively.
Enrofloxacin	12 mg/kg IM then 5 mg/kg PO SID × 3d [1]	Aardvarks	n = 1, 17 yr old male with intervertebral disc disease that underwent hemilaminectomy. Drug given perioperatively and postoperatively.
	5 mg/kg PO SID × 14d [3]	Aardvarks	n = 1, 23 yr old male underwent eyelid surgery, given postoperatively.
Linezolid	12 mg/kg BID PO × 10 weeks [1]	Aardvarks	n = 1, 17 yr old male with intervertebral disc disease that underwent hemilaminectomy, drug given postoperatively for osteomyelitis (treatment unsuccessful).
Metronidazole	10 mg/kg BID PO × 14d [3]	Aardvarks	n = 1, 23 yr old male underwent eyelid surgery, given postoperatively.
Procaine benzylpenicillin and benzathine benzyl penicillin (aka Peni LA)	600 000 IU/animal [4]	Aardvarks	n = 9 adult aardvarks, free-ranging, immobilized with 5 combinations of ketamine for anesthesia.

(*Continued*)

Drug name	Drug dose	Species	Comments
Analgesia			
Buprenorphine	0.01 mg/kg IM [2]	Aardvarks	n = 1, 5 yr old captive animal undergoing Caesarian section, given postoperatively.
Carprofen	1.9 mg/kg PO SID × 6d [2]	Aardvarks	n = 1, 5 yr old captive animal undergoing Caesarian section, given postoperatively.
	2 mg/kg PO BID × 3d then 4 mg/kg PO SID × 5d then PO EOD × 5d [3]	Aardvarks	n = 1, 23 yr old male underwent 2 eyelid surgeries 5 days apart, given postoperatively.
	4.4 mg/kg SC [1]	Aardvarks	n = 1, 17 yr old male with intervertebral disc disease that underwent hemilaminectomy, drug given perioperatively.
Fentanyl	6.27 μg/kg/hr IV as CRI [1]	Aardvarks	n = 1, 17 yr old male with intervertebral disc disease that underwent hemilaminectomy, drug given perioperatively.
	3 μg/kg topically applied to surgical incision prior to closure [1]	Aardvarks	n = 1, 17 yr old male with intervertebral disc disease that underwent hemilaminectomy, drug given perioperatively.
Fentanyl patch	100 mg transdermal patch (2 mg/kg/hr) [1]	Aardvarks	n = 1, 17 yr old male with intervertebral disc disease that underwent hemilaminectomy, drug given postoperatively for discomfort.
Hydromorphone	0.1–0.3 mg/kg IV [1]	Aardvarks	n = 1, 17 yr old male with intervertebral disc disease that underwent hemilaminectomy, drug given postoperatively for analgesia and with midazolam to control anxiety and dysphoria during recovery.
	0.3 mg/kg IV q8 rs for 2 hrs [1]	Aardvarks	n = 1, 17 yr old male with intervertebral disc disease that underwent hemilaminectomy, drug given postoperatively for discomfort.
Anesthesia and Sedation			Drug delivery via hand injection is often not wholly successful and darting is recommended [5].
Detomidine	D: 0.12–0.14 mg/kg [6]	Aardvarks	n = 4 captive animals, sedation.
Detomidine + ketamine	D: 0.09–0.18 mg/kg IM followed 15 min later by K: 4.3–8.2 mg/kg IM, antagonized with atipamezole 0.05–0.09 mg/kg IM [6]	Aardvarks	n = 6 captive animals, for anesthesia.
Diazepam	D: 0.25–0.45 mg/kg PO SID to BID [5]	Aardvarks	Some females are too restless to allow their offspring to nurse sufficiently or may injure them inadvertently. Oral diazepam appears to help with this and has allowed successful rearing of calves. The female is weaned off after 3–4 weeks once the infant is ambulatory and more effective at nursing.

Drug name	Drug dose	Species	Comments
	10 mg/animal [5]	Aardvarks	Given orally in the recovery period from anesthesia to prevent pacing to the point of bleeding toenails. Given in late afternoon.
Ketamine + diazepam	K: 11 mg/kg + Dia: 0.26 mg/kg IM [7]	Aardvarks	
Ketamine + medetomidine	K: 3 mg/kg + M: 0.03–0.07 mg/kg IM; antagonize with atipamezole 0.15–0.4 mg/kg [3, 5]	Aardvarks	Provides 30 min anesthesia, and rapid smooth inductions.
	K: 3 mg/kg + M: 0.08 mg/kg IM. Maintained on 1.5% halothane; antagonize with 0.4 mg/kg atipamezole [4]	Aardvarks	n = 6 adult free-ranging animals immobilized for intraabdominal radiotransmitter placement. Rapid smooth inductions and recoveries.
	K: 1.9 mg/kg + M: 0.019 mg/kg IM; antagonized with atipamezole 0.05 mg/kg IM then IV 15 min later, post intubation and was maintained on isoflurane [2]	Aardvarks	n = 1, 5 yr old captive animal undergoing Caesarian section.
Ketamine + medetomidine + midazolam	K: 3.8 mg/kg + M: 0.1 mg/kg + Mid: 0.25 mg/kg IM; antagonized with atipamezole 0.5 mg/kg IM [8]	Aardvarks	n = 7 adult, free-living, aardvarks weighing 33–45 kg. Within 7 min of drug administration animals were laterally recumbent, hypertensive, rectal temperature dropped significantly, and 4 animals had mild to moderate hypercapnia but not hypoxemia.
Ketamine + midazolam	K: 15–20 mg/kg + Mid: 0.28–0.68 mg/kg Supplemental medetomidine 0.04 mg/kg or ketamine 5.4–8.1 mg/kg required to maintain surgical plane [4]	Aardvarks	n = 2 adult free-ranging females immobilized for intraabdominal radiotransmitter placement. Multiple supplemental ketamine or medetomidine injections used to maintain anesthesia. One animal had pneumonia and died probably due to hypothermia. Other animal was more fully recovered before release and survived.
Ketamine + xylazine	K: 14 mg/kg + X: 0.94 mg/kg, Supplemental doses of 1.5–4.7 mg/kg ketamine IV and IM to maintain anesthesia; antagonize with atipamezole 0.3 mg/kg [4]	Aardvarks	n = 1 adult free-ranging male immobilized for intraabdominal radiotransmitter placement. Multiple supplemental ketamine injections used to maintain anesthesia. Animal not fully recovered when released and died in burrow.
Medetomidine + butorphanol + Isoflurane	M: 0.029 mg/kg + B: 0.17 mg/kg for sedation, induction with isoflurane via facemask; antagonized with atipamezole 0.14 mg/kg and naltrexone 0.1 mg/kg IM [1]	Aardvarks	n = 1, 17 yr old male with Intervertebral disc disease that underwent hemilaminectomy.
Midazolam	0.2 mg/kg IV [1]	Aardvarks	n = 1, 17 yr old male with Intervertebral disc disease that underwent hemilaminectomy, drug given postoperatively to control anxiety and dysphoria during recovery. For the first 24 hrs 0.2–0.4 mg/kg IV was given as needed to reduce anxiety.

(*Continued*)

Drug name	Drug dose	Species	Comments
Telazol	4–5 mg/kg; antagonize with flumazenil 0.01 mg/kg [5, 9]	Aardvarks	
Other			
Dopamine	5–10 µg/kg/min IV as CRI [1]	Aardvarks	n = 1, 17 yr old male with Intervertebral disc disease that underwent hemilaminectomy. During surgery used to treat hypotension.
Famotidine	0.5 mg/kg IV BID × 26d [1]	Aardvarks	n = 1, 17 yr old male with Intervertebral disc disease that underwent hemilaminectomy, drug given postoperatively. Paper actually indicates 5 mg/kg but 0.5 mg/kg is consistent with other mammals.
Gabapentin	10 mg/kg PO BID × 21d [1]	Aardvarks	n = 1, 17 yr old male with Intervertebral disc disease that underwent hemilaminectomy.
Gadodiamide contrast medium	0.1 mmol/kg IV once [1]	Aardvarks	n = 1 Used for MRI imaging contrast of an animal's lumbar vertebral area.
Iohexol	744 mg/kg IV once [1]	Aardvarks	n = 1 Used for CT imaging contrast of an animal's lumbar vertebral area.

Species	Weight [10, 11]
Aardvarks *(Orycteropus afer)*	50–70 kg

References

1 Nevitt, B.N., Adkesson, M.J., Jankowski, G. et al. (2018). Lumbar hemilaminectomy for treatment of diskospondylitis in an aardvark (*Orycteropus afer*). *Journal of the American Veterinary Medical Association* 252 (4): 464–472.

2 Mutlow, A.G. and Mutlow, H. (2008). Caesarian section and neonatal care in the aardvark (*Orycteropus afer*). *Journal of Zoo and Wildlife Medicine* 39 (2): 260–262.

3 Matas, M., Wise, I., Masters, N.J. et al. (2010). Unilateral eyelid lesion and ophthalmologic findings in an aardvark (*Orycteropus afer*): case report and literature review. *Veterinary Ophthalmology* 13 (s1): 116–122.

4 Nel, P.J., Taylor, A., Meltzer, D.G. et al. (2000). Capture and immobilisation of aardvark (*Orycteropus afer*) using different drug combinations. *Journal of the South African Veterinary Association* 71 (1): 58–63.

5 Buss, P.E. and Meyer, L.C.R. (2015). Tubulidentata. In: *Fowler's Zoo and Wild Animal Medicine*, vol. 8 (ed. R.E. Miller and M. Fowler), 514–516. St. Louis: Elsevier Saunders.

6 Vodicka, R. (2004). Chemical immobilization of captive aardvark (*Orycteropus afer*). *Journal of Zoo and Wildlife Medicine* 35 (4): 544–545.

7 Goldman, C.A. (1986). A review of the management of the aardvark (*Orycteropus afer*) in captivity. *International Zoo Yearbook* 24/25: 286–294.

8 Rey, B., Costello, M.A., Fuller, A. et al. (2014). Chemical immobilization and anesthesia of free-living aardvarks (*Orycteropus afer*) with ketamine-medetomidine-midazolam and isoflurane. *Journal of Wildlife Diseases* 50 (4): 864–872.

9 Langan, J. (2003). Managing dental disease in aardvarks (*Orycteropus afer*). *Proceedings of the American Association of Zoo Veterinarians* 93–95.

10 Kreeger, T.J., Arnemo, J.M., and Raath, J.P. (2012). *Handbook of Wildlife Chemical Immobilization*. Fort Collins, Colorado: Wildlife Pharmaceuticals Inc.

11 West, G., Heard, D., and Caulkett, N. (eds.) (2014). *Zoo Animal and Wildlife Immobilization and Anesthesia*, 2e. Ames, IA: Wiley Blackwell.

6

Bats

Drug name	Drug dose	Species	Comments
Antimicrobials and Antifungals			
Amikacin	5–10 mg/kg SC, IM, or IV TID [1]		Used in treating severe burns like those associated with electrocution when there is marked cellulitis or bacteremia.
	Toxic dose: 830 mg/kg SQ, divided into 4 injections 2 hrs apart [2]		Given in research animals to induce hearing loss at this dose.
Amoxicillin/ clavulanic acid	20–30 mg/kg PO BID × 7d [3, 4]	Megachiroptera	
	12.5 mg/kg of each component PO BID [1]		For treatment of pulmonary inflammation and secondary infection after aspiration of milk in hand-raised animals.
Enrofloxacin	5–10 mg/kg PO BID [1, 3]		For treatment of pulmonary inflammation and secondary infection after aspiration of milk in hand-raised animals.
	10 mg/kg IM or PO BID [4]	Wahlberg's epauletted fruit bats	For treatment of pneumonia, possible Pasteurella infection.
Fluconazole	10 mg/kg PO SID for 10–14d [1]	Pteropodids	Gastric yeast infection. Nystatin is also effective.
Metronidazole	25 mg/kg PO SID [1]		
Miconazole	Topical 10–14d [1]		
Nystatin	50 000 IU/100 g PO TID for 5–7d, BID × 2d, and SID for 3 more days [1]	Pteropodids	Gastric yeast infection. Fluconazole is also effective.

(*Continued*)

Zoo and Wild Mammal Formulary, First Edition. Alicia Hahn.

Drug name	Drug dose	Species	Comments
Terbinafine	20–60 mg/kg SC SID × 10d [5]	Little brown bats	n = 120 bats in 6 different groups treated with varying doses of Terbinafine. >200 mg/kg resulted in neurologic effects and death, <6 mg/kg did not reach presumed therapeutic levels. 20 and 60 mg/kg resulted in presumed therapeutic concentrations in skin and wing for 6 and 30 days respectively.
Trimethoprim sulfadiazine	30 mg/kg PO BID [1]		For treatment of pulmonary inflammation and secondary infection after aspiration of milk in hand-raised animals.
Trimethoprim sulfamethoxazole	20 mg/kg PO BID × 7d [4]	Megachiroptera	
Voriconazole	Toxicity: 4–20 mg/kg SQ or TO [6]	Little brown bats	Voriconazole at a minimum is not tolerated by bats at expected therapeutic dosages, and may be toxic causing increased mortality. Voriconazole is not a safe or effective drug in *Myotis lucifugus* and should not be used in further *in vivo* experiments in this species.
Analgesia			
Buprenorphine	0.03 mg/kg SC or IM q6–12 hrs [1, 7]	Megachiroptera	
	0.05–0.1 mg/kg SC or IM q6–12 hrs [7]	Microchiroptera	
Buprenorphine	0.01 mg/kg IM [8]	Livingstone's fruit bats	n = 2 animals that received a femoral head ostectomy and analgesia was provided perioperatively.
Butorphanol	0.4 mg/kg IM or SC q4 hr [7]	Megachiroptera	
	0.2 mg/kg SC or IM q4 hrs [4, 9]	Microchiroptera	
	0.4 mg/kg SC [10]	Vampire bats	n = 3 bats undergoing ovariohysterectomy. Received meloxicam and butorphanol perioperatively.
Carprofen	2 mg/kg SC [7]	Microchiroptera	
	1–4 mg/kg SC IM SID or PO BID [1, 7]	Megachiroptera	
	3–5 mg/kg SC, IM or PO BID [7]	Microchiroptera	
Copper indomethacin	0.1 ml/200 g, diluted to 1:10 for bats <100 g [1]		NSAID for pain relief.
Meloxicam	0.1–0.3 mg/kg SC, IM, or PO BID [3, 7]	Megachiroptera	

Drug name	Drug dose	Species	Comments
	0.2 mg/kg PO [11]	Malayan flying foxes	Due to rapid elimination frequent dosing may be required, peak plasma concentration was reached 1 hr post administration, with a 1–1.2 hr half-life indicating rapid metabolism of this medication in this species.
	1–2 mg/kg SC, IM or PO BID [7]	Microchiroptera	
	0.2 mg/kg SC × 7–14d [8]	Livingstone's fruit bats	n = 2 animals that received a femoral head ostectomy and analgesia was provided peri- and postoperatively.
	0.3 mg/kg SC [10]	Vampire bats	n = 3 bats undergoing ovariohysterectomy. Received meloxicam and butorphanol perioperatively. M: 0.2 mg/kg PO SID was given for an additional 7 days postoperatively.
Morphine	0.5–1 mg/kg SC or IM q4–6 hrs [7]	Megachiroptera	
	2–5 mg/kg SC or IM q4–6 hrs [7]	Microchiroptera	
Pentosan polysulphate	3 mg/kg SC weekly for 4 weeks [1]		For pain relief associated with degenerative disease.
Tramadol	0.5–2 mg/kg PO SID [1, 7]	Megachiroptera	
	2 mg/kg SC [8]	Livingstone's fruit bat	n = 1 bat with femoral head luxation that was replaced. Meloxicam was also given at 0.2 mg/kg PO SID for 14 days.
Anesthesia and Sedation			Some recommend to not reverse alpha-2 agonists when used with ketamine as rough recoveries result.
Diazepam	0.5–2 mg/kg IM or IV [1]		Sedation for 30 min to 4 hrs. Highly agitated or aggressive bats may require a higher dose than calm bats and the duration will be shorter. Higher dose for electrocuted bats with seizures and fasciculations repeated 3–4×/day as needed.
Halothane	Induction with 4–5% and maintain at 1–1.5% [7]	Megachiroptera	
Isoflurane	Induction with 5% and maintain at 2.5% [7, 12]	Megachiroptera	
Ketamine	30–37.5 mg/kg IM [7]	Variable flying foxes	Produced short-term restraint but poor muscle relaxation and struggling during recovery.

(*Continued*)

Drug name	Drug dose	Species	Comments
	40–50 mg/kg IM [7]	Megachiroptera	NOT RECOMMENDED as sole agent due to poor muscle relaxation and prolonged recovery with wing flapping.
	100 mg/kg [7]	Microchiroptera	NOT RECOMMENDED as sole agent due to poor muscle relaxation and prolonged recovery with wing flapping.
Ketamine + acepromazine	K: 10 mg/kg + A: 1 mg/kg IM [12].	Bats	
Ketamine + medetomidine	Combine equal volumes medetomidine 1 mg/ml and ketamine 100 mg/ml and use 0.5 ml/kg IM [7]	Captive Variable flying foxes	
	K: 2.5 mg/kg with M: 0.025 mg/kg or K: 5 mg/kg with M: 0.05 mg/kg [7, 13]	Free-living Variable flying foxes	
	K: 6 mg/kg + M: 0.06 mg/kg IM [1, 12]	Pteropodids	The eyes frequently remain open, so corneas need to be lubricated. Antagonize with atipamezole at 5 × the dose of medetomidine.
Ketamine + xylazine	K: 5 mg/kg + X: 0.05 mg/kg IM [7]	Variable flying foxes	Produces short-term immobilization of approximately 30 min with good muscle relaxation and quiet recovery.
	Combine equal volumes of ketamine (100 mg/ml) and xylazine 20 mg/ml) to create a solution and dose of 0.4 ml/kg IM OR 0.1 ml IV [7, 14]	Variable flying foxes, Australian flying foxes	n = 8 adult male flying foxes. Mean induction time was 60–100 seconds and immobilization time 16–36 min.
	K: 10–20 mg/kg + X: 2–4 mg/kg IM [1]	Pteropodids	Induction in 2–5 min, for a duration of 10–40 min, and recovery is quiet without wing flapping. Antagonizing is not recommended, to prevent stormy recoveries.
Ketamine + xylazine	K: 10 mg/kg + X: 2 mg/kg [12]	Bats	Supplement with ketamine 5 mg/kg as needed. Antagonist not recommended due to rough recovery.
Medetomidine	0.03 mg/kg IV [7]	Free-living Variable flying foxes	Provided safe short-term immobilization to collect biological samples.
	0.03–0.08 mg/kg IM [1]		A useful sedative but induces profound bradycardia, poor peripheral circulation, and altered thermoregulation; antagonize with atipamezole at 5 × the medetomidine dose.

Drug name	Drug dose	Species	Comments
Medetomidine + midazolam	M: 0.15 mg/kg + Mid: 1.5 mg/kg IM [15]	Egyptian fruit bats	Anesthesia; used atipamezole without incident.
Medetomidine + midazolam + fentanyl	M: 0.15 mg/kg + Mid: 1.5 mg/kg + F: 0.015 mg/kg IM [15]	Egyptian fruit bats	Anesthesia; used atipamezole without incident.
Medetomidine + midazolam + ketamine	M: 0.15 mg/kg + Mid: 1.5 mg/kg + K: 10 mg/kg IM [15]	Egyptian fruit bats	Anesthesia; used atipamezole without incident.
Medetomidine + midazolam + Morphine	Med: 0.15 mg/kg + Mid: 1.5 mg/kg + Mor: 1.5 mg/kg IM [15]	Egyptian fruit bats	Anesthesia; used atipamezole without incident.
Propofol	8–10 mg/kg IV [1, 7]	Megachiroptera	Provides 5–15 min of anesthesia if a vessel can be accessed. May be diluted 1:4 with saline to facilitate administration.
	6–8 mg/kg IV [1, 7]	Microchiroptera	Provides 5–15 min of anesthesia if a vessel can be accessed. May be diluted 1:4 with saline to facilitate administration.
Sevoflurane	Via facemask at 8% for induction and 4% for maintenance [16]	Livingstone's fruit bats	n = 104 animals included in the study 3 males with DCM and 1 pregnant female were excluded) Induction and recovery were smooth. There were significant differences in esophageal and rectal temperatures and a drop in blood glucose that was likely fasting and time related.
	Induction with 6–7% and maintain at 3–4% [7]	Megachiroptera	
Telazol	T: 10 mg/kg [12]	Bats	
	10–40 mg/kg IM [1, 7]	Megachiroptera	Produces immobilization but prolonged recovery and may be violent with wing thrashing and agitation. Drug is sprayed into the mouth to decrease risk of biting with aggressive or possibly rabid animals – 20 mg/kg generally works well.
Antiparasite			
Fenbendazole	25 mg/kg PO once and repeat in 14d, 20 mg/kg PO q24h × 3d [1, 17]		NOT for bats <100 g.
	10 mg/kg PO SID × 5d or 20 mg/kg PO SID × 3d [17]	Gray headed fruit bats	n = 2 of 5 bats with *Angiostrongylus cantonensis* infection. 3/5 died peracutely due to infestation, 2 survived with treatment and one relapsed later and was treated with higher dose a 2nd time.

(*Continued*)

Drug name	Drug dose	Species	Comments
Ivermectin 1%	NOT RECOMMENDED topically [1, 18]	Dog-faced fruit bats	Administered 1 drop of solution topically and this resulted in approximately 2 mg/kg/bat and clinical signs of death, inability to perch and minimal body movement. It is assumed that while grooming the bats consumed the solution. It is unknown if doses closer to the 0.2 mg/kg SC or IM dose used in other mammals would have had the same result.
Praziquantel	5–20 mg/kg PO as required [1]		For treatment of cestodes and trematodes.
Pyrantel	11 mg/kg PO once [1]		
Other			
Atropine	0.02 mg/kg SC [1]		Administered at or following induction to reduce pharyngeal secretions occasionally seen with inhalation anesthesia.
Calcionate syrup (calcium glubionate)	23 mg/ml, given 2 ml PO BID [4]	Vampire bats	To treat metabolic bone disease with curvature of long bones and flattened faces in pups. Product is often sold as a 360 mg/ml solution and may require compounding or dilution.
Calcium disodium edentate	100–200 mg/kg SID [1]		
Chlorhexidine solution 1–3%	Applied topically to treat cutaneous candidiasis [1]	Juvenile Pteropodids	Animal is washed with warm water and dried then Chlorhexidine solution applied and allowed to stay on. Direct sunlight for 10 min also assists recovery. Antifungal creams will likely be groomed off.
Dexamethasone	0.1–2 mg/kg IV or SC [1]		Dose depends on condition being treated.
Enalapril	0.5 mg/kg PO q72 hrs [19]	Flying foxes	A captive group of Flying foxes had 5 animals develop signs or histopathology consistent with dilated cardiomyopathy. Two bats were diagnosed antemortem and given enalapril. One detected before the onset of hepatomegaly and edema survived another 6 months. A second bat which had more advanced signs was euthanized shortly after starting treatment.
Fluids: Lactated Ringer's or Hartmann's solution	0.1–0.2 ml/5 g of body-weight PO or preferably or SC [3].	Microchiroptera	Fluids are warmed, and given up to 4 times per day for 2–3 days.

Drug name	Drug dose	Species	Comments
Furosemide	2–8 mg/kg IM (or PO SID for 3–5 d) [1]	Hand-raised Bats	Hand-raised bats with pulmonary edema secondary to aspiration of milk. Often given with antibiotics and NSAIDS if needed.
Furosemide	0.5–5 mg/kg 1–3× per day [20]	Livingstone's fruit bats	n = 11 bats treated for dilated cardiomyopathy, diagnosed on routine exam or with clinical signs. Often given with spironolactone, Imidapril and pimobendan depending on severity of signs.
Glucose syrup	5 ml diluted in 200 ml water. Given as 1–2 ml/100 g body weight or 5% dextrose saline given at 5–10 ml/100 g SC [1]	Tube nosed bats and others easily stressed by handling	Suggested to give to easily stressed species during handling to aid recovery.
Glycopyrrolate	0.01 mg/kg IM [19]		Administered prior to anesthesia induction may reduce pharyngeal secretions.
Imidapril	0.24–0.38 mg/kg PO SID [20]	Livingstone's fruit bats	n = 11 bats treated for dilated cardiomyopathy diagnosed on routine exam or with clinical signs. Often given with spironolactone, furosemide, and pimobendan depending on severity of signs.
Metoclopramide syrup	0.01 ml/g [1]	Hand-raised Bats with gastric dilation	Alternated with simethicone 0.01 ml/g is often effective for gastric dilation if the bat is still passing feces.
Melengesterol acetate	Implants (MGA) [21]	Rodrigues fruit bats	n = 48 placed implants, 20 results reported thus far: 4 lost, 4 females pregnant when implanted, 1 failure. A 2nd report described 93% efficacy in 15 animals with no behavioral effects but did see weight gain, retarded hair growth at incision site and 22% implant loss.
Pimobendan	0.2–0.5 mg/kg PO BID [20]	Livingstone's fruit bat *(Pteropus livinstonii)*	n = 11 bats treated for dilated cardiomyopathy diagnosed on routine exam or with clinical signs. Often given with spironolactone, furosemide, and imidapril depending on severity of signs.
Rabies vaccine (Defensor 3)	0.1 ml IM given as 2 doses 30 days apart [22]	Egyptian fruit bats	n = 12 animals, 6 given one dose and 6 given 2 doses, 30 days apart with the latter resulting in higher titers at 60 days.
Simethicone infant gas relief	0.01 ml/g or 400 mg/kg q8 h [1, 3]	Hand-raised bats with gastric dilation	Alternated with metoclopramide syrup 0.01 ml/g is often effective for gastric dilation if the bat is still passing feces.

(*Continued*)

Drug name	Drug dose	Species	Comments
Spironolactone	1–4 mg/kg PO 1–2× per day [20]	Livingstone's fruit bats	n = 11 bats treated for dilated cardiomyopathy diagnosed on routine exam or with clinical signs. Often given with furosemide, imidapril and pimobendan depending on severity of signs.
Soft nails	For treatment of thumbnail avulsion [4]	Megachiroptera	A plastic cap designed to use with surgical glue to glue on cat nails. Can also be used to protect the nailbed in megachiropterans. The cap will fall off when the nail starts growing.
Vitamin C	100 mg/kg PO × 3d then 50 mg/kg PO SID [23]	Vampire bats	A collection of captive bats developed non-healing subcutaneous hemorrhage and serum ascorbic acid levels were 0.08 mg/dl – bats receiving this dose of Vitamin C resolved in 10–60 days.
Vitamin E	levels in the diet >240 mg/kg	Megachiroptera	Diets including this level or above vitamin E appear to prevent dilated cardiomyopathy seen with hypovitaminosis E [4, 19].

Species	Weight
Hoary bat *(Lasiurus cinereus)*	20–35 g
Vampire bat *(Desmodus rotundus)*	15–50 g
Seba's short-tailed bat *(Carollia perspicillata)*	15 g
Little brown myotis/bat *(Myotis lucifugus)*	5–14 g
Wahlberg's epauletted fruit bat *(Epomorphus wahlbergi)*	54–124 g
Horsfield's fruit bat (aka Larger dog-faced fruit bats) *(Cynopterus horsfieldii)*	58 g
Malayan/Large flying foxes *(Pteropus vampyrus)*	0.6–1.1 kg
Indian flying fox *(Pteropus giganteus)*	0.6–1.6 kg
Rodrigues fruit bat/Flying fox *(Pteropus rodricensis)*	0.3–0.35 kg
Variable flying fox *(Pteropus hypomelanus)*	0.467–0.576 kg
Gray-headed flying fox *(Pteropus poliocephalus)*	0.6–1 kg
Egyptian fruit bat/Rousette *(Rousettus aegyptiacus)*	80–170 g
Straw-colored fruit bat *(Eidolon helvum)*	0.23–0.35 kg
Livingstone's fruit bat (aka Comoro black flying fox) *(Pteropus livingstonii)*	0.5–0.8 kg

References

1 Olsen, A. and Woods, R. (2008). Bats. In: *Medicine of Australian Mammals* (ed. L. Vogelnest and R. Woods), 45–502. Victoria, Australia: Csiro Publishing.
2 Kossl, M. and Vater, M. (2000). Consequences of outer hair cell damage for Otoacoustic emissions and audio-vocal feedback in the Mustached bat. *Journal of the Association for Research in Otoloaryngology* 1 (4): 300–314.
3 Bexton, S. and Couper, D. (2010). Handling and veterinary care of British bats. *In Practice* 32: 254–262.
4 Fleming, G.J. and Heard, D.J. (2001). Common medical problems of Megachiropterans in captivity. *Proceedings of the American Association of Zoo Veterinarians* 305–309.
5 Court, M.H., Robbins, A.H., Whitford, A.M. et al. (2017). Pharmacokinetics of terbinafine in little brown myotis (*Myotis lucifugus*) infected with *Pseudogymnoascus destructans*. *American Journal of Veterinary Research* 78 (1): 90–99.
6 Reeder, D.M. (2010). Laboratory and Field Testing of Treatments for White Nose Syndrome: Immediate Funding Need for the Northeast Region. https://rcngrants.org/content/laboratory-and-field-testing-treatments-white-nose-syndrome-immediate-funding-need-northeast (accessed 3 June 2019).
7 Heard, D. (2014). Chiropterans (bats). In: *Zoo Animal and Wildlife Immobilization and Anesthesia*, 2e (ed. G. West, D. Heard and N. Caulkett), 543–550. Ames, IA: Wiley Blackwell.
8 Barbon, A.R., Rushton-Taylor, P., Bell, E. et al. (2017). Femoral head resection in two Livingstone's fruit bats (*Pteropus livingstonii*). *Journal of Zoo and Wildlife Medicine* 48 (3): 941–944.
9 Lafortune, M., Canapp, S.O., Heard, D. et al. (2004). A vasectomy technique for Egyptian fruit bats (*Rousettus aegyptiacus*). *Journal of Zoo and Wildlife Medicine* 35 (1): 104–106.
10 Clarke, E.O. and DeVoe, R.S. (2011). Ovariohysterectomy of three vampire bats (*Desmodus rotundus*). *Journal of Zoo and Wildlife Medicine* 42 (4): 755–758.
11 Goodnight, A.L. and Cox, S. (2018). Pharmacokinetics of meloxicam following a single oral dose in Malayan flying foxes (*Pteropus vampyrus*). *Journal of Zoo and Wildlife Medicine* 49 (2): 307–314.
12 Kreeger, T.J. and Arnemo, J.M. (2012). *Handbook of Wildlife Chemical Immobilization*. China: Kreeger.
13 Heard, D., Towles, J., and Leblanc, D. (2006). Evaluation of Medetomidine/ketamine for short-term immobilization of variable flying foxes (*Pteropus hypomelanus*). *Journal of Wildlife Disease* 42 (2): 437–441.
14 Sohayati, A.R., Zaini, C.M., Hassan, L. et al. (2008). Ketamine and Xylazine combinations for short-term immobilization of wild variable flying foxes (*Pteropus hypomelanus*). *Journal of Zoo and Wildlife Medicine* 39 (4): 674–676.
15 Tuval, A., Las, L., and Shilo-Benjamini, Y. (2018). Evaluation of injectable anaesthesia with five Medetomidine-Midazolam based combinations in Egyptian fruit bats (*Rousettus aegyptiacus*). *Laboratory Animals* 52 (5): 515–525.
16 Barbon, A.R., Glendewar, G., Drane, A.L. et al. (2017). Sevoflurane anesthesia in Livingstone's fruit bats (*Pteropus livingstonii*). *Journal of Zoo and Wildlife Medicine* 48 (4): 1081–1085.
17 Reddacliff, L.A., Macarthur, E., and Hartley, W.J. (1999). *Angiostrongylus cantonensis* infection in Grey-headed fruit bats (*Pteropus poliocephalus*). *Australian Veterinary Journal* 77 (7): 466–468.

18 DeMarco, J.H., Heard, D.J., Fleming, G.J. et al. (2001). Toxicosis associated with topical administration of Ivermectin in dog-faced fruit bats (*Cyanopterus brachyotis*). *Proceedings of the American Association of Zoo Veterinarians* 123–126.

19 Heard, D.J. (1997). Medical management of Megachiropterans. *Proceedings of the American Association of Zoo Veterinarians* 240–244.

20 Killick, R., Barbon, A.R., Barrows, M. et al. (2017). Medical management of dilated cardiomyopathy in Livingstone's fruit bats (*Pteropus livingstonii*). *Journal of Zoo and Wildlife Medicine* 48 (4): 1077–1080.

21 Asa, C.S. and Porton, I.J. (2005). *Wildlife Contraception: Issues, Methods, and Applications.* The Johns Hopkins University Press.

22 Peters, C., Isaza, R., Heard, D.J. et al. (2004). Vaccination of Egyptian fruit bats (*Rousettus Aegyptiacus*) with monovalent inactivated rabies vaccine. *Journal of Zoo and Wildlife Medicine* 35 (1): 55–59.

23 Hausman, J.C., Manasse, J., Steinberg, H. et al. (2015). Non-healing subcutaneous hemorrhage in a colony of vampire bats (*Desmodus rotundus*) due to suspected vitamin C deficiency. *Proceedings of the American Association of Zoo Veterinarians* 70.

7

Rodents

Drug name	Drug dose	Species	Comments
Antimicrobials and Antifungals			
Amikacin	10–15 mg/kg BID SC, IM, IV [1]	Rodents	
Azytromycin	15–30 mg/kg SID PO [1]	Rodents	
Cephalexin	50 mg/kg IM BID [1]	Rodents	May cause dysbacteriosis.
Ceftiofur	1 mg/kg BID IM	Rodents	For pneumonia.
Chloramphenicol	20–50 mg/kg BID PO, IM [1]	Rodents	Ophthalmic ointments also safe in rodents.
Ciprofloxacin	10 mg/kg PO BID [1]	Rodents	May have less bacterial resistance possibility than enrofloxacin.
Doxycycline	2.5 mg/kg PO BID [1]	Rodents	Do not use in young animals. May cause dysbacteriosis.
Enrofloxacin	5 mg/kg PO or IM SID [2]	Naked mole rats	
	5–7.4 mg/kg PO BID [3]	Prehensile-tailed porcupines	n = 9 cases of gastroliths of which 7 animals were treated peri- and postoperatively with enrofloxacin for 5–14 days.
	5–10 mg/kg SID to BID, PO, IM, SC [1]	Rodents	May cause tissue necrosis if parenteral injections not diluted with saline. Higher dose used with less frequency.
	7 mg/kg PO BID × 14d [4]	Brazilian porcupines	n = 1 animal, 5 mo old, chronic diarrhea, failure to thrive, and anorexia. Cytologic exam of feces revealed blastocytosis. Treated with metronidazole for 30 days and enrofloxacin for 14 days and supportive care in hospital.
Gentamicin	2–24 mg/kg SID to BID, IM, SC [1]	Rodents	May give in combination with enrofloxacin for respiratory infections.
Griseofulvin	15–50 mg/kg PO SID for 14–28d [1]	Rodents	Antifungal for dermatophytosis.

(*Continued*)

Zoo and Wild Mammal Formulary, First Edition. Alicia Hahn.

Drug name	Drug dose	Species	Comments
	250 mg/kg on feed every 10 d × 4 treatments [1]	Prairie dogs	
Itraconazole	5–10 mg/kg PO SID × 6 weeks [1]	Rodents	Systemic candidiasis.
	25 mg/kg PO SID [1]	Chinchillas	Treatment of dermatophytosis.
Ketoconazole	10–40 mg/kg PO SID × 14d [1]	Rodents	Systemic mycoses and candidiasis.
Metronidazole	10–40 mg/kg PO BID (all species); 20–60 mg/kg PO BID Prairie dogs [1]	Rodents	Anaerobic and antiprotozoal. Taste may reduce food consumption, or use metronidazole benzoate (flavorless).
	17–20 mg/kg PO BID × 30d [4]	Brazilian porcupines	n = 1 animal, 5 mo old, chronic diarrhea, failure to thrive, and anorexia. Cytologic exam of feces revealed blastocytosis. Animal treated with metronidazole for 30 days and enrofloxacin for 14 days.
Oxytetracycline	5–50 mg/kg BID, PO, IM, SC [1]	Rodents	Toxicity reported in Guinea pigs and Chinchillas.
Terbinafine	10–30 mg/kg PO SID × 4–6 weeks [1]	Rodents	Antifungal.
	40 mg/kg PO SID × 83d [5]	North American porcupines	To treat dermatophytosis (cleared after 83 days).
Tetracycline	10–20 mg/kg BID to TID, PO [1]	Prairie dogs	Toxicity reported in Guinea pigs.
Trimethoprim sulfadiazine	15–30 mg/kg [1, 5]	Rodents	Tissue necrosis can occur if given SC.
	15–30 mg/kg PO SID to BID [2]	Naked mole rats	
Trimethoprim sulfamethoxazole	20 mg/kg PO BID × 14d [6]	Eastern gray squirrels	n = 1 animal treated for transitional cell carcinoma with radiation – which resulted in perineal erythema, treated with trimethoprim sulfamethoxazole.
	28 mg/kg SC once or PO BID [3]	Prehensile-tailed porcupines	n = 1 animal with gastrotomy, treated peri- and postoperatively with trimethoprim sulfamethoxazole.
Analgesia			
Buprenorphine	B: 0.01–0.03 mg/kg IM, SC q8–12 hr [1, 7]	Beavers, Capybaras, Porcupines	
	B: 0.05 mg/kg IM, SC q6–12 hr [7]	Prairie dogs	
	B: 0.05 mg/kg IM [3]	Prehensile-tailed porcupines	n = 9 cases of gastroliths of which 2 animals were treated peri- and postoperatively with buprenorphine.
Butorphanol	Bu: 0.5 mg/kg IM, SC q4 hr [1, 7]	Beavers, Capybaras, Porcupines	Weaker analgesic than buprenorphine.

Drug name	Drug dose	Species	Comments
	Bu: 2 mg/kg IM, SC q4 hrs [7]	Prairie dogs	
Carprofen	4 mg/kg IM, SC SID [7]	Prairie dogs	
Flunixin meglumine	F: 0.5 mg/kg IM, SC q12–24 hr [1, 7]	Beavers, Capybaras, Porcupines	Not recommended in smaller rodents due to potential renal damage.
	F: 2.5 mg/kg IM, SC q12–24 hrs [7]	Prairie dogs	
Ketoprofen	K: 1–3 mg/kg IM, SC SID [1]	Beavers, Capybaras, Porcupines	
Lidocaine	5 mg/kg epidural anesthesia of lumbosacral space [1]	Agoutis	n = 7 animals given 5 min after induction with azaperone, meperidine, xylazine, and ketamine. Analgesia was 64–96 min, no complications.
Meloxicam	M: 0.1 mg/kg [5]	North American porcupines	n = 1 adjunct treatment of skin disease.
	M: 0.1–0.2 mg/kg PO [2]	Naked mole rats	
	M: 0.1–0.3 mg/kg SC, PO q12–24 hr [1, 7]	Beavers, Capybaras, Porcupines	
	M: 0.5 mg/kg SC PO q12 hrs [7]	Prairie dogs	
	M: 0.1–0.2 mg/kg PO SID × 3d [3]	Prehensile-tailed porcupines	n = 9 cases of gastroliths of where 4 animals were treated peri- and postoperatively with meloxicam.
Meperidine	Mep: 10–20 mg/kg IM, SC q2–4 hrs [7]	Prairie dogs	
Morphine	M: 1–3 mg/kg IM, SC q4–6 hr [1, 7]	Beavers, Capybaras, Porcupines	Most commonly used as a single dose pre-operatively.
	M: 2–5 mg/kg IM, SC q4 hr [7]	Prairie dogs	
Oxymorphone	O: 0.1 mg/kg IM, SC q6–12 hr [7]	Beavers, Capybaras, Porcupines	
	O: 0.2–0.5 mg/kg IM, SC q6–12 hr [7]	Prairie dog	
Piroxicam	0.3 mg/kg PO SID [6]	Eastern gray squirrels	n = 1 treated for transitional cell carcinoma of the kidney with nephrectomy and postoperative piroxicam.
Tramadol	T: 0.5–5 mg/kg PO q12–24 hr [7]	Beavers, Capybaras, Porcupines	

(*Continued*)

Drug name	Drug dose	Species	Comments
	T: 2–5 mg/kg PO q12–24 hr [7]	Prairie dogs	
	T: 3 mg/kg PO BID × 3d [3]	Prehensile-tailed porcupines	n = 1 animal after gastrotomy surgery to remove gastrolith.
Anesthesia and Sedation			ET tube suggestions: size 6 for Capybara and 2–2.5 for Prairie dog [7]
Acepromazine	A: 0.1 mg/kg IM [1, 7]	Beavers, Capybaras, Porcupines	
	A: 0.5–2.5 mg/kg IM [7]	Prairie dogs	
Butorphanol + azaperone + medetomidine	B: 0.65 mg/kg + A: 0.22 mg/kg + M: 0.26 mg/kg IM + isoflurane inhalant as needed [8]	American beavers	Lower doses required. Isoflurane for full induction.
Diazepam	D: 0.1–1 mg/kg IM, IP, PO [7]	Beavers, Capybaras, Porcupines	Erratic results and irritation if given IM.
	D: 0.1–0.5 mg/kg IV or PO, or up to 1 mg/kg [7]	Rodents	Preanesthetic sedation and relaxation, minimal cardiopulmonary effects. If administering IV, monitor for hypotension caused by propylene glycol in the formulation.
Droperidol + fentanyl (Innovar-Vet)	DF: 0.3 ml/kg; antagonize with 0.2 mg/kg naloxone [9]	Hoary marmots	Innovar-Vet is a combination of droperidol and fentanyl.
Etomidate	E: 1 mg/kg IV [1]	Prairie dogs, Chinchillas, Guinea pigs	Nonbarbiturate, potent, short-acting hypnotic and anesthetic agent. Used for dental evaluation and trimming.
Fentanyl + xylazine	F: 0.16 mg/kg + X: 0.66 mg/kg; antagonize with naloxone 0.2 mg/kg + yohimbine 0.2 mg/kg [9]	Cape porcupines	
Isoflurane	3–5% induction via facemask or chamber induction, with 1.5–3% for maintenance [1, 7, 9]	Rodents	Some rodents are prone to apnea with inhalants. Doxapram 5–10 mg/kg IV or IM may assist with this.
Ketamine	K: 36 mg/kg [9]	Fox squirrels	
	K: 75 mg/kg	Bushy-tailed wood rats	Supplement with K: 35 mg/kg as needed [9].
	K: 80 mg/kg [9]	African ground squirrels	Supplement with ketamine 40 mg/kg as needed.
	K: 10–15 mg/kg IM [7]	Beavers	Successfully immobilized for handling.

Drug name	Drug dose	Species	Comments
	K: 50 mg/kg IM [9]	Yellow-bellied marmots	Supplement with K: 25 mg/kg as needed.
Ketamine + acepromazine	K: 15 mg/kg + A: 0.1 mg/kg [9]	Capybaras	
	K: 25 mg/kg + A: 0.125 mg/kg IM [9]	Pacas	Supplement with K: 15 mg/kg as needed.
	K: 11 mg/kg + A: 0.22 mg/kg IM [9]	Beavers	
Ketamine + acetylpromazine + atropine	K: 25 mg/kg + Ace: 0.125 mg/kg + At: 0.05 mg/kg IM [10]	Pacas	Rapid induction, good to excellent depth and muscle relaxation and duration of 26–88 min.
Ketamine + acepromazine + midazolam	K: 10 mg/kg + A: 0.05 mg/kg + Mid: 0.3 mg/kg [9]	Prehensile-tailed porcupines	Supplement with K: 5 mg/kg as needed. Tail muscles are the optimal injection site.
	K: 15 mg/kg + A: 0.1 mg/kg + Mid: 0.3 mg/kg [9]	New World/ Prehensile-tailed porcupines	Supplement with K: 10 mg/kg as needed.
Ketamine + diazepam	K: 30 mg/kg + D: 0.5 mg/kg [9]	Prairie dogs	Supplement with K: 15 mg/kg as needed.
Ketamine + diazepam + halothane	K: 25 mg/kg + D: 0.1 mg/kg IM + H inhalant [7]	Beavers	Safe and effective for handling and surgical implantation of intraperitoneal radiotransmitters. Recommend ventilation, and monitor for hypotension as was commonly seen.
Ketamine + fenothiazine	K: 4 mg/kg + F: 0.4 mg/kg IM [11]	Capybaras	Heavy sedation without full immobilization.
Ketamine + medetomidine	K: 4 mg/kg + M: 0.04 mg/kg IM [11]	Capybaras	Good immobilization without full anesthesia; risk of post anesthesia suffocation.
	K: 3–4 mg/kg + M: 0.03–0.04 mg/kg IM, IV [1, 7]	Beavers, Capybaras, Porcupines	
	K: 5 mg/kg + M: 0.05 mg/kg IM; antagonize with atipamezole 0.2 mg/kg IM [9]	Cape porcupine	Supplement with K: 2.5 mg/kg as needed.
	K: 5 mg/kg + M: 0.1 mg/kg IM [9]	Nutrias, Brown squirrels	Squirrel: Supplement with ketamine 3 mg/kg as needed. Antagonize with atipamezole 0.5 mg/kg 1/2 IV and 1/2 IM.
	K: 70 mg/kg + M: 0.5 mg/kg; antagonize with atipamezole 2 mg/kg IM [9]	Alpine marmots	Doses listed are for late summer or autumn, lower doses can be used for earlier in the year. Hypothermia was observed.

(Continued)

Drug name	Drug dose	Species	Comments
	K: 35 mg/kg + M: 0.25 mf/kg [12]	Alpine marmots	Spring doses for short surgery, double doses for longer surgery and recommended K: 60 mg/kg and M: 0.2 mg/kg for late summer/autumn. Significant decrease in heart rate.
Ketamine + medetomidine + midazolam + butorphanol	K: 5 mg/kg + M: 0.05 mg/kg + Mid: 0.25 mg/kg + B: 0.1 mg/kg IM; antagonize with atipamezole 0.25 mg/kg [7, 9]	European beavers	Study for surgical implantation of radiotransmitters may develop hypoxemia, supplement with oxygen.
Ketamine + midazolam	K: 3–4 mg/kg + Mid: 0.03–0.04 mg/kg IM, IV [1]	Beavers, Capybaras, Porcupines	Provided less cardiopulmonary depression and analgesia but good muscle relaxation.
Ketamine + xylazine	K: 4 mg/kg + X: 0.5 mg/kg IM [9]	Nutrias	
Ketamine + xylazine	K: 5 mg/kg + X: 1 mg/kg IM [9]	Cape porcupines	
	K: 5 mg/kg + X: 2 mg/kg; antagonize with yohimbine 0.15 mg/kg [9, 13]	North American porcupines	n = 345 immobilizations on 150 animals. Supplement with K: 5 mg/kg as needed. Tail muscles are the optimal injection site as decreased drug dose by 50% and need for multiple injections by 26%. <1% mortality rate.
	K: 5–10 mg/kg + X: 1–2 mg/kg IM [1, 7]	Beavers, Capybaras, Porcupines	Provides mild to severe dose-dependent hypotension, bradyarrythmias, and respiratory depression.
	K: 10 mg/kg + X: 0.5 mg/kg [7, 9, 11]	Capybaras	This combination was preferred over Telazol or Telazol + levomepromazine in one study. Combinations of alpha-2 agonists and ketamine or tiletamine can produce hypertension, bradycardia, arrhythmias and respiratory depression.
	K: 40 mg/kg + X: 3 mg/kg [12]	Alpine marmots	This dose was for short surgery in spring, for long surgery K: 80 mg/kg + X: 20 mg/kg. In late summer fall K: 60 mg/kg + X: 20 mg/kg. hypothermia.
	K: 10 mg/kg + X: 1 mg/kg IM [9]	Beavers	Supplement with K: 5 mg/kg as needed.
	K: 10 mg/kg + X: 2 mg/kg [9]	Crested porcupines	Supplement with ketamine 5 mg/kg only. Porcupines require high doses for complete immobilization. This dose may only heavily sedate the animal and additional ketamine may be required for surgery other manipulations.

Drug name	Drug dose	Species	Comments
	K: 10 mg/kg + X: 12 mg/kg IM [9]	Patagonian cavies	
	K: 20 mg/kg + X: 1 mg/kg [9]	Red squirrels	Supplement with ketamine 6.6 mg/kg as needed.
	K: 85 mg/kg + X: 10 mg/kg IM [9]	Richardson's ground squirrels	Supplement with ketamine 40 mg/kg as needed.
Midazolam	Mid: 1–2 mg/kg IM IP [7]	Prairie dogs	
	Mid: 0.1–2 mg/kg IM, IP, or SC (0.1–0.5 mg/kg IM lower dose for premedication) [1, 7]	Beavers, Porcupines, Capybaras	For preanesthetic sedation and relaxation. Good for debilitated patients due to minimal cardiorespiratory effects. Sedation for approximately 1 hr.
Propofol	P: 6–8 mg/kg IV [1, 7]	Beavers, Porcupines, Capybaras	
Sevoflurane	Induction with 5–6% via facemask or chamber induction, maintenance with 1.5–3% [1]	Rodents	Some rodents are prone to apnea with inhalants. Doxapram 5–10 mg/kg IV or IM may assist with this.
Telazol	T: 4.4 mg/kg IM [9]	Pacaranas	Supplement with ketamine 4.4 mg/kg as needed.
	T: 4.6–5 mg/kg [9, 11, 14]	Capybaras	Reported as a safe anesthetic combination. In higher doses may have produced longer anesthetic period. Minimal analgesia.
Telazol	T: 4–6 mg/kg IM [1, 7]	Beavers, Porcupines, Capybaras	
	T: 9–11 mg/kg IM [15]	Porcupines	
	T: 5 mg/kg IM [9]	Beavers, Nutrias, Flying squirrels	Nutria and Squirrel: Supplement with ketamine 5 mg/kg as needed.
	T: 6.6 mg/kg IM	Hispaniola hutias, Gray squirrels	Supplement with ketamine 6.6 mg/kg as needed.
	T: 7.25 mg/kg (6.87–7.61 mg/kg range) [9, 16]	Crested porcupines	n = 42 procedures with 31 animals. Porcupines require high doses for complete immobilization. May need to supplement T: 3–4 mg/kg for induction or maintenance sedation. Short induction time and small volume, overall safe but one death/abortion seen.
	T: 10 mg/kg IM [9]	Patagonian cavies, North American porcupines	Cavy: Supplement with T: 5 mg/kg as needed.

(*Continued*)

Drug name	Drug dose	Species	Comments
	T: 12 mg/kg [9]	Fox squirrels, Tricolored squirrels	Supplement with ketamine 12 mg/kg as needed.
	T: 20 mg/kg [9]	Prairie dogs	
	T: 20–40 mg/kg [1]	Australian brown rats	
Telazol ± butorphanol	T: 4–6 mg/kg ± B: 0.1 mg/kg [1]	Beavers, Porcupines, Capybaras	The addition of butorphanol is helpful for wound cleaning or tooth trimming. Can also be used as induction for longer anesthesias with the addition of gas anesthesia.
Telazol + levomepromazine	T: 5 mg/kg + L: 0.5 mg/kg [11]	Capybaras	Safe anesthetic combination with good analgesia.
Telazol + medetomidine	T: 1.6 mg/kg + M: 0.008 mg/kg [11, 14]	Capybaras	Safe anesthetic combination.
Telazol + medetomidine + butorphanol	T: 1.5 mg/kg + M: 0.0075 mg/kg + B: 0.075 mg/kg IM [7, 11, 14]	Capybaras	Safe anesthetic combination with good analgesia. Preferable to Telazol alone or Telazol + medetomidine.
Telazol + morphine + azaperone	T: 3 mg/kg + M: 0.3 mg/kg + A: 1.2 mg/kg IM [11]	Capybaras	Sedation for ophthalmic evaluation and diagnostics.
Telazol + xylazine	T: 20 mg/kg + X: 10 mg/kg IM; antagonize with tolazoline 2 mg [9]	Alpine marmots	Supplement with T: 10 mg/kg and X: 5 mg/kg or isoflurane as needed. Doses listed are for late summer or autumn or long-term surgery. Lower doses can be used for earlier in the year or short procedures. Hypothermia was observed.
	T: 15 mg/kg + X: 3 mg/kg [12]	Alpine marmots	For a short surgery in spring. For longer procedure/surgery in spring K: 20 mg/kg + X: 10 mg/kg. For a short surgery in late summer/autumn K: 15 mg/kg + X: 10 mg/kg.
Xylazine	X: 1–5 mg/kg SC [1, 7]	Beavers, Porcupines, Capybaras	Sedative
	X: 5–10 mg/kg IP SC [7]	Prairie dogs	
Antiparasitic			
Amitraz	0.3% solution topically [1]	Rodents	Use with caution, not recommended in young animals.
	1.4 ml/l topically, q7–14d for 3–6 treatments [1]	Rodents	For demodecosis.
Carbaryl powder	5% topical q7d × 3 treatments [1]	Rodents	Ectoparasites.
Fenbendazole	20–50 mg/kg PO SID × 5d [1]	Rodents	For Giardia and endoparasites. Adverse side effects reported in North American porcupines.

Drug name	Drug dose	Species	Comments
	MAY NOT BE SUITABLE FOR SPECIES [17]	North American porcupines	n = 4 cases (2 died) that received 50 mg/kg of fenbendazole and within 10 days had moderate to severe diarrhea, and or neutropenia. Previous animals had been treated with 25–50 mg/kg without clinical effect. 2/4 animals were treated supportively and recovered after 9–33 days.
Imidacloprid	1/2 kitten dose topically [1]	Prairie dogs	
Advantage (Bayer)	20 mg/kg, Topically q30d [1]	Rodents	Flea control.
Ivermectin	0.2–0.4 mg/kg SC q7–14d [1, 5]	Rodents	Ecto- and endoparasites; preferred dose appears to be 0.4 mg/kg q7d.
Permethrin	0.25% dust in cage [1]	Rodents	Ectoparasites.
Piperazine	200–600 mg/kg PO SID × 7d, off 7d, on 7d [1]	Rodents	Nematodes
Ponazuril	30 mg/kg PO × 2 treatments 48 hrs apart [18]	Black-tailed prairie dogs	n = 7 animals, passing Eimeria in feces without clinical signs, negative after treatment.
Praziquantel	6–10 mg/kg PO, SC, repeat in 10 days [1]	Rodents	Cestodes
Pyrantel pamoate	50 mg/kg PO SID [1]	Rodents	Nematodes
Pyrethrin powder	Topical q7d × 3 treatments [1]	Rodents	Ectoparasites.
Selamectin (Revolution, Bayer)	15–30 mg/kg Topically q21–28 d × 2 treatments [1]	Rodents	Give every 14 days for demodecosis, and 30 mg/kg with Sarcoptes mites.
Sulfadimethoxine	10–15 mg/kg PO BID [1]	Rodents	Coccidiosis.
Thiabendazole	100 mg/kg PO SID × 5d [1]	Rodents	Acariasis
Toltrazuril	10 mg/kg PO SID × 3d, off 3d, on 3d [1]	Rodents	Drug of choice to treat coccidiosis.
Other			
Atropine	0.03 mg/kg SC, IM [1, 7]	Beavers, Capybaras, Porcupines	
	0.05 mg/kg SC, IM [7]	Prairie dogs	
Doxapram	5–10 mg/kg IV or IM [1]	Rodents	Some rodents are prone to apnea with inhalants, doxapram can keep respirations regular.

(*Continued*)

Drug name	Drug dose	Species	Comments
Famotidine	0.5 mg/kg PO SID [6]	Eastern gray squirrels	n = 1 animal treated for transitional cell carcinoma of the kidney with nephrectomy and postoperative piroxicam and famotidine.
	0.6–1.2 mg/kg PO SID × 5d [3]	Prehensile-tailed porcupines	n = 2 animals were treated postoperatively after gastrotomy for gastroliths.
Glycopyrrolate	0.01 mg/kg SC IM [1, 7]	Beavers, Capybaras, Porcupines	
	0.01–0.02 mg/kg SC, IM [7]	Prairie dogs	
Leuprolide Acetate	NOT EFFECTIVE at 0.075–0.225 mg/kg q28d [19]	African crested porcupines	NOT effective in lowering testosterone or controlling intermale aggression behavior.
Melengesterol acetate (MGA implant)	0.15 mg/kg SC [2]	Naked mole rats (Heterocephalus glaber)	n = 1 successful for 24 months, but pregnancy detected at 26 months.
Porcine Zona Pellucida Vaccine (PZP)	P: 0.2 ml emulsion (50 µg) given IP, 1 injection followed by a 2nd 2 wks later, then annual booster [2]	Naked mole rats (H. glaber)	n = 1 animal receiving this protocol for contraception with success for more than 3 yrs.
Oxbow Critical Care Formula	Syringe fed per directions [3, 4]	Multiple species of herbivorous rodents	Fed to debilitated, anorexic, and postoperative animals to stimulate GI motility.
Sucralfate	70 mg/kg PO BID × 3d [4]	Brazilian porcupines (Coendou prehensilis)	n = 1 5 mo old, chronic diarrhea, failure to thrive, and anorexia. Cytologic exam of feces revealed blastocytosis. Treated with metronidazole and enrofloxacin, supportive care including sucralfate.
Sucralfate	122 mg/kg PO BID × 2d [3]	Prehensile-tailed porcupines	n = 1 cases of gastrolith surgically removed and treated postoperatively with sucralfate.

Species	Weight
Acouchi (*Myoprocta achouchy*)	0.6–1.3 kg
Agouti (*Dasyprocta spp.*)	3–6 kg
Beaver (*Castor canadensis*)	9–30 kg
Beaver (*Castor fiber*)	18–25 kg
Capybara (*Hydrochoerus spp.*)	30–100 kg
Coendou (*Coendou spp.*)	1.5–2 kg
Hispaniola Hutia (*Plagiodontia aedium*)	1–1.3 kg
Marmot, Alpine (*Marmota marmota*)	1–4 kg
Marmot, Hoary (*Marmota caligata*)	3–7.5 kg

Species	Weight
Marmot, Yellow-bellied (*Marmota flaviventris*)	2–5 kg
Muskrat (*Ondatra zibethicus*)	0.5–1.8 kg
Naked mole rat (*Heterocephalus glaber*)	avg 35 g
Nutria/Coypu (*Myocastor coypus*)	5–10 kg
Paca *(Agouti paca)*	6–10 kg
Pacarana *(Dinomys branickii)*	10–15 kg
Patagonian Hare/Cavy *(Dolichotis patagonum)*	9–16 kg
Porcupine, Cape *(Hystrix africaeaustralis)*	12–18 kg
Porcupine, Crested *(Hystrix cristata)*	9–15 kg
Porcupine, North American *(Erethizon dorsatum)*	3.5–11 kg
Porcupine, Prehensile tailed *(Coendou prehensilis)*	1–5 kg
Porcupine, New world/Prehensile tailed *(Sphiggurus spinosus)*	0.5–1.3 kg
Prairie Dog *(Cynomys spp.)*	0.5–2.2 kg
Rat, Plains *(Pseudomys australis)*	50–80 g
Rock Cavy *(Kerodon rupestris)*	1 kg
Spinifex Hopping mouse *(Notomys spp.)*	27–45 g
Springhaas *(Pedetes capensis)*	4 kg
Squirrel, African Ground *(Xerus inauris)*	375–800 g
Squirrel, Brown *(Sciurus vulgaris)*	200–800 g
Squirrel, Flying *(Glaucomys volans)*	50–185 g
Squirrel, Fox *(Sciurus niger)*	600–800 g
Squirrel, Giant *(Ratufa spp.)*	1.5–2 kg
Squirrel, Gray *(Sciurus carolinensis)*	0.4–0.7 kg
Ingram's Squirrel *(Sciurus ingrami)*	0.25 kg
Squirrel, Red *(Tamiascirus hudsonicus)*	141–312 g
Squirrel, Richardson's Ground *(Spermophilus richard-sonii)*	290–345 g
Squirrel, Tricolored *(Callosciurus erythraeus)*	150–500 g
Viscacha *(Lagostomus maximus)*	5–8 kg
Water Rat *(Hydromys chrysogaster)*	340–1275 g
Woodchuck *(Marmot monax)*	3–7 kg
Wood rat, Bushy-tailed *(Neotoma cinerea)*	115–350 g

References

1 Yarto-Jaramillo, E. (2014). Rodentia. In: *Fowler's Zoo and Wild Animal Medicine*, vol. 8 (ed. R.E. Miller and M. Fowler), 384–422. St. Louis, MO: Elsevier.

2 Raines, J. (2019). Naked mole rat management and medicine. In: *Fowler's Zoo and Wild Animal Medicine Current Therapy*, vol. 9 (ed. R.E. Miller, N. Lamberski and P.P. Calle), 514–518. St. Louis, MO: Elsevier.

3 Spriggs, M., Thompson, K.A., Barton, D. et al. (2014). Gastrolithiasis in prehensile-tailed porcupines (*Coundou prehensilis*): nine cases and pathogenesis of stone formation. *Journal of Zoo and Wildlife Medicine* 45 (4): 883–891.

4 Goe, A.M., Heard, D.J., Easley, J.R. et al. (2016). Blastocystis spp and Blastocystis Ratti in a Brazilian porcupine (*Coendou prehensilis*) with diarrhea. *Journal of Zoo and Wildlife Medicine* 47 (2): 640–644.
5 Hackworth, C.E., Eschar, D., Nau, M. et al. (2017). Diagnosis and successful treatment of a potentially zoonotic Dermatophytosis caused by Microsporum gypseum in a Zoo-housed North American porcupine (*Erethizon dorsatum*). *Journal of Zoo and Wildlife Medicine* 48 (2): 549–553.
6 Childs-Sanford, S.E., St-Vincent, R., and Hiss, A. (2015). Radiation therapy of a presumptive urethral transitional cell carcinoma in an eastern gray squirrel (*Sciurus carolinensis). Journal of Zoo and Wildlife Medicine* 46 (4): 918–920.
7 Heard, D. (2014). Rodents. In: *Zoo Animal and Wildlife Immobilization and Anesthesia*, 2e (ed. G. West, D. Heard and N. Caulkett), 893–903. Ames, IA: Wiley Blackwell.
8 Roug, A., Talley, H., Davis, T. et al. (2018). A mixture of butorphanol, azaperone, and medetomidine for the immobilization of American beavers (*Castor canadensis*). *Journal of Wildlife Diseases* 54 (3): 617–621.
9 Kreeger, T.J. and Arnemo, J.M. (2012). *Handbook of Wildlife Chemical Immobilization*. China: Kreeger.
10 Pachaly, J.R. and Werner, P.R. (1998). Restraint of the Paca (*Acouti paca*) with ketamine hydrochloride, Acetylpromazine maleate, and atropine sulfate. *Journal of Zoo and Wildlife Medicine* 29 (3): 303–306.
11 Monsalve, S. (2019). Immobilization, health, and current status of knowledge of free-living capybaras. In: *Fowler's Zoo and Wild Animal Medicine Current Therapy*, vol. 9 (ed. R.E. Miller, N. Lamberski and P.P. Calle), 519–526. St. Louis, MO: Elsevier.
12 Beiglbock, C. and Zenker, W. (2003). Evaluation of three combinations of anesthetics for use in free-ranging alpine marmots (*Marmota marmota*). *Journal of Wildlife Diseases* 39 (3): 665–674.
13 Morin, P. and Berteaux, D. (2003). Immobilization of North American porcupines (*Erethizon dorsatum*) using Ketamine and Xylazine. *Journal of Wildlife Diseases* 39 (3): 675–682.
14 King, J.D., Congdon, E., and Tosta, C. (2010). Evaluation of three immobilization combinations in the capybara (*Hydrochoerus hydrochaeris*). *Zoo Biology* 29 (1): 59–67.
15 Hale, M.B., Grisemer, S.J., and Fuller, T.K. (1994). Immobilization of porcupines with tiletamine hydrochloride and zolazepam hydrochloride (Telazol). *Journal of Wildlife Diseases* 30 (3): 429–431.
16 Massolo, A., Sforizi, A., and Lovari, S. (2003). Chemical immobilization of crested porcupines with tiletamine HCl and zolazepam HCl (Zoletil) under field conditions. *Journal of Wildlife Diseases* 39 (3): 727–731.
17 Weber, M.A., Miller, M.A., Neiffer, D. et al. (2006). Presumptive fenbendazole toxicosis in North American porcupines. *Journal of the American Veterinary Medical Association* 228 (8): 1240–1242.
18 Gardhouse, S. and Eschar, D. (2015). Diagnosis and successful treatment of Eimeria infection in a group of zoo-kept black-tailed prairie dogs (*Cynomys ludovicianus*). *Journal of Zoo and Wildlife Medicine* 46 (2): 367–369.
19 Stremme, D.W. (2010). Lupron (Leuprolide Acetate) Depot use in African Crested porcupines (*Hystrix africaeaustralis*) to control intermale aggression. *Annual Proceedings of the American Association of Zoo Veterinarians*. 263–264.

8

Primates

Drug name	Drug dose	Species	Comments
Antimicrobials and Antifungals			
Prosimians			
Amoxicillin	10–20 mg/kg PO BID [1]	Prosimians	
Ampicillin	10–30 mg/kg SC, IM, IV q6–8 hrs [1]	Prosimians	
Amoxicillin/ clavulanic acid (Clavamox)	12.9–15.4 mg/kg PO BID [2]	Coquerel's sifakas, Ring tailed lemurs, Black and white ruffed lemurs	For treatment post dental extraction and for upper respiratory infection.
	13.75 mg/kg PO BID [3]	Red ruffed lemurs	n = 1 postoperative antibiotics for 30 days.
Azithromycin	5–10 mg/kg PO SID [1]	Prosimians	
Cefadroxil	20 mg/kg PO BID [1]	Prosimians	
Cefazolin	10–30 mg/kg IM, IV q8 hr [1]	Prosimians	
	20 mg/kg IV [4]	Ring-tailed lemurs	n = 1, 10 yr old 3.4 kg, female with arteriovenous fistula that was surgically repaired, given intraoperative medications.
	22 mg/kg IV intraoperatively [3]	Red ruffed lemurs	n = 1, 3.54 kg female with surgical repair of metacarpal fractures.
Cefdinir	14 mg/kg PO SID × 5 wk [4]	Ring-tailed lemurs	n = 1, 10 yr old 3.4 kg, female with arteriovenous fistula that was surgically repaired, postop developed hyperesthesia of skin and secondary staph spp. infection that resolved.
Ceftazidime	30–50 mg/kg IM, IV q8 hr [1]	Prosimians	
Ceftiofur	1.1–2.2 mg/kg IM SID [1]	Prosimians	

(*Continued*)

Drug name	Drug dose	Species	Comments
Ceftiofur crystalline free acid (Excede)	6 mg/kg SC [4]	Ring-tailed lemurs	n = 1, 10 yr old 3.4 kg female with arteriovenous fistula that was surgically repaired, given intraoperative medications.
Doxycycline	5–10 mg/kg PO BID [1]	Prosimians	
Enrofloxacin	5 mg/kg PO, SC, IM SID [1]	Prosimians	
	5 mg/kg PO SID [2]	Black lemurs	n = 1 for treatment of cystitis.
Metronidazole	25 mg/kg PO SID [1]	Prosimians	
Oxytetracycline (LA 200)	20–33 mg/kg IM SID [5]	Black and white ruffed lemurs, Ring-tailed lemurs, Brown lemurs and Thick tailed bush babies	n = captive collection of primates with outbreak of tularemia and remaining asymptomatic animals treated with tetracycline or oxytetracycline if refused oral dose.
Penicillin G procaine/benzathine	40 000 IU/kg SQ [2]	Coquerel's sifakas	n = 1 treated perioperatively for dental extraction.
	45 000 IU/kg SQ [2]	Black lemurs	n = 1 with renal failure and periosteal hyperostosis.
Tetracycline	16.5–20 mg/kg PO BID [5]	Black and white ruffed lemurs, Ring-tailed lemurs, Brown lemurs and Thick tailed bush babies	n = captive collection of primates with outbreak of tularemia and remaining asymptomatic animals treated with tetracycline for 14 days or oxytetracycline if refused oral dose.
Trimethoprim sulfamethoxazole	25 mg/kg PO, IM BID [1]	Prosimians	
Monkeys and Lesser Apes			
Amikacin	2–3 mg/kg IM SID [6]	Callitrichids, Cebids and Lemurs	
Amoxicillin	11 mg/kg PO BID or SC/IM SID [6, 7]	Callitrichids, Cebids and Lemurs	Pediatric suspension available.
Amoxicillin/clavulanic acid (Clavamox)	12.9–15.4 mg/kg PO BID [2]	Allen's swamp monkeys, Goeldi's monkeys, Golden lion tamarins, White-face sakis	For treatment post dental extraction, facial abscesses, and for upper respiratory infections.
	15 mg/kg PO BID [6]	Callitrichids, Cebids and Lemurs	
Azithromycin	40 mg/kg PO SID [7]	Nonhuman primates	
Cephalexin	20 mg/kg PO BID [6]	Callitrichids, Cebids and Lemurs	
Cefazolin	25 mg/kg IM/IV BID [7]	Nonhuman primates	

Drug name	Drug dose	Species	Comments
Cefovecin	8 mg/kg SC [8, 9]	Olive baboons, Cynomolgus macaques, Rhesus macaques, Squirrel monkeys	Protein binding is much lower than in carnivores with half-lives of 5–10 hrs compared to dogs and cats with 133 or 166 hrs. Area under the curve values are much lower than in dogs and cats.
Ceftazidime	50 mg/kg IM/IV QID [6]	Callitrichids, Cebids and Lemurs	
Cefuroxime	50 mg PO SID × 14d [10]	Brown capuchins	n = 1 given postoperatively following perineal urethrostomy.
Cephalexin	100 mg PO BID × 7d [10]	Brown capuchins	n = 1 given postoperatively following perineal urethrostomy.
	15 mg PO TID × 28d [11]	Squirrel monkeys	n = 1 with traumatic luxation of left radial head and mid-diaphyseal fracture of ulna. Preoperatively started on penicillin G, then postoperatively treated with cephalexin.
Ceftriaxone	25 mg/kg IM/IV SID [7]	Nonhuman primates	
Ciprofloxacin	20 mg/kg PO BID [6]	Callitrichids, Cebids and Lemurs	Possible side effects: hallucinations seen in humans, presumably possible in primates.
Clindamycin	10 mg/kg PO BID [6]	Callitrichids, Cebids and Lemurs	
Doxycycline	2.5 mg/kg PO SID [7]	Nonhuman primates	
	3–4 mg/kg PO BID [6]	Callitrichids, Cebids and Lemurs	
Enrofloxacin	5 mg/kg PO/SC/IM SID [6, 7]	Callitrichids, Cebids and Lemurs	Possible side effects: hallucinations seen in humans, presumably possible in primates.
	5 mg/kg PO SID [2]	Black-handed spider monkeys	
Erythromycin	30–50 mg/kg IM BID [7]	Nonhuman primates	
	75 mg/kg PO BID × 10d [6]	Callitrichids, Cebids and Lemurs	For treatment of campylobacter-associated diarrhea and clostridial gastroenteritis.
Fluconazole	18 mg/kg PO BID [6]	Callitrichids, Cebids and Lemurs	For systemic mycoses.

(Continued)

Drug name	Drug dose	Species	Comments
Gentamicin	3 mg/kg q6–8 hrs IM [12]	Baboons	n = 6 animals administered a single dose of IM gentamicin. For Pseudomonas give every 6 hrs. In a preliminary study 4.4 mg/kg proved toxic.
	3–5 mg/kg IM/SC SID [7]	Nonhuman primates	
Griseofulvin	25 mg/kg PO for 3–4 wks [7]	Nonhuman primates	For treatment of ringworm (*Microphyton* and *Trichophyton spp*).
	20 mg/kg PO SID or 200 mg/kg PO q10d [6]	Callitrichids, Cebids and Lemurs	
Itraconazole	10 mg/kg PO SID	Callitrichids, Cebids and Lemurs [6]	For fungal/yeast gastroenteritis.
Ketoconazole	5–10 mg/kg PO for 3–4 wks [7]	Nonhuman primates	For treatment of ringworm (*Microphyton* and *Trichophyton spp*).
Metronidazole	25 mg/kg PO BID [6]	Callitrichids, Cebids and Lemurs	Clostridial gastroenteritis. Metronidazole benzoate is flavorless and more palatable.
Nystatin	200 000 IU PO q6 hrs [6, 7]	Callitrichids, Cebids and Lemurs	GI candidiasis. Continue for 48 hrs after clinical resolution.
Oxytetracycline	10 mg/kg SC//IM SID [6]	Callitrichids, Cebids and Lemurs	
Penicillin G	40 000 IU/kg IM once [11]	Squirrel monkeys	n = 1 animal with traumatic luxation of left radial head and middiaphyseal fracture of ulna. Preoperatively started on penicillin G.
Penicillin G Procaine	20 000 IU/kg IM BID [6]	Callitrichids, Cebids and Lemurs	
Penicillin G procaine/ benzathine	35 000 IU/kg SQ [2]	Goeldi's monkeys	n = 1 animal treated for facial abscess.
	45 000 IU/kg SQ [2]	Dusky leaf monkeys	n = 1 animal treated post dental extraction.
	20–60 000 IU/kg IM SID to BID [7]	Nonhuman primates	
Trimethoprim sulfadiazine	15 mg/kg PO BID or 30 mg/kg SC/IM SID [6]	Callitrichids, Cebids and Lemurs	
	25 mg/kg PO BID [2]	Goeldi's monkeys	n = 1 animal treated post dental extraction.
Trimethaprim sulfamethoxazole	24 mg/kg PO BID [7]	Nonhuman primates	
Great Apes			
Amoxicillin	15 mg/kg PO BID [13]	Chimpanzees	n = 1 female adult 68 kg, postoperative antibiotics after cholecystotomy, combined with ciprofloxacin 10 mg/kg PO BID.

Drug name	Drug dose	Species	Comments
	20 mg/kg PO BID × 10d [14]	Chimpanzees	n = 30 captive animals with human respiratory syncytial virus and Streptoccus pneumonia – 19 took oral amoxicillin, 1 received 15 mg/kg IM EOD for 2 doses then took oral, and the remaining 10 animals took ciprofloxacin 20 mg/kg PO SID for 10 days. 3 animals died. After 17 days, remaining 14 animals survived and no longer had clinical signs.
	500 mg PO BID [2]	Chimpanzees, Gorillas	For treatment of traumatic wounds.
Amoxicillin/clavulanic acid (Clavamox)	15.6 mg/kg PO BID [2]	Orangutans	n = 1 female with diarrhea.
Azithromycin	500 mg PO once, then 250 mg PO SID [2]	Chimpanzees, Gorillas	n = 2 animals, treated for wounds.
Cefazolin	1–2 g IV [2]	Gorillas, Chimpanzees	Used in multiple animals during surgery prophylactically.
Ceftazidime	500 mg IM [15]	Chimpanzees	n = 1 postoperative management of bilateral compound metatarsal fractures. Ceftazidime given IM during bandage changes daily or every 2–3 days.
Cephalexin	500 mg PO BID [2]	Chimpanzees, Gorillas	For treatment of traumatic wounds.
Cephalexin monohydrate	1000 mg PO BID for 2 weeks [15]	Chimpanzees	n = 1 postoperative management of bilateral compound metatarsal fractures.
Ciprofloxacin	10 mg/kg PO BID [13]	Chimpanzees	n = 1 female adult 68 kg, postoperative antibiotics after cholecystotomy, combined with amoxicillin 15 mg/kg PO BID.
Gentamicin	3.5 mg/kg IV TID or 50 mg nebulized for 30 min [16]	Sumatran orangutans	n = 1, 2 yr old female undergoing surgical repair of atrial septal defect with secondary complications postoperatively of adult respiratory distress syndrome. Gentamicin was administered via nebulization for tracheal infection, but stopped at 30 min due to accumulation of gas in laryngeal air sacs. IV gentamicin was initiated based on culture results.
Marbofloxacin	200 mg IM SID [17]	Sumatran orangutans	n = 1 post dilation of bile duct for 14 days.

(*Continued*)

Drug name	Drug dose	Species	Comments
Piperacillin sodium	500 mg intralesional during bandage changes, 500 mg IV, 1 g on gel foam and placed into the wounds, Added to Lactated Ringer's solution at 4 g/l and given IV [15]	Chimpanzees	n = 1 postoperative management of bilateral compound metatarsal fractures.
Streptomycin + Penicillin G	400 mg IM [18]	Mountain gorillas	n = 1 juvenile female, 30 kg estimated, perioperative treatment of necrotic rectal prolapse resection.
Sulfasalazine	1000 mg PO BID [2]	Gorillas	n = 1 male, treated for colitis.
Trimethoprim sulfadiazine	15 mg/kg PO BID [2]	Gorillas	n = 1 male, treated for wounds.
Analgesia			
Prosimians			
Acetominophen	A: 10–15 mg/kg PO q8–12 hrs [19]	Prosimians	
Aspirin	Asp: 10–20 mg/kg PO q8–12 hrs [19]	Prosimians	
	10 mg/kg PO SID for 7 mo [20]	Ruffed lemur	n = 1 with chronic focal osteomyelitis.
Buprenorphine	Bup: 0.01–0.02 mg/kg SC, IM, IV q8–12 hrs [19]	Prosimians	
Butorphanol	B: 0.1–0.4 mg/kg SC, IM, IV q3–4 hrs [19]	Prosimians	
Flunixin meglumine	0.25–0.5 mg/kg SC, IM, IV SID [19]	Prosimians	
Gabapentin	5 mg/kg PO BID [2]	Black lemurs	n = 1 treated for periarticular hyperostosis.
	15 mg/kg PO BID [2]	Black and white Ruffed lemurs	For treatment of suspected nerve trauma of front limb.
Ibuprofen	10 mg/kg PO q8–12 hrs [19]	Prosimians	
	14 mg/kg PO BID × 10d [4]	Ring-tailed lemurs	n = 1, 10 yr old 3.4 kg female with arteriovenous fistula that was surgically repaired, given in intra- and perioperative medications.
Ketoprofen	2 mg/kg once, then 1 mg/kg PO, SC, IV, IM SID [19]	Prosimians	
Meloxicam	0.2 mg/kg once, then 0.1 mg/kg PO, SC, IV SID [19]	Prosimians	

Drug name	Drug dose	Species	Comments
	0.2 mg/kg SC once, then 0.1 mg/kg PO SID [3]	Red ruffed lemurs	n = 1 for postoperative pain, for a total of 19 days, combined with tramadol.
Morphine	0.5 mg/kg IV [3]	Red ruffed lemur	n = 1 animal, 3.54 kg, treated for perioperative pain control.
Tramadol	1–4 mg/kg PO BID [19]	Prosimians	
	1.3 mg/kg PO BID [3]	Red ruffed lemurs	n = 1 animal, 3.54 kg, postoperative pain control for 5 days, combined with meloxicam. 2 mg/kg resulted in lethargy and anorexia.
Monkeys and Lesser Apes			
Aspirin	5–10 mg/kg PO q4–6 hrs [6]	Callitrichids, Cebids and Lemurs	Anti-inflammatory and antipyretic.
Buprenorphine	0.01–0.02 mg/kg IM BID [6]	Callitrichids, Cebids and Lemurs	Antagonize with naltrexone if needed.
	0.05 mg IM [21]	Siamangs	Postoperative analgesia.
Buprenorphine sustained release (SR)	0.2 mg/kg SC once [22]	Cynomologous and Rhesus macaques	n = 5 of each species, remained at hypothesized therapeutic levels for 5 days, 4/10 had mild injection site reactions.
Butorphanol	0.02 mg/kg IM q3–4 hrs [6]	Callitrichids, Cebids and Lemurs	May cause profound respiratory depression. Antagonize with naloxone if needed.
Carprofen	2–4 mg/kg PO/SC SID to BID [6]	Callitrichids, Cebids and Lemurs	Anti-inflammatory and antipyretic. Variation in half life with species. Cox-1 selectivity may be an issue.
Fentanyl	1.3 or 2.6 mg/kg Topical application [23]	Rhesus macaques	Provided efficacious analgesia and reduced stress, discomfort and risk to animals and personnel.
	Transdermal patch 25 µg/h or transdermal fentanyl solution 1.95 mg/kg topically [23, 24]	Cynomolgus macaques	Marked interanimal variability and 3/4 animals given 2.6 mg/kg transdermal solution had life threatening side effects that improved after naloxone administration.
Flunixin meglumine	0.3–1 mg/kg SC. IV SID [6]	Callitrichids, Cebids and Lemurs	Anti-inflammatory and antipyretic.
Ibuprofen	20 mg/kg PO SID [6]	Callitrichids, Cebids and Lemurs	Anti-inflammatory.
	4 mg PO BID [11]	Squirrel monkeys	n = 1 postoperative administration after repair of left radial luxation and ulnar fracture.
Ketoprofen	1 mg/kg IM [11]	Squirrel monkeys	n = 1 administration for left radial luxation and ulnar fracture prior to surgical repair.

(*Continued*)

Drug name	Drug dose	Species	Comments
	2 mg/kg IV/IM SID [7]	Nonhuman primates	
Morphine	1 mg/kg PO/SC/IM/IV q4 hrs [6]	Callitrichids, Cebids and Lemurs	May cause profound respiratory depression. Antagonize with naloxone as needed.
Naloxone	0.01–0.05 mg/kg IM/IV [6]	Callitrichids, Cebids and Lemurs	Opiod antagonist.
Oxymorphone	0.15 mg/kg IV/IM/SC q4–6 hrs [7]	Nonhuman primates	Monitor for respiratory depression.
Paracetamol	5–10 mg/kg PO q6 hrs [6]	Callitrichids, Cebids and Lemurs	Antipyretic and minimally anti-inflammatory.
Great Apes			
Acetominophen (Infant Tylenol syrup)	360 mg PO as needed for pain [15]	Chimpanzees	n = 1 postoperative management of bilateral compound metatarsal fractures.
Acetominophen (Tylenol)	300 mg PO TID [25]	Chimpanzees	Postoperative management of an appendectomy.
	10 mg/kg PO via nasogastric tube [16]	Sumatran orangutans	n = 1, 2 yr old female received prior to administration of a whole blood transfusion.
Buprenorphine	B: 0.005 mg/kg IM [25]	Chimpanzees	n = 1 perioperatively for an appendectomy,.
Butorphanol	But: 0.01 mg/kg IM [25]	Chimpanzees	n = 1 postoperative administration following an appendectomy.
Diclofenac	75 mg IM [25]	Chimpanzees	n = 1 perioperative removal of retained placenta.
Ibuprofen	200–800 mg PO BID to TID [25]	Western lowland gorillas, Chimpanzees	
	900 mg PO SID [17]	Sumatran orangutans	n = 1 animal post procedure for dilation of bile duct.
Ketoprofen	2 mg/kg IM [25]	Western lowland gorillas	
	2 mg/kg SC once [26]	Orangutans	n = 1 postoperative administration following tubal ligation.
Meloxicam	7.5 mg PO or SC SID [2]	Chimpanzees	Human dose used in a Chimpanzee.
Morphine	0.15 mg/kg PO BID [13]	Chimpanzees	n = 1 animal 68 kg, 40 yr., with suspected biliary obstruction, pre and postoperatively.
Tramadol	1 mg/kg PO BID [2, 25]	Western lowland gorillas	Appeared to have a mild sedative effect. Human dose is 50–100 mg PO SID to QID as needed and is useful in Great Apes.

Drug name	Drug dose	Species	Comments
Anethesia and Sedation			
Prosimians			
Butorphanol	B: 0.1–0.4 mg/kg IM, IV, SC; antagonize with naloxone 0.02 mg/kg IM [19]	Prosimians	Duration of 3–4 hrs.
Butorphanol + dexmedetomidine + ketamine	B: 0.3–0.4 mg/kg + Dexmed: 0.02 mg/kg + K: 3–5 mg/kg IM [1, 19]	Prosimians	Complete immobilization, duration 15–30 min.
Butorphanol + dexmedetomidine + midazolam	B: 0.3–0.4 mg/kg + Dexmed: 0.02 mg/kg + Mid: 0.2–0.3 mg/kg IM [1, 19]	Prosimians	Complete immobilization, duration 20–50 min.
Dexmedetomidine	Dexmed: 0.02 mg/kg IM; antagonize with atipamezole 0.2 mg/kg IM [1, 19]	Prosimians	Duration 30–60 min.
Dexmedetomidine + ketamine	Dexmed: 0.02 mg/kg + K: 3–5 mg/kg IM [1, 19]	Prosimians	Heavy sedation to complete immobilization. Duration 10–20 min.
Dexmedetomidine + midazolam	Dexmed: 0.02 mg/kg + Mid: 0.2 mg/kg IM [1, 19]	Prosimians	Light to moderate sedation, duration 30 min.
Diazepam	D: 0.25–0.5 mg/kg PO, IV; antagonize with flumazenil 0.02 mg/kg IV [1]	Prosimians	
	D: 0.5–2.5 mg/kg IV, Antagonize with flumazenil 0.02 mg/kg IV [21]	Prosimians	Duration of 30 min.
Fentanyl	F: 0.001–0.03 mg/kg/hr IV CRI; antagonize with naloxone 0.02 mg/kg IM [1, 19]	Prosimians	
Ketamine	K: 5–15 mg/kg IM, IV [1, 19]	Prosimians	Duration of 30 min, not recommended for use alone.
	K: 11 mg/kg [27]	Slow loris	Supplement with ketamine 5 mg/kg as needed.
	K: 12 mg/kg IM [27]	Black lemurs, Ring-tailed lemurs, Ruffed lemurs	
	K: 15 mg/kg IM [27]	Galagos	
Ketamine + diazepam	K: 12.2–40.5 mg/kg + D: 0.05–1.19 mg/kg IM [28]	Ring-tailed lemurs	n = 70 free-ranging animals. Weights not known prior to darting thus the wide range of doses once weight obtained.

(*Continued*)

Drug name	Drug dose	Species	Comments
Ketamine + medetomidine	K: 4 mg/kg + M: 0.04 mg/kg; antagonize with atipamezole 0.2 mg/kg [27]	Ring-tailed lemurs	
Ketamine + midazolam	K: 5–10 mg/kg + Mid: 0.2 mg/kg IM [1]	Prosimians	Heavy sedation to complete immobilization. Duration 20–30 min.
Ketamine + xylazine	K: 10 mg/kg + X: 1 mg/kg; antagonize with tolazoline 1 mg/kg [27]	Ring-tailed lemurs	
Midazolam	0.1–0.3 mg/kg IM, IV; antagonize with flumazenil 0.02 mg/kg IV [1, 19]	Prosimians	Duration of 30 min.
Propofol	P: 3–6 mg/kg IV [1, 19]	Prosimians	Duration 10–15 min.
Telazol	T: 10 mg/kg [27]	Galagos, Thick-tailed galagos/ Greater bush babies	Supplement with ketamine 10 mg/kg as needed.
	T: 3–5 mg/kg IM; antagonize zolazepam with flumazenil 0.02 mg/kg IV [19]	Prosimians	
Telazol	T: 5 mg/kg IM [27]	Ruffed lemurs	Supplement with ketamine 5 mg/kg as needed.
	T: 5–10 mg/kg SC, IM; can antagonize with flumazenil 0.02 mg/kg IV [1]	Prosimians	
	T: 10 mg/kg IM [27]	Black lemurs	Supplement with ketamine 5 mg/kg as needed.
	T: 10 mg/kg IM [29, 30, 31, 32]	White-fronted brown lemurs, Red ruffed lemurs, Black lemurs, Decken's sifakas, Red-fronted brown lemurs, Ring-tailed lemurs	n = 37 White-fronted brown lemurs and 22 Red ruffed lemurs, 25 Black lemurs (range 1.1–2.2 kg), 20 Decken's Sifaka, 20 Red-fronted brown lemurs, 20 adult Ring-tailed lemurs, free-ranging individuals for biomedical evaluation.
	T: 20 mg/kg IM [27]	Ring-tailed lemurs	Young lemurs <5 yr may require 30 mg/kg.
Monkeys and Lesser Apes			
Acepromazine	0.5–1 mg/kg PO [6]	Callitrichids, Cebids and Lemurs	Tranquilization, no reversal.
Detomidine + ketamine	D: 0.44 mg/kg + K: 10.2 mg/kg PO [33]	Mandrills, Baboons	n = 7 animals were given oral DK but only 3 received complete doses and were more sedated at earlier times. All animals required supplemental drugs for induction and safe handling.

Drug name	Drug dose	Species	Comments
Diazepam	0.5–1 mg/kg PO [6]	Callitrichids, Cebids and Lemurs	Sedation, give in small amounts of food or drink 30–60 min prior to anesthesia. Variable effect and recovery prolonged unless reversed.
Fentanyl + midazolam + ketamine	F: 15 µg/kg + Mid: 0.3 mg/kg + K: 5 mg/kg IM [21]	Japanese macaques	n = 8 animals, administered either the Fentanyl-Midazolam-Ketamine (FMK) protocol or ketamine (5 mg/kg) + medetomidine (0.05 mg/kg) (KM) IM. Both resulted in rapid smooth induction, but required supplemental oxygen, FMK duration was 32–52 min and KM was 54–79 min; KM had lower heart rates and higher arterial pressure, but woke up more rapidly.
Ketamine	K: 5 mg/kg IM [27]	Hanuman langurs	Better relaxation when not used alone.
	K: 6–10 mg/kg IM [34]	For medium to large species	
	K: 9 mg/kg IM [27]	Douroucoulis/Owl monkeys	Supplement with 4.5 mg/kg ketamine as needed.
Ketamine	K: 10 mg/kg IM [27]	Colobus monkeys, Debrazza's monkeys/Guenons, Patas monkeys	Better relaxation when not used alone.
	K: 10 mg/kg IM [27]	Siamangs, Uakaris	
	K: 11 mg/kg IM [27]	Gelada baboons	
	K: 12 mg/kg IM [27]	Chacma baboons, Hamadryas baboons, White-handed gibbons, Vervet monkeys	
	K: 12.5 mg/kg IM [27]	Sooty mangabeys	
	K: 15 mg/kg IM [27]	Olive baboons, Barbary macaques, Mandrills, Monkeys/Guenons, Green	
	K: 16 mg/kg IM [27]	White-cheeked gibbons	
	K: 20 mg/kg [27]	Crab-eating/cynomologous macaques	
	K: 22 mg/kg [27]	Japanese macaques, Lion-tail macaques, Pig-tail macaques, Rhesus macaques, Stump-tailed macaques	

(*Continued*)

Drug name	Drug dose	Species	Comments
	K: 22 mg/kg [27]	Douroucoulis/Owl monkeys, Proboscis monkeys	Supplement with ketamine 11 mg/kg as needed.
Ketamine + acepromazine	K: 5 mg/kg + A: 0.2 mg/kg IM [27]	Western baboons	Be aware of possible aggression among males during recovery.
Ketamine + dexmedetomidine	K: 2–4 mg/kg + Dexmed: 0.02–0.03 mg/kg IM [34]	For medium to large species	Antagonize with atipamezole at 10 × the dose of dexmedetomidine.
	K: 5–10 mg/kg + Dexmed: 0.01–0.02 mg/kg IM [21]	Golden lion tamarins	Higher K doses increase duration of anesthesia.
Ketamine + diazepam	K: 10 mg/kg + D: 0.2–0.36 mg/kg IM [21, 27]	Olive baboons	
	K: 15 mg/kg + D: 1 mg/kg IM [6]	Callitrichids, Cebids and Lemurs	Surgical anesthesia for 30–40 min, improved muscle relaxation compared with ketamine alone.
Ketamine + medetomidine	K: 2–4 mg/kg + M: 0.04–0.06 mg/kg IM [34]	For medium to large species	Antagonize with atipamezole at 5 × the dose of medetomidine.
Ketamine + medetomidine	K: 5–8 mg/kg + M: 0.02–0.04 mg/kg IM [21]	For most species of monkeys	For induction or short duration of anesthesia.
	K: 3 mg/kg + M: 0.15 mg/kg [21]	Cynomolgus macaques	
	K: 2 mg/kg + M: 0.075 mg/kg IM [21]	Rhesus macaques	
	K: 3 mg/kg + M: 0.07 mg/kg IM; antagonize with atipamezole 0.35 mg/kg half IV and half IM [27]	White-handed gibbons	Supplement with ketamine 1.5 mg/kg as needed.
	K: 4 mg/kg + M: 0.15 mg/kg; antagonize with atipamezole 0.75 mg/kg [27]	Howler monkeys	Supplement with ketamine 2 mg/kg as needed.
	K: 4 mg/kg + M: 0.15 mg/kg IM [21]	Capuchin monkeys/Guenons	
	K: 5 mg/kg + M: 0.05 mg/kg [35]	Japanese macaques	Mean induction time of 4 min, duration of 65 min, give supplemental oxygen to combat hypoxemia.
	K: 5 mg/kg + M: 0.07 mg/kg IM; antagonize with atipamezole 0.35 mg/kg IM [27]	Olive baboons, Yellow baboons, Barbary macaques	Supplement with ketamine 3 mg/kg as needed.

Drug name	Drug dose	Species	Comments
	K: 5 mg/kg + M: 0.08 mg/kg IM; antagonize with atipamezole 0.4 mg/kg IM [27]	Lesser white-nosed monkeys/Guenons	Supplement with ketamine 3 mg/kg as needed.
	K: 5–7.5 mg/kg + M: 0.05–0.1 mg/kg IM; antagonize with atipamezole 0.5 mg/kg half IV and half IM [6, 27]	Hamadryas baboons, Japanese macaques, Common marmosets, Cotton-headed/topped tamarins, Emperor tamarins, Red-bellied tamarins	Supplement with ketamine 3 mg/kg as needed. May not induce complete immobilization and require additional ketamine. Use higher doses in smaller primates. Anesthesia of 45–60 min. Deepen with gas anesthesia. Excellent muscle relaxation.
	K: 6 mg/kg + M: 0.09 mg/kg; antagonize with atipamezole 0.45 mg/kg [27]	Bonnet macaques, Pig-tail macaques, Rhesus macaques	Supplement with ketamine 3 mg/kg as needed.
	K: 7 mg/kg + M: 0.1 mg/kg; antagonize with atipamezole 0.5 mg/kg [27]	Black mangabeys	Supplement with ketamine 3 mg/kg as needed.
	K: 8 mg/kg + M: 0.1 mg/kg; antagonize with atipamezole 0.5 mg/kg [27]	Crab-eating/cynomologous macaques, Monkeys/Guenons, Green	Supplement with ketamine 3 mg/kg as needed.
	K: 9 mg/kg + M: 0.1 mg/kg; antagonize with atipamezole 0.5 mg/kg [27]	Blue monkeys/Guenons	Supplement with ketamine 3 mg/kg as needed.
	K: 5– 10 mg/kg + M: 0.1 mg/kg; antagonize with atipamezole 0.5 mg/kg half IV and half IM [27]	Golden lion tamarins	Supplement with ketamine 3 mg/kg as needed.
Ketamine + medetomidine	K: 10 mg/kg + M: 0.02 mg/kg; antagonize with atipamezole 0.5 mg/kg [27]	Capuchin monkeys/Guenons	Supplement with ketamine 3 mg/kg as needed.
Ketamine + midazolam	K: 10 mg/kg + Mid: 0.2 mg/kg [2]	White-cheeked gibbons, Black mangabeys, Golden-bellied mangabeys, Squirrel monkeys, Howler monkeys, and Spider monkeys	

(Continued)

Drug name	Drug dose	Species	Comments
Ketamine + midazolam	K: 10 mg/kg + Mid: 1 mg/kg [21, 27]	Black-tufted marmosets, Common marmosets	Supplement with ketamine 5 mg/kg as needed, duration of 30–45 minutes.
Ketamine + xylazine	K: 5.25 mg/kg + X: 0.45 mg/kg [21]	Rhesus macaques	Duration 23–63 min, anesthetic emergence was fast, pedal reflex preceded end of anesthesia by 2–3 min.
	K: 2.5 mg/kg + X: 2 mg/kg [21, 27]	Rhesus macaques	Minimum effective ketamine dose was 2.5 mg/kg but 5 mg/kg also produced safe anesthesia. Xylazine minimum effective dose was 0.25 mg/kg but up to 2 mg/kg increased duration of anesthesia to 60–80 min.
	K: 5 mg/kg + X: 1 mg/kg IM [21]	Japanese macaques	
	K: 10–11 mg/kg + X: 0.5 mg/kg IM [21, 27]	Yellow Baboons	Easily intubated and duration of anesthesia 90–125 min.
	K: 10–15 mg/kg + X: 1 mg/kg IM [21]	Wild Savanna baboons	
	K: 18 mg/kg + X: 1.8 mg/kg [27]	Black-cheeked monkeys/Guenons	Supplement with ketamine 9 mg/kg as needed.
Medetomidine + midazolam	M: 0.06 mg/kg + Mid: 0.3 mg/kg; antagonize with atipamezole 0.25 mg/kg [21, 27]	Japanese macaques	Most likely only used for captive animals, provided deep sedation with rapid reversal.
Midazolam	0.5 mg/kg PO [6]	Callitrichids, Cebids and Lemurs	Half-life 1–4 hrs, more applicable for larger species.
Propofol	1 mg/kg IV induction, 0.3–0.5 mg/kg/min CRI [7]	Nonhuman primates	
Telazol	T: 1.3 mg/kg IM [27]	Hamadryas baboons	
	T: 2 mg/kg IM [27]	Lesser white-nosed monkeys/Guenons	Supplement with 2 mg/kg ketamine as needed.
Telazol	T: 2.2 mg/kg IM [27]	Mandrills, Common marmosets, Allen's monkeys, Cotton headed/topped tamarins, Emperor tamarins, Golden lion tamarins, Red-bellied tamarins	Supplement with ketamine 2.2 mg/kg as needed.
	T: 2.5 mg/kg IM [27]	Gelada baboons	Supplement with ketamine 2.5 mg/kg as needed.
	T: 2.6 mg/kg IM [27]	Toque macaques	Supplement with ketamine 2.6 mg/kg as needed.
	T: 2–5 mg/kg IM [34]	For medium to large species	Considerably longer recoveries, than ketamine + alpha-2 agonist.

Drug name	Drug dose	Species	Comments
	T: 3 mg/kg IM [27]	Chacma baboons, Gray-cheeked mangabeys, Sykes monkeys/Guenons	Supplement with ketamine 3 mg/kg as needed.
	T: 3.2 mg/kg IM [27]	Uakaris	Supplement with ketamine 3.2 mg/kg as needed.
	T: 3.3 mg/kg IM [27]	White-cheeked gibbons, Hanuman langurs	Supplement with ketamine 3.3 mg/kg as needed.
	T: 4.4 mg/kg IM [27]	Howler monkeys, White-nosed monkeys/Guenons	Supplement with ketamine 4.4 mg/kg as needed.
	T: 5 mg/kg IM [27]	Mona monkeys, Patas monkeys	Supplement with ketamine 5 mg/kg as needed.
	T: 4.4 mg/kg IM [27]	Celebes apes, Olive baboons, Yellow baboons, Siamangs, White-handed gibbons, Barbary macaques, Lion-tail macaques, Pig-tail macaques, Sooty mangabeys, Colobus monkeys	Supplement with ketamine 4.4 mg/kg as needed.
Telazol	T: 5 mg/kg IM [27]	Western baboons, Bonnet macaques, Japanese macaques, Stump-tailed macaques, Debrazza's monkeys/Guenons, Diana Monkeys/Guenons, Monkeys/Guenons, Green,	Supplement with ketamine 2.5–5 mg/kg as needed.
	T: 5–10 mg/kg IM [21]	Cynomolgus macaques, Vervet monkeys	Adequate for ophthalmologic surgery. Rapid onset, duration of 30–50 min, excellent muscle relaxation, no ocular movement, and gradual emergence with no adverse effects.
	T: 5–10 mg/kg IM [21]	Commonly used for many species	High therapeutic index and large variation in dosage. Can use flumazenil to reverse zolazepam. Prolonged recoveries can be seen.
	T: 6.6 mg/kg [27]	Rhesus macaques	6.6 mg/kg ketamine.
	T: 7 mg/kg IM [27]	Grivet monkeys/Guenons	Supplement with ketamine 4 mg/kg as needed.
	T: 7 mg/kg IM [27]	Wooly monkeys, White-lipped tamarins, Vervet monkeys	Supplement with ketamine 7 mg/kg as needed.

(Continued)

Drug name	Drug dose	Species	Comments
	T: 5–10 mg/kg [27]	Crab-eating/ cynomologous Macaques	Supplement with 5 mg/kg ketamine as needed.
	T: 11.6–18 mg/kg IM [21, 36]	Wild black spider monkeys	Higher doses resulted in more reliable and stable planes of anesthesia, duration of 80–150 min,.
	T: 10–12 mg/kg [27]	Squirrel Monkeys	Supplement with ketamine 6–10 mg/kg as needed.
	T: 10–15 mg/kg IM [27]	Capuchin monkeys/ Guenons, Spider monkeys	Supplement with up to 10 mg/kg ketamine as needed.
	T: 22.5 mg/kg IM [21]	Wild red howler monkeys	Adults 22.5 mg/kg, juveniles 30.5 mg/kg. Induction time was 1–6 min, duration of 40–300 min, no apparent adverse effects.
Telazol + medetomidine	T: 1 mg/kg + M: 0.02 mg/kg IM; antagonize with atipamezole 0.1 mg/kg IM [27]	Gibbons, Gray	Supplement with 0.5 mg/kg Telazol as needed.
	T: 0.8–2.3 mg/kg + M: 0.02–0.06 mg/kg IM; antagonize with atipamezole 0.1–0.25 mg/kg [21]	Bornean gibbons, Long-tailed and Pig-tailed macaques	Monitor for blood pressure and respirations, provide oxygen support.
Great Apes			
Alprazolam	0.25 mg/kg PO BID [2]	Chimpanzees	n = 1 female, treated postoperatively for wounds.
Alprazolam	0.5 mg/kg PO BID [2]	Chimpanzees	n = 1 male, treated for aggression.
Buprenorphine	0.01–0.02 mg/kg IM, IV; antagonize with naloxone 0.02 mg/kg IM, IV [37]	Orangutans	May be used in combination with other drugs for inductions. May produce respiratory depression.
Butorphanol	0.1–0.2 mg/kg IM, IV; antagonize with naloxone 0.02 mg/kg IM, IV [37]	Orangutans	May be used in combination with other drugs for inductions.
Clonidine	0.05–0.1 PO, or titrated up to 0.2 mg/kg SID to BID [22]	Chimpanzees	To treat different forms of aggression, Guanfacine may also be used but with less sedation.
Diazepam	D: 0.2 mg/kg PO; antagonize with flumazenil 0.02–0.1 mg/kg IV [37]	Gorillas	May reduce anxiety, may be used in combination with other drugs.
	5 mg PO [25]	Juvenile Gorillas	Given to juveniles orally 2 hrs prior to hand injection with ketamine.
	D: 0.2 mg/kg PO [33, 25]	Gorillas	Given 90–120 min prior to anesthetic induction.

Drug name	Drug dose	Species	Comments
	D: 0.5–1 mg/kg PO IM IV; antagonize with flumazenil 0.02–0.1 mg/kg IV [37]	Orangutans	May reduce anxiety, may be used in combination with other drugs.
	5–30 mg SID to BID [22]	Chimpanzees	Anxiolytic for short-term use, rapid effect and well tolerated for animals that display inappropriate fear, anxiety, or mild forms of self-injury during introductions or in general. Appears to work better than lorazepam 0.5–3 mg SID to BID.
	10–40 mg total in juice 1–2 hrs prior to anesthesia [22]	Chimpanzees	Given to decrease anxiety prior to anesthesia.
Detomidine + ketamine	D: 0.32 mg/kg + K: 9.6 mg/kg PO [33]	Gorillas	n = 6 one received complete dose and was laterally recumbent then received 1 mg/kg Telazol for safe handling, 5 animals receiving partial doses required supplemental Telazol for induction. No screaming or charging in response to darting. One animal had complications including regurgitation and difficulty maintaining suitable plane of anesthesia.
Droperidol + carfentanil	Dro: 1.25 mg for juvenile and 2.5 mg for Adults, PO + C: 2 µg/kg transmucosal [25]	Chimpanzees	Provided effective premedication with profound sedation prior to IM Telazol for induction. Carfentanil was administered onto oral mucosa with a syringe, which produced heavy sedation 25 min after administration. Naltrexone at 100 × carfentanil dose in mg was given concurrently with Telazol. Provide supplemental oxygen. Facial pruritis noted in some.
Fentanyl	10–15 µg/kg in lollipop [25]	Orangutans, Chimpanzees, Gorillas	Trained for 4–6 weeks to suck slowly and Orangutans and Gorillas accepted lollipops and displayed adequate sedation in 30–45 min and responded minimally to darting. Chimpanzees were minimally accepting of the lollipops.

(Continued)

Drug name	Drug dose	Species	Comments
Haloperidol	2–4 mg/day PO [22]	Chimpanzees	n = 1 female successfully treated for generalized anxiety and intermittent self-mutilation. Previous doses of 5–10 mg/day PO were discontinued due to bradykinesia in 5 males.
Ketamine	K: 5–20 mg/kg IM [25, 37]	Chimpanzees	Rapid induction, minimal cardiovascular and respiratory changes, not reversible, short duration of action.
	K: 6–10 (up to 14) mg/kg IM [25, 37]	Orangutans, Gorillas	Rapid induction, minimal cardiovascular and respiratory changes, not reversible, short duration of action.
	K: 7 mg/kg IM via dart [25]	Free-ranging mountain gorillas	Induction of 5 min and recovery 42 min,.
	K: 10–15 mg/kg IM [27]	Gorillas	Better relaxation when not used alone.
	K: 15 mg/kg IM [27]	Chimpanzees	Better relaxation when not used alone.
	K: 20 mg/kg IM [27]	Orangutans	Better relaxation when not used alone.
Ketamine + medetomidine	K: 2–5 mg/kg + M: 0.02–0.05 mg/kg IM [25]	Chimpanzees	Antagonize with atipamezole 0.1–0.25 mg/kg IM.
	K: 2–5 mg/kg + M: 0.03–0.05 mg/kg IM [25]	Gorillas	Antagonize with atipamezole 0.1–0.25 mg/kg IM.
	K: 3 mg/kg + M: 0.02–0.03 mg/kg IM [25]	Orangutans	Antagonize with atipamezole 0.1–0.25 mg/kg IM.
	K: 2–5 mg/kg + M: 0.02–0.05 mg/kg IM; antagonize with atipamezole 0.1–0.5 mg/kg [37]	Chimpanzees, Gorillas	Spontaneous arousal, potential for cardiovascular effects, reversible.
	K: 2–7 mg/kg + M: 0.03–0.04 mg/kg IM; antagonize with atipamezole 0.1–0.5 mg/kg [37]	Orangutans	Spontaneous arousal, potential for cardiovascular effects, reversible.
	K: 5 mg/kg + M: 0.05 mg/kg IM; antagonize with atipamezole 0.2 mg/kg half IV and half IM [27]	Chimpanzees	Supplement with ketamine 3 mg/kg as needed.
	K: 5 mg/kg + M: 0.05 mg/kg IM; antagonize with atipamezole 0.25 mg/kg half IV and half IM [27]	Gorillas	Supplement with ketamine 2.5 mg/kg as needed.

Drug name	Drug dose	Species	Comments
	K: 5.5 mg/kg + M: 0.056 mg/kg IM via hand injection [13]	Chimpanzees	n = 1 immobilization for a 40 yr old 68 kg female with a biliary calculus.
Ketamine + midazolam + atropine	K: 2.28 mg/kg total + Mid: 0.03 mg/kg + Atr: 0.01 mg/kg [26]	Orangutans	n = 1 animal undergoing tubal ligation, initially given K: 1 mg/kg + atropine, then 10 min later an additional 1 mg/kg ketamine IM and midazolam IM, then ketamine given 0.28 mg/kg IV for intubation and maintained on isoflurane.
Ketamine + midazolam	K: 1–2 mg/kg + Mid: 0.03 mg/kg IM, antagonize with flumazenil 0.02–0.2 mg/kg IV [25, 37]	Orangutans	Shorter duration of effect than Telazol, drug volume may be an issue.
Ketamine + midazolam	K: 2.5 mg/kg + Mid: 0.25 mg/kg IM [25]	Chimpanzees	Antagonize with flumazenil 0.02–0.1 mg/kg IV.
	K: 9 mg/kg + Mid: 0.05 mg/kg IM; antagonize with flumazenil 0.02–0.1 mg/kg IV [25, 37]	Gorillas	Shorter duration of effect than Telazol, drug volume may be an issue.
Ketamine + xylazine	K: 5–7 mg/kg + X: 1–1.4 mg/kg IM; antagonize with yohimbine 0.125–0.25 mg/kg [25, 37]	Orangutans	Rapid induction, cardiovascular stable, longer anesthetic times.
	K: 5–10 mg/kg + X: 1 mg/kg IM; antagonize with yohimbine 0.125–0.25 mg/kg [37]	Chimpanzees	Rapid induction, cardiovascular stable, longer anesthetic times.
	K: 6.5 mg/kg + X: 0.8 mg/kg IM [27]	Orangutans	
	K: 10 mg/kg + X: 1 mg/kg IM [27]	Chimpanzees	
	K: 15–20 mg/kg + X: 1 mg/kg IM [25]	Chimpanzees	
Medetomidine	M: 0.02–0.05 mg/kg IM given 3–15 min prior to ketamine or Telazol for induction [22]	Chimpanzees	
	50–100 µg/kg in marshmallow creme prior to injection with ketamine [25]	Chimpanzees	Some sedation in animals with no anesthesia experience but little to no effect in experienced animals.

(Continued)

Drug name	Drug dose	Species	Comments
Medetomidine + Telazol	M: 0.1 mg/kg PO in marshmallow creme or applesauce prior to immobilization or with 3 mg/kg Telazol given IM [22, 25]	Chimpanzees	Animals receiving oral M exhibited less excitatory behavior and agitation with darting than those that did not receive premedication.
Midazolam	0.05–0.15 mg/kg IM, IV, PO; antagonize with flumazenil 0.02–0.1 mg/kg IV [37]	Orangutans	May reduce anxiety, may be used in combination with other drugs.
Midazolam	M: 0.7–1.2 mg/kg PO given in orange juice [25]	Chimpanzees and Orangutans	Used as premedication with slight to marked sedation.
Propofol	25–100 µg/kg/min IV or 50 mg/kg total dose [37]	Orangutans	Monitor for blood pressure and respirations, may be used for unexpected arousals.
Risperidone	0.02–0.07 mg/kg (or 1–6 mg/animal) divided BID PO for 6 months to 2 yrs [22]	Chimpanzees	n = 7 aggressive males to integrate a group, no side effects and weaned at 6–12 mo, one animal intermittently treated for 2 yrs.
Telazol	T: 2.2 mg/kg [27]	Gorillas	
	T: 2–6 mg/kg IM; antagonize with flumazenil 0.02–0.1 mg/kg IV [25, 37]	Chimpanzees, Gorillas	Smooth induction, may have prolonged recovery.
	T: 2–6.9 mg/kg IM; antagonize with flumazenil 0.02–0.1 mg/kg IV [25, 37]	Orangutans	Smooth induction, may have prolonged recovery.
	T: 3.5 mg/kg IM [27]	Orangutans	Supplement with ketamine 3.5 mg/kg as needed.
Telazol	16 mg/kg PO once [38]	Chimpanzees	n = 1 male, 62 kg, with bullet wounds after escaping enclosure. Telazol given orally in 30 ml Coca-Cola. Within 7 min animal was recumbent and non-responsive. Respiration and heart rate stable and maintained laryngeal reflexes. Chimp began to respond to external stimuli at 40 min.
Telazol + ketamine	T: 3 mg/kg + K: 2 mg/kg IM [2]	Chimpanzees, Gorillas, Orangutans	Likely need supplements of additional ketamine as animals frequently need supplementation.
	T: 3.4 mg/kg + K: 5.66 mg/kg IM [25, 39]	Orangutans	n = 1 female captive animal immobilized for MRI and exam after lameness, ultimately diagnosed with baylisascaris infection on histopathology.

Drug name	Drug dose	Species	Comments
Telazol + medetomidine	T: 0.8–2.3 mg/kg + M: 0.02–0.06 mg/kg IM; antagonize with atipamezole 0.1–0.25 mg/kg [37]	Orangutans	Monitor for blood pressure and respirations, provide oxygen support.
	T: 1.25 mg/kg + M: 0.03–0.04 mg/kg IM; antagonize with atipamezole 0.1–0.25 mg/kg [37]	Chimpanzees	Monitor for blood pressure and respirations, provide oxygen support.
	T: 1 mg/kg IM + M: 0.02 mg/kg; antagonize with atipamezole 0.1 mg/kg [27]	Orangutans	Captive animals.
	T: 0.8–2.3 mg/kg + M: 0.02–0.06 mg/kg IM [25]	Orangutans	
	T: 1.25–3 mg/kg + M: 0.03–0.05 mg/kg IM [25]	Chimpanzees	
	T: 3 mg/kg IM + M: 0.05 mg/kg; antagonize with atipamezole 0.25 mg/kg [27]	Chimpanzees	
Zuclopenthixol	Z: 0.1–0.36 mg/kg PO BID [25]	Gorillas	Used during a prolonged journey. Animals were calm, traveled well and maintained good appetites during the transport.
Antiparasitic			
Prosimians			
Albendazole	5 mg/kg PO TID, treat for 2 week, then off for 2 weeks, for a total of 4 months [39]	Black and white ruffed lemurs	n = 2 successful reported treatment of neural larval migrans due to baylisascaris.
Albendazole	10 mg/kg PO BID [40]	White-headed lemurs	n = 1 animal treated successfully for clinical baylisascaris, initially daily with 37 mg/kg PO SID, but changed to BID with better results.
Fenbendazole	50 mg/kg PO SID × 3d [41]	Prosimians	For treatment of Physaloptera stomach worms, up to 8 days of treatment for Intestinal nematodes infestation.
Fipronil	0.2 ml of 9.8% solution/kg body weight, topically q6 wks [1]	Prosimians	To treat *Cuterebra sp.* and ticks.
Ivermectin	0.2–0.4 mg/kg SC, IM or PO q7d [41]	Prosimians	Some have tried as treatment for cerebral larval migrans, also can be used for intestinal nematodes.

(*Continued*)

Drug name	Drug dose	Species	Comments
	0.6 mg/kg TO, PO, or SC daily for 3–10 months [42]	Galagos	n = 8 captive animals treated successfully for demodicosis.
Levamisole	2.5 mg/kg PO SID × 14d [41]	Prosimians	For treatment of Physaloptera stomach worms.
Metronidazole	25 mg/kg PO SID × 7d [1]	Prosimians	Protozoa treatment.
Nitazoxanide	25 mg/kg PO SID for 5–7d [1, 41]	Prosimians	Protozoa treatment, 3 days of treatment for intestinal nematodes.
Paromomycin	15 mg/kg PO BID × 7d [41]	Prosimians	For treatment of protozoa such as Balantidium, Giardia, Entamoeba, and Cryptosporidia.
Pyrantel pamoate	5–10 mg/kg PO q14d [1]	Prosimians	Nematode treatment.
Thiabendazole	50 mg/kg PO SID × 3–5d [1]	Prosimians	Nematode treatment.
Tinidazole	40–45 mg/kg PO SID × 6d [1]	Prosimians	To treat protozoa.
Monkeys and Lesser Apes			
Albendazole	25 mg/kg PO BID × 5d [6, 34]	New World and Old World monkeys	For, GI nematodes, Filaroides and Giardia infestations.
Amitraz	250 ppm solution Topical bath for 2–5 min, repeat q2 wks for 4 treatments or until lesions resolve [6, 34, 43]	Tamarins	Demodectic mange, dry but do not rinse. Transient ataxia may be seen.
Azithromycin	25–50 mg/kg SQ for 3–10d [34]	Macaques	For malaria, in humans is combined with chloroquine.
Azithromycin	40 mg/kg IM SID once, then 20 mg/kg SID for 2–5d [34]	New World and Old World monkeys	For Malaria, in humans is combined with chloroquine.
Bunamidine (Scolaban)	25–100 mg/kg PO once [34]	New World and Old World monkeys	For cestodes.
Chloroquine phosphate (Arelan)	2.5–5 mg/kg IM SID 4–7d, then 0.75 mg/kg primaquine PO SID × 14d [34]	New World and Old World monkeys	For *Plasmodium sp.* give chloroquine and primaquine separately to prevent toxicity.
	5 mg/kg PO, IM SID × 14d [34]	New World and Old World monkeys	For Entamoeba histolytica.
	10 mg/kg PO, IM once, then 6 hrs later 5 mg/kg, and 24 hrs later 5 mg/kg SID × 2d, then primaquin 0.3 mg/kg SID × 14d or mefloquine 25 mg/kg PO once [34, 41]	New World and Old World monkeys	For *Plasmodium sp.* Give chloroquine and primaquine separately to prevent toxicity.

Drug name	Drug dose	Species	Comments
Clindamycin (Antirobe)	12.5–25 mg/kg PO, IM BID × 28d [34]	New World and Old World monkeys	For toxoplasmosis.
Dichlorvos (Atgard-V)	10 mg/kg PO SID for 1–2d [34]	New World and Old World monkeys	For *Trichuris spp.*
	10–15 mg/kg PO SID for 2–3d [34]	New World and Old World monkeys	For gastrointestinal nematodes.
Diethycarbamazine citrate (Filaribits)	6–20 mg/kg PO SID for 6–15d [34]	Owl monkeys	For filariasis *(Dipetalonema).*
	20–40 mg/kg PO SID for 7–21d [34]	Owl monkeys	For filariasis *(Dipetalonema).*
	50 mg/kg PO SID × 10d [34]	Squirrel monkeys	For filariasis (adults and microfilaria).
Diiodohydroxyquin (iodoquinol/Yodoxin)	10–13.3 mg/kg PO TID for 10–20d [34]	New World and Old World monkeys	For *Entamoeba histolytica*, with metronidazole in severe cases.
	13.3 mg/kg PO TID for 14–21d [34]	New World and Old World monkeys	For *Balantidium coli.*
	20 mg/kg PO BID × 21d [34]	New World and Old World monkeys	
	30 mg/kg PO SID × 10d [34]	New World and Old World monkeys	
Dithiazanine sodium (Dizan)	10–20 mg/kg PO SID for 3–10d [34]	New World and Old World monkeys	For strongyloides.
Doxycycline	5 mg/kg PO BID × 1d, then 2.5 mg/kg PO SID [6, 34]	New World and Old World monkeys	For *Balantidium coli.*
Fenbendazole	10–25 mg/kg PO SID for 3–10d [34]	New World and Old World monkeys	For *Anatrichosoma cynomolgi*, may result in remission.
	20 mg/kg PO SID × 14d [6, 34]	New World and Old World monkeys	For Strongyloides and Filaroides.
	20 mg/kg PO SID × 7d [34]	Marmosets	For *Prosthenorchis spp.*
	25 mg/kg PO q7d for 2 treatments [34]	New World and Old World monkeys	For *Ancyclostoma spp.*
	50 mg/kg PO SID for 3–14d [6, 34]	New World and Old World monkeys	For Filaroides treat for 14 days, later dose scheme for Baboons with GI nematodes, Filaroides, *Trichuris trichura*, and in New World primates *Capillaria hepatica.*
	50 mg/kg PO SID × 3d, repeat in 14d [7]	Nonhuman primates	
Fenbendazole	50 mg/kg PO SID × 3d [44]	Baboons	n = 3 captive animals treated for *Trichuris trichura*, all 3 stopped shedding oocysts within 6 days and were still negative at 65 days post treatment. Treatment with milbemycin oxime was not as effective.

(*Continued*)

Drug name	Drug dose	Species	Comments
	50 mg/kg PO SID × 14d [41]	Callitrichids	For treatment of *Trichospirura leptosoma* infestations and prevent cockroaches in habitat.
Fipronil	Feline doses [41]	All primates	For treatment of fleas.
Flubendazole 5%	27–50 mg/kg PO BID × 5d [34]	Baboons	For *Trichuris spp.*
Fluralaner	30–35 mg/kg PO once [45]	Red-handed tamarins	Demodicosis.
Imidacloprid	Feline doses [41]	All primates	For treatment of fleas.
Ivermectin	0.2 mg/kg IM/SC [7]	Nonhuman primates	
	0.2 mg/kg PO q30d [41]	Monkeys	May be protective against heartworm *Dirofilaria immitis.*
	0.2 mg/kg PO, IM, SC once then repeat in 10–14d [6, 34]	New world and Old World Monkeys	For *strongyloides sp., Gonglyonema sp., Pneumonussus sp.,* Anoplura.
	0.2 mg/kg IM, repeat in 21 days if needed [34]	New World and Old World monkeys	For *Ancyclostoma duodenale.*
	0.2 mg/kg SC or Topically once, repeat in 4 weeks [45]	Common marmosets	Anatrichosoma, Sarcoptes, Demodex, Dipetalonema, pentastomids.
	0.2–0.4 mg/kg PO, repeat in 21 days [41]	Monkeys	For strongyloides and pinworm infestations.
	0.3 mg/kg PO q7d × 4 treatments [41]	Callitrichids	*Gonglyonema sp.*
	0.2–0.4 mg/kg SC or PO with repeated treatments [41]	Macaques, Guenons, Baboons	For treatment of scabies *(Sarcoptes scabei),* and *Psorergates pitheci,* and respiratory mites.
	0.4 mg/kg IM once then every 7–14 days [55]	Siamangs	n = 1 captive adult male, with clinical with *Psorobia* mite infestation. Initial treatment was once IM then every 2 weeks for 4 treatments PO. Following reoccurrence, treatment was increased to every 7 days and a lime sulfur dip was performed, resulting in resolution.
	0.4 µg/kg IM [34]	Macaques	For strongyloides, dilute with propylene glycol.
	0.5 µg/kg SC SID × 3d [34]	New World and Old World monkeys	For *Ptergodermatites sp.,* Dilute in sterile water for smaller species (Marmosets).
Levamisole	4–5 mg/kg PO SID × 6d [34]	Saki monkeys	For oral spiruidiasis.

Drug name	Drug dose	Species	Comments
	5 mg/kg PO once, repeat in 21 days [6, 34]	New World and Old World monkeys	For spiruids, strongyloides, and Trichuris.
Levamisole	7.5 mg/kg SC, repeat in 2 weeks [34]	New World and Old World monkeys	For *Trichuris sp.* and *Ancyclostoma sp.*
	10 mg/kg PO [34, 41]	New World and Old World monkeys	For Strongyloides, Filaroides, Oesophagostomum, and Trichuris. PO or SC for 2–3 days for Strongyloides.
	10 mg/kg [34]	Spider monkeys	For Physaloptera give for 3 d.
	11 mg/kg [34]	Tamarins	For filariasis give for 10 days in combination with thiacetarsamide sodium at 0.22 ml/kg BID × 2d.
Mebendazole	3 mg/kg PO SID × 10d [34]	New World and Old World monkeys	For Ancyclostoma sp.
	15 mg/kg PO SID × 3d [34]	New World and Old World monkeys	For Strongyloides, Necator, Pterogodermatitis, and Trichuris.
	22 mg/kg PO SID × 3d then repeat in 14 days or in 3 weeks [7, 34, 45]	New World and Old World monkeys	
	40 mg/kg PO SID × 3d repeated 3–4 × per year [6, 34]	New World and Old World monkeys	For *Pterygodermatites sp.*, Trichuris, Strongyloides, and Acanthocephalans.
	40 mg/kg PO SID × 30d [6]	New World and Old World monkeys	Strongyloides, Trichuris, Pterygodermatites.
	70 mg/kg PO SID × 3d [34]	New World monkeys	For oral spiruidiasis.
	100 mg/kg PO q14d or 100 mg/kg PO SID for alternating weeks post surgical removal of worms [34, 41]	Callitrichids	For Acanthocephalans, use as preventative and along with surgical removal of parasite.
Mefloquine (Lariam)	25 mg/kg PO once [34]	New World and Old World monkeys	Antimalarial.
Metronidazole	10–16.7 mg/kg PO TID for 5–10d [34]	New World and Old World monkeys	For Giardia intestinalis. Flagyl-S or metronidazole benzoate may be compounded with flavored syrup to increase palatability.
	11.7–16.7 mg/kg PO TID × 10d [34]	New World and Old World monkeys	For *Balantidium coli.* Flagyl-S or metronidazole benzoate may be compounded with flavored syrup to increase palatability.
	17.5–25 mg/kg PO BID × 10d [34, 41]	New World and Old World monkeys	For enteric amoebas and flagellates. Flagyl-S or metronidazole benzoate may be compounded with flavored syrup to increase palatability.

(*Continued*)

Drug name	Drug dose	Species	Comments
	20 mg/kg PO BID or 30–50 mg/kg PO SOD × 5–10d [46]	Common marmosets	Entamoeba, Giardia.
Metronidazole	25 mg/kg PO BID for 5–10d [6, 34]	New World and Old World monkeys	For *Giardia lamblia* and *Tritrichomonas mobilensis, Balantidium coli* and *Entamoeba histolytica.* Flagyl-S or metronidazole benzoate may be compounded with flavored syrup to increase palatability.
	30–50 mg/kg PO SID × 5d [7]	Nonhuman primates	
	30–50 mg/kg PO BID for 5–10d [34]	New World and Old World monkeys	For *B. coli.* Flagyl-S or metronidazole benzoate may be compounded with flavored syrup to increase palatability.
Milbemycine oxime	1 mg/kg PO SID every 30d for 3 months [44]	Baboons	n = 3 captive animals treated for *Trichuris trichura.* Although the number of eggs per gram decreased significantly after the 2nd treatment, this regimen never totally eliminated egg shedding. Fenbendazole was 100% successful.
Moxidectin (Proheart)	0.5 mg/kg PO, IM [34]	New world and Old World monkeys	For *Strongyloides sp.*, give one dose.
Niclosamide (Yomensan)	100 mg/kg PO once [34]	New World and Old World monkeys	For intestinal cestodiasis. For Owl monkeys give 150 mg/kg PO, and New World species 166 mg/kg PO for cestodes and anoplocephalids.
Paromomycin	10–20 mg/kg PO BID for 5–10d [34]	New World and Old World monkeys	For *Balantidium coli.*
	12.5–15 mg/kg PO BID for 5–10d [34]	New World and Old World monkeys	For amoebae and *Entamoeba histolytica*: minimal absorption so need to use additional drugs for invasive disease.
	25–30 mg/kg PO BID for 5–10d [34]	Owl monkeys	For enteric amoebiasis.
	100 mg/kg PO SID × 10d [34]	Cercopithecids	
Piperazine	605 mg/kg PO SID × 10d [41]	Old World monkeys	For treatment of pinworm infestation.
Praziquantel	5 mg/kg IM [7]	Nonhuman primates	
	15–20 mg/kg PO, IM [34, 41]	New World and Old World monkeys	Treatment for trematodes, may need multiple treatments at 10-day intervals.

Drug name	Drug dose	Species	Comments
	20 mg/kg PO/IM once [6]	Callitrichids, Cebids and Lemurs	Cestodes
	30–40 mg/kg PO or SC repeated at 2–3 wk intervals [41]	Monkeys	Hydatid disease/*Echinococcus spp.* cysts in abdomen and SC, after removal treat with praziquantel.
	40 mg/kg PO, IM once [6, 34, 41]	New world and Old World monkeys	For *Schistosoma sp.*, other cestodes and trematodes, may need to repeat for respiratory flukes (*Dinobdella ferox*); for liver flukes repeat in 14 days.
Primaquine (primaquine phosphate)	0.3 mg/kg PO SID × 14d [34]	New World and Old World monkeys	For *Plasmodium sp.* Use with chloroquine.
Pyrantel pamoate (Strongid T)	11 mg/kg PO once then repeat in 10d [34, 41]	New World and Old World monkeys	For oxyurids. Better than thiabendazole for *Trypanoxyuris micron* in Owl monkeys. For pinworm and Trichuris infestations in Old World monkeys.
Pyrimethamine	0.5 mg/kg PO BID [46]	Common marmosets	Encephalitozoon cuniculi, treat concurrently with trimethoprim sulfamethoxazole and folic acid for encephalitozoonosis or toxoplasmosis.
	10 mg/kg PO SID [34]	New World and Old World monkeys	For *Plasmodium sp.* Monitor for signs of folate acid deficiency and treat if needed.
Pyrvinium pamoate (Novan)	5 mg/kg PO Once q6 months [34]	New World and Old World monkeys	
Quinacrine (Atabrine)	2 or 10 mg/kg PO TID for 5–7d [34]	New World and Old World monkeys	For Giardia, lower dose may cause GI upset in Squirrel monkeys, at higher dose reported to be 70–95% effective.
Ronnel (Ectoral)	55 mg/kg PO, Topical [34]	New World and Old World monkeys	For lung and ectoparasite mites: give q72 hrs for 4 treatments then q7d for 3 months topically.
Sulfadiazine	100 mg/kg PO [34]	New World and Old World monkeys	For toxoplasma, treat along with Pyrimethamine.
Sulfadimethoxine (Albon)	50 mg/kg PO once, then 25 mg/kg/day [34]	New World and Old World monkeys	Coccidiosis.
Thiabendazole (Thibenzole)	50 mg/kg PO SID × 2d [34, 41]	New World and Old World monkeys	For Strongyloides and hookworms *Necator sp.* May need to repeat in 21 days.
	75–100 mg/kg PO once then repeat in 21d [7, 34]	New World and Old World monkeys	For strongyloides.

(*Continued*)

Drug name	Drug dose	Species	Comments
Tinidazole (Tindamax)	150 mg/kg PO SID once, then 4d later 77 mg/kg PO SID once [48]	Marmosets	n = 13 animals in a captive colony with Giardia. All were cleared after treatment. Initially animals received 1/4 tablet and 4 days later 1/8th tablet. Used 250 mg tablets divided and crushed, then dissolved in 2 ml warm water and delivered via gastric lavage via a pediatric feeding tube. Human pediatric dose is 50 mg/kg and adult dose 2 g but a higher dose given to humans did not result in adverse effects. Based on allometric scaling the first dose at 900 mg/m2 was lower than human pediatric 1250 mg/m2 and adult 960 mg/m2 doses.
Toltrazuril	7 mg/kg PO SID × 2d [46]	Common marmosets	Toxoplasmosis: Treat concurrently with trimethoprim sulfamethoxazole.
Trimethoprim sulfadiazine	15 mg/kg PO BID [6]	New world and Old World monkeys	Toxoplasmosis: Treat concurrently with trimethoprim sulfamethoxazole.
Trimthoprim sulfamethoxazole	30 mg/kg PO BID for at least 3 weeks [45]	Common marmosets	*Encephalitozoon cuniculi*, treat concurrently with pyrimethamine and folic acid for encephalitozoonosis or toxoplasmosis.
Great Apes			
Diiodohydroxyquin	12–16 mg/kg PO q8 hrs [41]	Infant and Juvenile Great apes	Balantidium.
	20 mg/kg PO BID × 21d [41]	Adult Great apes	Balantidium, use with metronidazole 30–50 mg/kg PO BID × 5–10 d.
Diiodohydroxyquin	30–40 mg/kg PO SID × 3–21d (used alone) [41]	Adult Great apes	Balantidium.
Doxycycline	5 mg/kg PO BID once, then 2.5 mg/kg PO SID [41]	Infant and juvenile Great apes	To treat Balantidium.
	100 mg BID × 10d [22]	Chimpanzees	To treat Balantidium.
	500–1000 mg PO TID × 10–14d [41]	Adult Great apes	To treat Balantidium.
Fenbendazole	10 mg/kg PO [22]	Chimpanzees	To treat internal parasites.
Ivermectin	0.17 mg/kg SC [18]	Mountain gorillas	n = 1 juvenile free-ranging female for potential parasitic enteritis.
	0.2 mg/kg PO q14d [22]	Chimpanzees	

Drug name	Drug dose	Species	Comments
	0.2 mg/kg PO monthly [2]	Orangutans	Per AZA SSP recommendations for strongyloides prevention.
Metronidazole	25 mg/kg PO BID × 10d [41]	Great apes	For treatment of Giardia.
	30–50 mg/kg PO BID × 5–10d [41]	Adult Great apes	To treat Balantidium – use with Diiodohydroxy-quin 20 mg/kg PO BID × 21 d.
Oxibendazole	10 mg/kg PO SID for several weeks [41]	Squirrel monkeys	Unproven suggestion for treatment of *Encephalitozoon cuniculi*.
Quinacrine	2 mg/kg PO TID × 7d (max 300 mg/d) [41]	Great apes	For treatment of Giardia.
Sulfadiazine	50 mg/kg PO q6 hrs [41]	Great apes	Toxoplasmosis: max dose of 6 g/day/animal, treat concurrently with pyrimethamine 2 mg/kg PO SID × 3d then 1 mg/kg PO SID × 28 d.
Prosimians			
Furosemide	0.5 mg/kg PO SID (4 mg/kg IV) [4]	Ring-tailed lemurs	n = 1 10 yr old 3.4 kg, female with congestive heart failure, treated pre (PO) and intraoperatively (IV) with furosemide.
Glipizide	0.38–2 mg/kg PO BID [49]	Ring-tailed lemurs, Bengal slow loris	n = 4 animals, 3 ring-tailed lemurs and 1 loris. Loris and 1 lemur benefited from glipizide. 2 others received glipizide, Metformin hydrochloride 48 mg/kg PO BID, and acarbose 1.9–3.7 mg/kg PO BID with no improvement.
Leuprolide acetate (Depo lupron)	3.75 mg/kg IM [50]	Collared lemurs	Treated during one breeding season, not successful at reducing aggression, but testosterone levels in fecal samples did decrease.
Medroxyprogesterone acetate (MGA implants)		Prosimians	Contraception. See https://www.stlzoo.org/files/9213/1429/7259/MGA_Primates.pdf [1].
Progesterone (Depo-Provera)	5 mg/kg IM q40d in Ring-tailed lemurs, q60 in other species [1]	Prosimians	Contraception.
Tetanus vaccine	Recommend: 40 IU of human tetanus toxoid IM 3 times at intervals of 2–3 months, then boostered at 5 and 10 yrs of age [6]	Primates	

(*Continued*)

Drug name	Drug dose	Species	Comments
Tuberculin (Old mammalian tuberculin OMT)	0.1 ml (0.05 ml smallest species) intradermal in eyelid [6]	Primates	For testing of mycobacterial infection due to clinical signs, as part of routine exam or prior to shipment.
Monkeys and Lesser Apes			
Deslorelin	1–2 (6 mg) implants SC [51]	Lion-tailed macaques	n = 3 males, 10, 12, and 32 yrs of age. Given implants to reduce aggression and allow for a bachelor group. At 1 yr post injection, successfully together as a group, serum testosterone and motile sperm were significantly decreased over time as well as muscle and weight loss similar to castrated males.
Famotidine	0.5 mg/kg PO SID [2]	Goeldi's monkeys	n = 1 monkey with chronic renal failure.
Measles vaccine	Has been given at 6 months and boostered at 12 months [6]	New World primates	Recommend killed vaccine if possible.
Polysulfated glucosaminoglycan	3 mg SC q48 hrs × 4d then q7d [11]	Squirrel Monkeys	n = 1 postoperative treatment of animal with traumatic luxation of left radial head and mid diaphyseal fracture of ulna.
Tuberculin (Old mammalian tuberculin OMT)	0.1 ml (0.05 ml smallest species) intradermal in eyelid [6]	Primates	For testing of mycobacterial infection due to clinical signs, as part of routine exam or prior to shipment.
Tetanus vaccine	Recommend: 40 IU of human tetanus toxoid IM 3 times at intervals of 2–3 months, then boostered at 5 and 10 yrs of age [6]	Primates	
Vitamin C	3–6 mg/kg PO SID [7]	Nonhuman primates	To prevent scurvy.
Vitamin C	25–50 mg/kg PO SID [7]	Nonhuman primates	To treat scurvy, to treat until signs resolve.
Great Apes			
Aspirin	81 mg PO SID [2]	Chimpanzees	n = 1 female, diagnosed with mitral valve regurgitation and left atrial enlargement to prevent thromboembolic disease.
Acyclovir	400 mg PO q6 hrs [22]	Chimpanzees	For ocular pain/blepharospasm and photophobia secondary to Herpes simplex 1 and 2. Treatment decreases duration of clinical signs from weeks to days.

Drug name	Drug dose	Species	Comments
Betamethasone	1 mg subconjunctival [52]	Gorillas	n = 2 gorillas undergoing bilateral cataract phacoemulsification and lens replacement.
Bismuth subsalicylate (Pepto Bismol)	525 mg PO BID [2]	Gorillas, Chimpanzees, Orangutans	n = 3 one female chimpanzee, One male gorilla, and one female orangutan with dyspepsia.
Carbamazepine	50 mg PO BID [53]	Gorillas	n = 1 younger animal with seizures secondary to hydrochephalus controlled well at this dose.
Dexamethasone	1 mg/kg/day IV [16]	Sumatran orangutans	n = 1, 2 yr old female undergoing surgical repair of atrial septal defect with secondary complications postoperatively of adult respiratory distress syndrome. Given dexamethasone postop during while on ventilatory support.
Ethinyl estradiol + norethindrone	E: 35 µg + N: 1 mg/daily [54]	Bonobos	n = 13 captive females. No contraceptive failures reported and 4 reversals. Most crushed pill and mixed with juice or food. Most had hormone-free intervals of at least 5 days and seldom experienced breakthrough estrus or bleeding. All exhibited some perineal swelling, and overall less sexual behavior, dominant females became subordinate and no appreciable change in weight.
Famotidine	20 mg PO SID [2]	Gorillas, Chimpanzees	n = 2 one chimpanzee and one gorilla for inappetence.
Furosemide	1 mg/kg IV TID [16]	Sumatran orangutans	n = 1, 2 yr old female undergoing surgical repair of atrial septal defect with secondary complications postoperatively-given furosemide postoperatively during while on ventilatory support.
Gadodiamide contrast (Omniscan)	0.1 mmol/kg IV [39]	Orangutans	n = 1 female during MRI scan.
Heparin sodium	400 units/kg IV [16]	Sumatran orangutans	n = 1, 2 yr old female undergoing surgical repair of atrial septal defect with secondary complications postoperatively of adult respiratory distress syndrome. Given heparin intraoperatively to prevent clotting. Antagonized later with protamine 40 mg IV.

(*Continued*)

Drug name	Drug dose	Species	Comments
Iron + Vitamin B12	0.5 ml [18]	Gorillas	n = 1 supportive therapy for a juvenile female, free-ranging Mountain gorilla during rectal prolapse resection.
Levetiracetam	125–250 mg PO BID [53]	Bonobos	n = 1 animal with seizures coinciding with ovulation. 250 mg initially resulted in fatigue and abdominal distension. Additional seizure was seen on 125 mg so increased back to 250 mg with no further side effects seen. Oral contraceptive was also given.
Lisinopril	10 mg/kg PO SID [2]	Gorillas, Chimpanzees	n = 3 one male gorilla with ventricular hypertrophy and fibrosis; one male chimpanzee with myocardial fibrosis; one female chimpanzee for mitral valve regurgitation and left atrial enlargement.
Phenobarbitol + acetazolamide	P: 100 mg PO BID + A 250 mg PO BID [53]	Bonobos	n = 1 animal with seizures prior to menses. Phenobarbital dose was increased for a few days prior to known menses when cycles were predictable. Was started on oral contraceptive during perimenopause.
Prednisone	10–60 mg PO SID [2]	Chimpanzees	n = 1 female chimpanzee with hyperkeratosis and immune mediated dermatitis.
Ramipril	2.5 mg SID [55]	Bonobos	n = 1 male diagnosed with concentrically hypertrophied heart, treated for 18 months with an improvement of ejection fraction of 10%.
Tetanus vaccine	Recommend: 40 IU of human tetanus toxoid IM 3 times at intervals of 2–3 months, then boostered at 5 and 10 yrs of age [6]	Primates	
Tropicamide + cyclpentolate ophthalmic drops	Used topically intraoperatively [52]	Gorillas	n = 2 gorillas undergoing bilateral cataract phacoemulsification and lens replacement. Eyes were dilated with tropicamide and cyclopentolate drops intraoperatively.

Drug name	Drug dose	Species	Comments
Tuberculin (old mammalian tuberculin OMT)	0.1 ml (0.05 ml smallest species) intradermal in eyelid [6]	Primates	For testing of mycobacterial infection due to clinical signs, as part of routine exam or prior to shipment.
Valacyclovir	1 g PO BID [22]	Chimpanzees	For ocular pain/ blepharospasm and photophobia secondary to Herpes simplex 1 and 2. Treatment decreases clinical signs from weeks to days.

Species	Weight
Prosimians [19]	0.6–1.3 kg
Aye-aye *(Daubentonia spp.)*	2.5–3 kg
Black Lemur *(Eulemur macacao)*	2–2.5 kg
Brown Lemur *(Eulemur fulvus)*	2–2.7 kg
Crowned Lemur *(Eulemur coronatus)*	1.5–2 kg
Coquerel's Sifaka *(Propithecus coquereli)*	3.3–4.5 kg
Eastern Lesser Bamboo lemur *(Hapalemur griseus)*	0.75–2.5 kg
Fat-tailed dwarf lemur *(Cheirogaleus medius)*	0.16–0.25 kg
Galago *(Galago senegalensis)*	120–300 g
Giant Mouse lemur *(Mirza spp.)*	0.028–0.320 kg
Indri *(Indri indri)*	6–7.25 kg
Mongoose lemur *(Eulemur mongoz)*	1.4–1.6 kg
Mouse Lemur *(Microcebus murinus)*	0.06–0.09 kg
Potto *(Perodicticus potto)*	0.85–1.6 kg
Pygmy loris *(Nycticebus pygmaeus)*	0.35–0.45 kg
Ring-tailed lemur *(Lemur catta)*	2–3 kg
Ruffed lemur *(Varecia sp.)*	3–3.8 kg
Slender loris *(Loris tardigradis)*	0.15–0.25 kg
Slow loris *(Nycticebus coucang)*	0.8–1.3 kg
Southern Lesser Bush baby *(Galago moholi)*	0.15–0.25 kg
Thick-tailed greater bush baby/Thick tailed galago *(Otole-mur crassicaudatus)*	0.7–0.85 kg
Woolly lemur *(Avahi)*	1–1.5 kg
Monkeys and lesser apes [27]	
Ape, Celebes (*Cynopithecus niger)*	6–15 kg
Baboon, Chacma *(Papio ursinus)*	8–30 kg
Baboon, Gelada *(Theropithecus gelada)*	13–20 kg
Baboon, Hamadryas *(Papio hamadryas)*	10–18 kg

(*Continued*)

Species	Weight
Baboon, Olive *(Papio anubis)*	14–41 kg
Baboon, Western *(Papio papio)*	10–30 kg
Baboon, Yellow *(Papio cynocephalus)*	14–41 kg
Douroucoulis/Owl Monkey *(Aotus spp.)*	0.6–1 kg
Gibbon, Gray *(Hylobates muelleri)*	2–4 kg
Gibbon, Siamang *(Hylobates syndactylus)*	8–13 kg
Gibbon, White-cheeked *(Hylobates concolor)*	4–8 kg
Gibbon, White-handed *(Hylobates lar)*	4–8 kg
Langur, Hanuman/Indian *(Semnopitehcus entellus)*	10–23.6 kg
Macaque Barbary *(Macaca sylvanus)*	6–15 kg
Macaque, Bonnet *(Macaca radiata)*	5–15 kg
Macaque, Crab-eatig/Cynomologous *(Macaca fascicularis)*	5–15 kg
Macaque, Japanese *(Macaca fuscata)*	5–15 kg
Macaque, Lion-tail *(Macaca silensis)*	5–15 kg
Macaque, Pig-tailed *(Macaca nemestrina)*	5–15 kg
Macaque, Rheses (*Macaca mulatta)*	9–12 kg
Macaque, Stump-tailed *(Macaca arctoides)*	5–15 kg
Macaque, Toque *(Macaca sinica)*	2.5–6.1 kg
Mandrill *(Mandrillus sphinx)*	20–54 kg
Mangabey, Black *(Lophocebus arterrimus)*	4–11 kg
Mangabey, gray-cheeked *(Cercocebus albigena)*	5–20 kg
Mangabey, Sooty *(Cercocebus torquatus)*	5–20 kg
Marmoset, Black-tufted *(Callithrix penicillata)*	230–453 g
Marmoset, Common *(Callithrix jacchus)*	230–453 g
Monkey, Allen's *(Allenopithecus nigroviridis)*	3.5–6 kg
Monkey/Guenon black-cheeked *(Cercopithecus ascanius)*	1.8–6.4 kg
Monkey/Guenon, Blue (*Cercopithecus mitis)*	6–12 kg
Monkey, Capuchin *(Cebus spp.)*	1.1–3.3 kg
Monkey, Colobus *(Colobus spp.)*	5.4–14.5 kg
Monkey/Guenon, Debrazza's *(Cercopithegus neclectus)*	4.5–7.8 kg
Monkey/Guenon, Diana (*Cercopithecus diana)*	3–6 kg
Monkey/Guenon, Green *(Chlorocebus sabaeus)*	3–7 kg
Monkey/Guenon, Grivet *(Cercopithecus aethiops)*	5–9 kg
Monkey, Howler (*Alouatta spp.)*	4–10 kg
Monkey/Guenon, Lesser white-nosed *(Cercopithecus petaurista)*	4–8 kg
Monkey/Guenon, Mona (*Cercopithecus mona)*	3–6 kg
Monkey, Patas *(Erythrocebus patus)*	4–13 kg
Monkey, Proboscis *(Nasalis larvatus)*	7–11 kg Female, 16–22.5 kg Male
Monkey, Spider *(Ateles spp.)*	4–6 kg
Monkey, Squirrel *(Saimiri spp.)*	0.7–1.1 kg

Species	Weight
Monkey/Guenon, Sykes *(Cercopithecus albogularis)*	3–6 kg
Monkey/Guenon, White-nosed *(Cercopithecus nictitans)*	2–8 kg
Monkey, Wooly *(Lagothrix spp.)*	5.5–10.8 kg
Tamarin, Cotton-headed *(Saguinus oedipus)*	225–900 g
Tamarin, Emperor *(Saguinus imperator)*	225–900 g
Tamarin, Golden Lion *(Leontopithecus rosalia)*	0.6–0.8 kg
Tamarin, Red-bellied *(Saguinus labiatus)*	225–900 g
Tamarin, White-lipped *(Saguinus nigricollis)*	225–900 g
Uakari *(Cacajao Spp.)*	5–10 kg
Vervet (monkey) *(Cercopithecus pygerythrus)*	3–8 kg
Great apes [27]	
Bonobo *(Pan paniscus)*	25–45 kg
Chimpanzee *(Pan troglodytes)*	35–70 kg
Gorilla *(Gorilla gorilla)*	70–140 kg Female, 135–275 kg Male
Sumatran Orangutan *(Pongo abelii)*	33–45 kg Female, 80–90 kg Male
Bornean Orangutan *(Pongo pygmaeus)*	30–50 kg Female, 50–100 kg Male

References

1 Williams, C.V. (2015). Prosimians. In: *Fowler's Zoo and Wild Animal Medicine*, vol. 8 (ed. R.E. Miller and M. Fowler), 291–301. St. Louis, MO: Elsevier Saunders.
2 Cerveny, S., DVM DACZM (2018). Personal communication.
3 Cerveny, S.N., Harper, J., Voges, A. et al. (2013). Surgical and medical management for fractures of the second through fifth metacarpals in a red ruffed lemur (*Varecia rubra*). *Journal of Zoo and Wildlife Medicine* 44 (1): 215–219.
4 Boedeker, N.C., Guzzetta, P., Rosenthal, S.L. et al. (2014). Surgical correction of an arteriovenous fistula in a ring-tailed lemur (*Lemur catta*). *Comparative Medicine* 64 (1): 71–74.
5 Calle, P.P., Bowerman, D.L., and Pape, J.W. (1993). Nonhuman primate tularemia (*Francisella tularensis*) epizootic in a zoological park. *Journal of Zoo and Wildlife Medicine* 24 (4): 459–468.
6 Masters, N. (2010). Primates. In: *BSAVA Manual of Exotic Pets* (ed. R.A. Meredith and C.J. Delaney), 148–166. Gloucester, UK: BSAVA.
7 Kahn, C.M. (2010). Nonhuman primates. In: *Merck Veterinary Manual*, vol. 10 (ed. C.M. Kahn), 1681–1687. London: Merck.
8 Papp, R., Popovic, A., Kelly, N. et al. (2010). Pharmacokinetics of Cefovecin in Squirrel Monkey (*Saimiri sciureus*), Rhesus Macaques (*Macaca mulatta*), and Cynomolgus Macaques (*Macaca fascicularis*). *Journal of the American Association for Laboratory Animal Science* 49 (6): 805–808.
9 Raabe, B.M., Lavaglio, J., Grover, G.S. et al. (2011). Pharmacokinetics of Cefovecin in Cynomolgus Macaques (*Macaca fascicularis*), Olive Baboons (*Papio Anubis*), and Rhesus Macaques (*Macaca mulatta*). *Journal of the American Association for Laboratory Animal Science: JAALAS* 50 (3): 389–395.

10 Ranen, E., Freidman, T., and Aizenberg, I. (2006). Perineal urethrostomy in a brown capuchin monkey (*Cebus apella*). *Journal of Zoo and Wildlife Medicine* 37 (1): 40–43.

11 Wellehan, J.F., Lafortune, M., and Heard, D.J. (2004). Traumatic elbow luxation repair in a common squirrel monkey (*Saimiri sciureus*) and a bonnet macaque (*Macaca radiata*). *Journal of Zoo and Wildlife Medicine* 35 (2): 197–202.

12 Watson, J.R., Stoskopf, M.K., Rozmiarek, H. et al. (1991). Kinetic study of serum gentamicin concentrations in baboons after single-dose administration. *American Journal of Veterinary Research* 52 (8): 1285–1287.

13 Chatterton, J., Unwin, S., Rehman, I.U. et al. (2015). Successful surgical treatment of obstructive liver disease caused by a biliary calculus in a captive chimpanzee (*Pan troglodytes*). *Journal of Zoo and Wildlife Medicine* 46 (4): 925–928.

14 Unwin, S., Chatterton, J., Chantrey, J. et al. (2013). Management of severe respiratory tract disease caused by human respiratory syncytial virus and streptococcus pneumonia in captive chimpanzees (*Pan troglodytes*). *Journal of Zoo and Wildlife Medicine* 44 (1): 105–115.

15 Dumonceaux, G., Greene, T., Burton, M. et al. (2000). Management of bilateral compound metatarsal fractures in a male chimpanzee (*Pan troglodytes*). *Proceedings of International Association of Aquatic Animal Medicine.*

16 Greenberg, M.J., Janssen, D.L., Jamieson, S.W. et al. (1999). Surgical repair of an atrial septal defect in a juvenile Sumatran orangutan (*Pongo pygmaeus sumatraensis*). *Journal of Zoo and Wildlife Medicine* 30 (2): 256–261.

17 Schuele, A., Fritsch, G., Holtze, S. et al. (2018). First detection of cholestasis and treatment with an endoscopic retrograde cholangiopancreatography in a Sumatran orangutan (*Pongo pygmaeus abelii*). *Annual Proceedings of the American Association of Zoo Veterinarians.* 36–37.

18 Kalema-Zikusoka, G. and Lowenstine, L. (2001). Rectal prolapse in a free-ranging mountain gorilla (*Gorilla beringe iberingei*): clinical presentation and surgical management. *Journal of Zoo and Wildlife Medicine* 32 (4): 509–513.

19 Williams, C.V. and Junge, R.E. (2014). Prosimians. In: *Zoo Animal and Wildlife Immobilization and Anesthesia*, 2e (ed. G. West, D. Heard and N. Caulkett), 551–559. Ames, IA: Wiley Blackwell.

20 Backues, K.A., Hoover, J.P., Bahr, R.J. et al. (2000). Chronic recurrent multifocal osteomyelitis in a Ruffed lemur (*Varecia variegata variegate*). *Proceedings of International Association of Aquatic Animal Medicine.*

21 Olberg, R.A. and Sinclair, M. (2014). Monkeys and gibbons. In: *Zoo Animal and Wildlife Immobilization and Anesthesia*, 2e (ed. G. West, D. Heard and N. Caulkett), 561–572. Ames, IA: Wiley Blackwell.

22 Bezner, J. (2019). Medical aspects of chimpanzee rehabilitation and sanctuary medicine. In: *Fowler's Zoo and Wild Animal Medicine Current Therapy*, vol. 9 (ed. R.E. Miller, N. Lamberski and P.P. Calle), 574–580. St. Louis, MO: Elsevier Saunders.

23 Emerson, J.A. and Guzman, D.S. (2019). Sustained-release and long-acting opiod formulations of interest in Zoological Medicine. In: *Fowler's Zoo and Wild Animal Medicine Current Therapy*, vol. 9 (ed. R.E. Miller, N. Lamberski and P.P. Calle), 574–580. St. Louis, MO: Elsevier Saunders.

24 Carlson, A.M., Kelly, R., Fetterer, D.P. et al. (2016). Pharmacokinetics of 2 formulations of transdermal fentanyl in cynomolgus macaques (*Macaca fascicularis*). *Journal of the American Association for Laboratory Animal Science* 55 (4): 436–442.

25 Cerveny, S. and Sleeman, J. (2014). Great apes. In: *Zoo Animal and Wildlife Immobilization and Anesthesia*, 2e (ed. G. West, D. Heard and N. Caulkett), 573–584. Ames, IA: Wiley Blackwell.

26 Hendrix, P.K. (2006). Anesthetic management of an orangutan (*Pongo abelii/pygmaeus*) undergoing laparoscopic tubal ligation. *Journal of Zoo and Wildlife Medicine* 37 (4): 531–534.
27 Kreeger, T.J. and Arnemo, J.M. (2012). *Handbook of Wildlife Chemical Immobilization*. China: Kreeger.
28 Miller, D.S., Sauther, M.L., Hunter-Ishikawa, M. et al. (2007). Biomedical evaluation of free-ranging ring-tailed lemurs (*Lemur catta*) in three habitats at the Beza Mahafaly Special Reserve, Madagascar. *Journal of Zoo and Wildlife Medicine* 38 (2): 201–216.
29 Dutton, C.J., Junge, R.E., and Louis, E.E. (2003). Biomedical evaluation of free-ranging ring-tailed lemurs (*Lemur catta*) in Tsimanampetsotsa Strict Nature Reserve, Madagascar. *Journal of Zoo and Wildlife Medicine* 34 (1): 16–24.
30 Dutton, C.J., Junge, R.E., and Louis, E.E. (2008). Biomedical evaluation of free-ranging red ruffed lemurs (*Varecia rubra*) within the Masoala National Park, Madagascar. *Journal of Zoo and Wildlife Medicine* 39 (1): 76–85.
31 Junge, R.E. and Louis, E.E. (2007). Biomedical evaluation of black lemurs (*Eulemur macaco macaco*) in Lokobe Reserve, Madagascar. *Journal of Zoo and Wildlife Medicine* 38 (1): 67–76.
32 Junge, R.E., Dutton, C.J., Knightly, F. et al. (2008). Comparison of biomedical evaluation for white-fronted brown lemurs (*Eulemur fulvus albifrons*) from four sites in Madagascar. *Journal of Zoo and Wildlife Medicine* 39 (4): 567–575.
33 Miller, M., Weber, M., Mangold, B. et al. (2000). Use of oral detomidine and ketamine for anesthetic induction in nonhuman primates. *Annual Proceedings of the International Association of Aquatic Animal Medicine*.
34 Calle, P.P. and Joslin, J.O. (2015). New world and old world monkeys. In: *Fowler's Zoo and Wild Animal Medicine*, vol. 8 (ed. R.E. Miller and M. Fowler), 301–336. St. Louis, MO: Elsevier Saunders.
35 Olberg, R., Sinclair, M., Barker, I.K. et al. (2018). Comparison of intramuscular Fentanyl-Midazolam, Fentanyl-Midazolam-Ketamine, and Ketamine-Medetomidine for immobilization of Japanese Macaques (*Macaca fuscata*). *Journal of Zoo and Wildlife Medicine* 49 (1): 99–107.
36 Karesh, W.B. and Olson, T.P. (1985). Hematology and serum chemistry values of juvenile and adult ruffed lemurs (*Varecia variegata*). *Journal of Medical Primatology* 14 (1): 5–12.
37 Murphy, H.W. (2015). Great apes. In: *Fowler's Zoo and Wild Animal Medicine*, vol. 8 (ed. R.E. Miller and M. Fowler), 336–354. St. Louis, MO: Elsevier Saunders.
38 Knottenbelt, M.K. and Knottenbelt, D.C. (1990). Use of an oral sedative for immobilisation of a chimpanzee (*Pan troglodytes*). *Veterinary Record* 126 (16): 404.
39 Hanley, C.S., Simmons, H.A., Wallace, R.S. et al. (2006). Visceral and presumptive neural baylisascariasis in an orangutan (*Pongo pygmaeus*). *Journal of Zoo and Wildlife Medicine* 37 (4): 553–557.
40 Jimenez Martinez, M.A., Cano, E.V., and Rois, J.L. (2015). Baylisascaris procyonis larva migrans in two white-headed lemurs (*Eulemur albifrons*) in Spain and response to treatment from a human derived pediatric protocol. *Veterinary Parasitology* 210: 246–249.
41 Johnson-Delaney, C.A. (2009). Parasites of captive nonhuman primates. *Veterinary Clinics Exotic Animal Practice* 12: 563–581.
42 Kuznetsova, E., Vysokikh, A., and Bourdeau, P. (2012). First description of demodicosis in 12 galagos (*Galago senegalensis*). *Veterinary Dermatology* 23 (1): 61–64.
43 James, S.B. and Raphael, B.L. (2000). Demodicosis in red-handed tamarins (*Saguinus midas*). *Journal of Zoo and Wildlife Medicine* 31 (2): 251–254.
44 Reichard, M.V., Wolf, R.F., Carey, D.W. et al. (2007). Efficacy of fenbendazole and Milbemycin oxime for treating baboons (*Papio cynocephalus anubis*) infected with *Trichuris trichiura*. *Journal of the American Association for Laboratory Animal Science* 46 (2): 42–45.

45 Churgin, S.M., Lee, F.K., Groenvold, K. et al. (2018). Successful treatment of generalized demodicosis in red-handed tamarins (*Saguinus midas*) using a single administration of oral fluralaner. *Journal of Zoo and Wildlife Medicine* 49 (2): 470–474.

46 Jepson, L. (2016). *Exotic Animal Medicine: A Quick Reference Guide*. St. Louis, MO: Elsevier.

47 Atkins, A., Heard, D.J., Mertins, J.W. et al. (2008). Hyperplastic dermatitis associated with acariasis in a siamang (*Symphalangus syndactylus*). *Journal of Zoo and Wildlife Medicine* 39 (4): 638–641.

48 Kramer, J.A., Hachey, A.M., Wachtman, L.M. et al. (2009). Treatment of giardiasis in common marmosets (*Callithrix jacchus*) with tinidazole. *Comparative Medicine* 59 (2): 174–179.

49 Singleton, C., Wack, R.F, Larsen, R.S. (2006). Use of oral hypoglycemic drugs for the management of diabetes mellitus in prosimians. *Proceedings of American Association of Zoo Veterinarians*. 379.

50 Ferrie, G.M., Becker, K.K., Wheaton, C.J. et al. (2011). Chemical and surgical interventions to alleviate intraspecific aggression in male collared lemurs (*Eulemur collaris*). *Journal of Zoo and Wildlife Medicine*. 42 (2): 214–221.

51 Norton, T.M., Penfold, L.M., Lessnau, B. et al. (2000). Long-Acting Deslorelin Implants to control aggression in Male Lion-tailed Macaques (*Macaca silenus*). *Proceedings of International Association of Aquatic Animal Medicine*.

52 de Faber, J.T., Pameijer, J.H., and Schaftenaar, W. (2004). Cataract surgery with foldable intraocular lens implants in captive lowland gorillas (*Gorilla gorilla gorilla*). *Journal of Zoo and Wildlife Medicine* 35 (4): 520–524.

53 Gerlach, T., Clyde, V.L., Morris, G.L. et al. (2011). Alternative therapeutic options for medical management of epilepsy in apes. *Journal of Zoo and Wildlife Medicine* 42 (2): 291–294.

54 Agnew, M.K., Asa, C.S., Clyde, V.L. et al. (2016). A survey of bonobo (*Pan paniscus*) oral contraceptive pill use in North American zoos. *Zoo Biology* 35 (5): 444–453.

55 Knauf-Witzens, T., Schuelfele, T., Weigold, A. et al. (2018). Pharmacological treatment of a male Bonobo (*Pan paniscus*) with suspected dilated cardiomyopathy under echocardiographic control at Wilhelma, Stuttgart, Germany, a single center experience. *Annual Proceedings of the American Association of Zoo Veterinarians*. 31.

9

Nondomestic Canids

Drug name	Drug dose	Species	Comments
Antimicrobials and Antifungals			
Amoxicillin	10 mg/kg PO BID [1]	Red wolves	n = 1 treatment of dermatitis.
Amikacin	2 mg/kg IM BID × 1 day, then 4 mg/kg SQ SID × 13d [2]	Red wolves	n = 1 treatment of degloving injury.
Cefazolin	20 mg/kg IV BID [3]	Red foxes	n = 1 pre-operative for repair of limb fractures.
Clavulanate-amoxicillin	5–10 mg/kg PO BID × 7d [2]	Red wolves	n = 1 treatment of degloving injury.
	12.75 mg/kg PO BID × 7d [4]	Red foxes	n = 1 peri-operative analgesia for laparoscopic ovariectomy.
Enrofloxacin	5 mg/kg SC; 4 mg/kg PO BID × 10d [2]	Red wolves	n = 1 treatment of degloving injury.
Doxycycline	0.3 mg/kg PO BID in a pulsatile 30d on and 30d off for 1–8 cycles [5]	Bat-eared foxes	n = 2 captive animals treated with low dose doxycycline to treat periodontal disease.
Penicillin G	30 g/kg [2]	Red wolves	n = 1 treatment of degloving injury.
Analgesia			
Butorphanol	0.1 mg/kg IV; 0.16 mg/kg IM [2]	Red wolves	n = 1 treatment of degloving injury (n = 1).
	0.1 mg/kg IM [6]	Eastern wolves	n = 53 peri-operative analgesia for intraperitoneal radiotransmitter placement.
	0.2 mg/kg IM [4]	Red foxes	n = 1 peri-operative analgesia for laparoscopic ovariectomy.
Carprofen	4.4 mg/kg SID × 3d [4]	Red foxes	n = 1 postoperative analgesia for laparoscopic ovariectomy.
Meloxicam	0.3 mg/kg IM [6]	Eastern wolves	n = 53 peri-operative analgesia for IP radiotransmitter placement.
	0.1–0.2 mg/kg IV SID [3]	Red foxes	n = 1 Pre-operative and postoperative analgesia for multiple limb fracture repair.

(*Continued*)

Drug name	Drug dose	Species	Comments
Morphine + lidocaine + bupivicaine epidural	M: 0.1 mg/kg + L: 2.5 mg/kg + B: 0.625 mg/kg, intrathecal at lumbosacral junction [3]	Red foxes	n = 1 pre-operative epidural for multiple limb fracture repair.
Anethesia and Sedation			
Acepromazine	5 mg/kg PO [7]	Canids	Tranquilizer to calm trapped canids. Drug interferes with thermoregulation, so should not be used with high ambient temperatures.
Dexmedetomidine + butorphanol	D: 0.02 mg/kg + B: 0.4 mg/kg IM [8]	Maned wolves	
Ketamine + dexmedetomidine	K: 8–10 mg/kg + D: 0.025 mg/kg IM [9]	African wolves	n = 14 induction of trapped wolves; calm induction with smooth recoveries. Antagonized with 10 mg Atipmezole/1 mg dexmedetomidine.
Ketamine + dexmedetomidine + midazolam	K: 3 mg/kg + D: 0.025 mg/kg + Mid: 0.15 mg/kg; antagonize with atipamezole and flumazenil [10]	African wild dogs	Generally larger dart volume.
Ketamine + medetomidine	K: 2.5 mg/kg + M: 0.05 mg/kg [11]	Arctic foxes	n = 6 Induction in 1–2 min; anesthesia for 13–25 min. Antagonized with 0.25 mg/kg atipamezole.
	K: 2 mg/kg + M: 0.11 mg/kg IM [12]	Golden jackals	
	K: 3–4 mg/kg + M: 0.04–0.07 mg/kg IM [8]	Coyotes	
	K: 3–4 mg/kg + M: 0.06–0.08 mg/kg [13, 14]	Gray wolves	Antagonize with atipamezole 0.3–0.4 mg/kg IM.
	K: 2 mg/kg + M: 0.04 mg/kg [15]	Red wolves	Antagonize with atipamezole 0.2 mg/kg.
	K: 2.5 mg/kg + M: 0.08 mg/kg IM [14]	Maned wolves	Antagonize with atipamezole 0.4 mg/kg IM.
	K: 3–5 mg/kg + M: 0.05–0.1 mg/kg IM [16, 17]	African wild dogs	Antagonize with atipamezole 0.15 mg/kg IM.
	K: 2.5–3.1 mg/kg + M: 0.05–0.06 mg/kg IM [18]	Chilla foxes	Antagonize with atipamezole 0.25 mg/kg (n = 28).
	K: 2–4 mg/kg + M: 0.04–0.07 mg/kg IM [19, 20]	Red foxes	Antagonize with atipamezole 0.2–0.35 mg/kg IM.
	K: 5 mg/kg + M: 0.05 mg/kg IM [21]	Bush dogs	
Ketamine + medetomidine + butorphanol	K: 1 mg/kg + M: 0.04 mg/kg + B: 0.4 mg/kg IM [8]	Gray wolves	
	K: 2 mg/kg + M: 0.02 mg/kg + B: 0.2 mg/kg [15]	Red wolves	Antagonize with atipamezole 0.2 mg/kg.

Drug name	Drug dose	Species	Comments
	K: 4 mg/kg + M: 0.02 mg/kg + B: 0.04 mg/kg IM [22]	Red foxes	Antagonize with atipamezole 0.1 mg/kg IM.
Ketamine + medetomidine ± midazolam ± butorphanol	K: 2.5–3 mg/kg + M: 0.025–0.04 mg/kg ± Mid: 0.1–0.15 mg/kg ± B: 0.1–0.2 mg/kg IM; antagonize with atipamezole 0.14–0.24 mg/kg ± flumazenil 0.01–0.05 mg/kg ± naloxone 0.02 mg/kg IM [10]	African wild dogs	Excellent muscle relaxation, quick recovery.
Ketamine + medetomidine	K: 2 mg/kg + M: 0.07 mg/kg [20]	Red foxes	Provided 20–25 min of anesthesia.
Ketamine + midazolam	K: 5–10 mg/kg + Mid: 0.1–0.4 m/kg IV after manual restraint [8]	Gray wolves	
Ketamine + midazolam + butorphanol	K: 2–4 mg/kg + Mid: 0.15–0.3 mg/kg + B: 0.3–0.4 mg/kg IM, antagonize with flumazenil and naloxone [10]	African wild dogs	Suggested alternative for cardiac cases. Supplement with propofol 0.4–0.5 mg/kg IV or gas anesthesia.
Ketamine + xylazine	K: 1.6 mg/kg + X: 2.2 mg/kg IM [23]	African wild dogs	Antagonize with yohimbine 0.2 mg/kg IM.
	K: 3–5 mg/kg + X: 0.6–0.8 mg/kg IM [24]	Hoary foxes	
	K: 4 mg/kg + X: 2 mg/kg [7]	Coyotes	Antagonize with yohimbine 0.15 mg/kg.
	K:4–10 mg/kg + X: 1–3 mg/kg; antagonize with yohimbine 0.15 mg/kg IV [8, 25]	Gray Wolves	
	K: 5–8 mg/kg + X: 0.5 mg/kg [25]	Short-eared dogs, Bat-eared foxes, Cape foxes	
	K: 6–9 mg/kg + X: 0.5–2 mg/kg IM, Antagonize with yohimbine 0.1–0.2 mg/kg IM [8, 25]	Maned wolves	
	K: 7.5 mg/kg + X: 1 mg/kg [25]	Dingos	
	K: 8–10 mg/kg + X: 2 mg/kg. Antagonize with yohimbine 0.1 mg/kg [25]	Red wolves	
	K: 9.3–17.7 mg/kg + X: 1.2–2 mg/kg IM [8]	Chillas	
	K: 10 mg/kg + X: 0.5–1 mg/kg IM [25]	Crab-eating foxes	

(*Continued*)

Drug name	Drug dose	Species	Comments
	K: 10 mg/kg + X: 1 mg/kg IM [25, 26]	Swift foxes	Antagonize with yohimbine 0.125 mg/kg IM.
	K: 11–15 mg/kg + X: 2–3 mg/kg IM [25]	Gray foxes	
Ketamine + xylazine	K: 15.5–18.6 mg/kg + X: 11.9–12.7 mg/kg IM [27]	Red foxes	n = 83 free-ranging, 15 pups and 68 adults, mean induction time was 1.6 min and first reaction 22.5 min for pups and 3.8 min and 39.4 min respectively for adults. Recommend for adults of unknown weight: 75 mg ketamine and 20 mg xylazine.
	K: 20–23 mg/kg + X: 1–1.2 mg/kg IM, antagonize with yohimbine 0.15 mg/kg [25]	Red foxes	
Medetomidine	0.05 mg/kg; antagonize with atipamezole 0.25 mg/kg IM [25]	Gray wolves	Habituated animals, complete immobilization.
	0.025–0.1 mg/kg IM [25]	Arctic foxes	Farmed animals, complete immobilization.
	0.06–0.12 mg/kg; antagonize with atipamezole 0.6 mg/kg [25]	Coyotes	Free-ranging, immobilization.
	0.14 mg/kg IM; antagonize with atipamezole 0.8 mg/kg IM [25]	Red foxes	Free-ranging, immobilization.
Medetomidine + butorphanol	M: 0.04 mg/kg + B: 0.4 mg/kg IM; antagonized with atipamezole 0.2 mg/kg and naltrexone 0.02 mg/kg IM [8, 25, 28]	Red wolves, Maned wolves	n = 24 wolves; 23 required minimal visual and auditory stimulation. A second group received supplemental diazepam 0.2 mg/kg IV, and a third group received 1 mg/kg ketamine IV 30 min post induction. A few experienced bradycardia and hypertension was seen in all groups but resolved by 30 min. The group that received ketamine had significant elevations in heart rate and transient hypertension after ketamine was given. Most wolves had mild to moderate acidemia. Hypoxemia, sinus arrythmia or second-degree heart block. Flumazenil was given 0.02–0.04 mg/kg IM to those who received diazepam.

Drug name	Drug dose	Species	Comments
Medetomidine + midazolam + butorphanol	M: 0.03 mg/kg + Mid: 0.3 mg/kg + B: 0.3 mg/kg IM [10]	African wild dogs	Completely reversible.
Medetomidine + butorphanol + midazolam	M: 0.04–0.06 mg/kg + B: 0.18–0.3 mg/kg + Mid: 0.18–0.4 mg/kg IM; antagonize with atipamezole 3 mg, naltrexone 10 mg, and flumazenil 0.2 mg [8, 25].	African wild dogs	
	M: 0.04 mg/kg + B: 0.1 mg/kg + Mid: 0.3 mg/kg IM; antagonize with atipamezole 0.15 mg/kg IM [25]	Red foxes	
Medetomidine + midazolam	M: 0.07 mg/kg + Mid: 0.8 mg/kg IM; antagonize with atipamezole 0.35 mg/kg IM [25]	Red foxes	
	M: 0.07–0.1 mg/kg + Mid: 0.39–0.55 mg/kg IM [8]	Golden jackals	
	M: 0.09 mg/kg + Mid: 0.5 mg/kg; antagonize with atipamezole 0.45 mg/kg [25]	Short-eared dogs	
Telazol	T: 1–4 mg/kg IM [8, 25]	African wild dogs	Wild dogs are more sensitive than captive ones.
	T: 1.2–5 mg/kg IM, supplement with ketamine 25–50 mg or isoflurane [25]	Maned wolves	
	T: 1.6–8 mg/kg IM [8]	Chillas	
	2–7 mg/kg IM [8, 25]	Ethiopian wolves	
	3–4 mg/kg [25]	Short-eared dogs	6–8 mg/kg if free-range.
	T: 3–5 mg/kg [8]	Maned wolves	
	3–10 mg/kg [25]	Gray wolves	For helicopter captures use 10–13 mg/kg.
	T: 4–10 mg/kg [8, 25]	Red foxes, Dholes	
Telazol	T: 5 mg/kg IM [25]	Bat-eared foxes, Cape foxes	
	T: 5–10 mg/kg IM [8]	Red wolves	
	7–10 mg/kg [25]	Dingos	
	9 mg/kg IM [25]	Gray foxes	

(Continued)

Drug name	Drug dose	Species	Comments
	10 mg/kg IM [25]	Arctic foxes, Kit foxes, Pale foxes, Swift foxes, Fennec foxes, Bush dogs	
	10 mg/kg IM [29]	Red foxes	n = 22 pups and 49 free-ranging red foxes. Induction times were 2–2.5 min, and recovered in 18–78 min in pups and in adults 3.5–3.9 min and 13–90 min respectively. For adults of unknown weight an initial dose of 60–70 mg of Telazol should allow for approximately 40 min of handling time.
	10–11 mg/kg [8, 25]	Coyotes, Red wolves, Crab-eating foxes, South American foxes, Bush dogs	
	10–13 mg/kg IM [8]	Gray wolves	For helicopter captures.
Telazol + ketamine	T: 2 mg/kg + K: 2 mg/kg IM [8]	Dholes	
	T: 3 mg/kg + K: 3 mg/kg IM [8]	Bush dogs	
Telazol + medetomidine	T: 1–2 mg/kg + M: 0.04 mg/kg [25]	Dingos	
	T: 2 mg/kg + M: 0.04 mg/kg IM; antagonize with atipamezole 0.2 mg/kg IM [25]	Red foxes	
Telazol + xylazine	T: 7 mg/kg [25]	Raccoon dogs	
	T: 10 mg/kg + X: 1.5 mg/kg [25]	Gray wolves	
Tolazoline	8 mg/kg [25]	Canids	To antagonize xylazine in anesthetic combinations.
Xylazine	2 mg/kg captive, or 3–4 mg/kg for free-ranging; antagonize with yohimbine 0.15 mg/kg IM [25]	Gray wolves	
Xylazine + butorphanol	X: 2 mg/kg + B: 0.4 mg/kg IM [14]	Gray wolves	Induction in 20 min, bradycardia, respiratory depression and normotension observed. Antagonized with yohimbine and naloxone.

Drug name	Drug dose	Species	Comments
Xylazine + fentanyl	X: 0.7–1 mg/kg + F: 0.1 mg/kg IM; antagonize with yohimbine 0.125 mg/kg + naloxone (0.04 mg/kg) or 1.2 mg/animal [25].	Canids, especially African wild dogs	Supplement with xylazine 10 mg, fentanyl 0.5 mg. Animals were recumbent in 5–7.5 min. As with all animals receiving alpha-2 agonists, the animal should be left alone for at least 10 min prior to approaching. Effects generally last 45–60 min.
Yohimbine	0.1–0.2 mg/kg IV IM or a combination of both [25]	Canids	To antagonize Xylazine in anesthetic combinations. Doses higher than 0.2 mg/kg do not hasten recovery, rather result in ataxia, hyperreflexion, tachycardia, and hypersalivation.
Antiparasitic			
Clindamycin hydrochloride	10 mg/kg SC BID SC × 30d [30]	Red foxes	n = 1 treatment of Neospora caninum.
Doxycycline	5 mg/kg PO BID × 10d [31]	Timber wolves	n = 1 treatment of acute granulocytic anaplasmosis.
Selamectin	6 mg/kg topically once [32]	San Joaquin kit foxes	n = 3 treatment of sarcoptic mange.
Other			
Blood transfusion	45 ml IV via filter [33]	Island foxes	n = 1 presumptive rattlesnake envenomation in an 11 yr old male fox, given 45 ml canine blood after supportive care, no reactions seen and patient made a full recovery 5 days later.
Canine Distemper Virus vaccine	Galaxy-d modified live vaccine 1 ml SC [34]	Red wolves	n = 32 adult wolves, captive, given CDV and a canine parvovirus vaccine (Recombitek parvovirus modified live 1 ml SC) and 100% of wolves developed and maintained a positive titer to CDV and 96.9% to CPV for 3 yrs.
Canine Distemper Vaccine	Purevax canary pox vectored Canine distemper vaccine [35]	Fennec foxes, Meerkats	n = 5 fennec foxes and 6 meerkats. All foxes had been vaccinated 5 yr prior with Durammune MLV CDV vaccine and only 1 meerkat given Galaxy-d 6 yr before. All given 1 ml Purevax IM, meerkats were also boostered with a second dose, and rechecked titers at 3,6,9, and 12 months and all maintained neutralizing antibody titers for at least a year.

(*Continued*)

Drug name	Drug dose	Species	Comments
Canine Distemper Vaccine (Purevax Ferret distemper)		African wild dogs	Has been shown to produce measurable titers after a series of 3 injections at 2–3 wk intervals. In one study protective titers persisted in 39–85% of dogs for a minimum of 1 yr. Another study indicated that dogs maintained presumably protective titers for 1 year but few for 2–3 yrs. Recommend to begin series at 6–9 wks of age, booster SC q2–3 wks through 16–20 wks of age and repeat annually [10].
Chlorambucil + prednisone	C: 0.26 mg/kg PO q48 hrs + P: 1.26 mg/kg PO q48 hr [36]	Bat-eared foxes	n = 1, 10 yr old, with regional alopecia and severe leukocytosis with bone marrow cytology and serology strongly suggestive of chronic lymphocytic leukemia, responsive to a degree to protocol, lived another 22 mo when euthanized for osteoarthritis with no neoplasia identified on necropsy.
Cyclosporine	10% matrix implant [37]	Red wolves	Treatment of idiopathic dry eye (n = 1).
Dantrolene (Revonto) for IV or dantrolene sodium capsule for oral	1.6 mg/kg IV TID × 2d, 2 mg/kg PO × 3d [38]	Coyotes	n = 1 captive adult 12.5 kg female coyote. Observed laterally recumbent after fighting, immobilized and given supportive care as well as dantrolene IV TID × 2d and oral SID for 3 more days at which point appeared fully recovered clinically. Dantrolene is a hydantoin analog that suppresses the release of calcium from the sarcoplasmic reticulum in striated and cardiac muscle. This prevents the excitation contraction coupling within the muscle and may allow a more precise treatment of Exertional myopathy in veterinary patients, compared to centrally acting muscle relaxants. Also, the intravenous formulation contains 3000 mg mannitol per 20 mg dantrolene, which may be beneficial for myoglobinuric acute renal failure by increasing renal perfusion.

Drug name	Drug dose	Species	Comments
Deslorelin	6 mg SC implant q12 months [39]	African wild dogs	n = 21 African wild dogs (6.15), where a 6 mg implant was given. Hormone levels, vaginal cytology, and semen evaluation occurred post implant. Males responded consistently and the implant was successful for approximately 12 months. In females, it was less consistent and one female conceived 4 weeks later. However in 9 females, mating was postponed until the next season.
Deslorelin Acetate (Suprelorin)		African wild dogs	Recommended by the AZA Reproduction Management Center. Have been used for contraception and behavioral alteration in males with variable results [10].
Leuprolide acetate (Lupron depot)	4.7 mg implant [10]	African wild dogs	Recommended by the AZA Reproduction Management Center.
Melengesterol acetate implant (MGA)		African wild dogs	Associated with uterine pathology. Suprelorin or Lupron Depot are recommended instead [10].
Rabies Killed Vaccine (Imrab 3)		African wild dogs	One study showed that a single vaccination of dogs older than 14 wks provided persistent protective titers. Another study indicated that dogs maintained presumably protective titers for a minimum of 1 year, but few animals maintained for up to 2–3 yrs [10].
Tiopronin	0–35 mg/kg PO BID	Fennec foxes	n = 1 captive male treated for cystine crystalluria and repeated urolithiasis, to prevent further crystals/stones. Started at 35 mg/kg PO BID along with removing purine from diet. Resulted in decreased rate of stone formation but not complete resolution and did not dissolve stones. Maintained at 20–28 mg/kg PO BID. Castration was ultimately effective in preventing further crystalluria and animal was slowly weaned off tiopronin over a year after surgery. Author's experience.
Zinc sulfate	10 mg/kg PO SID × 10 weeks [1]	Red wolves	n = 1 Treatment of zinc-responsive dermatosis.

Species	Weight [8, 14, 25]
Arctic fox *(Alopex lagopus)*	2.4–5.4
Short eared dog *(Atelocynus microtis)*	9–10 kg
Side-striped jackal *(Canis adustus)*	7–12 kg
Golden jackal *(Canis aureus)*	6.5–9.8 kg
Coyote *(Canis latrans)*	7.7–15 kg
Gray wolf *(Canis lupus)*	23–60 kg
Dingo *(Canislupus dingo)*	7–22 kg
Black-backed jackal *(Canis mesomelas)*	6–12 kg
Red wolf *(Canis rufus)*	20–34 kg
Ethiopian wolf *(Canis simiensis)*	11–19 kg
Crab-eating fox *(Cerdocyon thous)*	4.5–8.5 kg
Maned wolf *(Chrysocyon brachyurus)*	21–30 kg
Dhole *(Cuon alpinus)*	10–20 kg
African hunting/wild dog *(Lycaon pictus)*	19–35 kg
Raccoon dog *(Nyctereutes procyonoides)*	3–13 kg
Bat-eared fox *(Otocyon megalotis)*	3.2–5.4 kg
Culpeo (Andean fox) *(Pseudalopex culpaeus)*	3.4–14 kg
Darwin's fox *(Pseudalopex fulvipes)*	1.8–4 kg
Chilla *(Pseudaopex griseus)*	2.5–5 kg
Pampas fox *(Pseudoalopex gymnocercus)*	3–8 kg
Sechuran fox *(Pseudalopex sechurae)*	2.6–4.2 kg
Hoary fox *(Pseudalopex vetulus)*	3–4 kg
Bush dog *(Speothos venaticus)*	5–8 kg
Gray fox *(Urocyon cinereoargenteus)*	2–5.5 kg
Island gray fox *(Urocyon littoralis)*	1.3–2.5 kg
Indian fox *(Vulpes bengalensis)*	1.8–3.2 kg
Blanford's fox *(Vulpes cana)*	0.8–1.5 kg
Cape fox (*Vulpes chama)*	2–4.2 kg
Corsac fox *(Vulpes corsac)*	1.6–3.2 kg
Tibetan sand fox *(Vulpes ferrilata)*	3–4.6 kg
Kit fox *(Vulpes macrotis)*	1.6–2.7 kg
Pale fox *(Vulpes pallida)*	2–3.6 kg
Sand fox *(Vulpes rueppelli)*	1.1–2.3 kg
Swift fox *(Vulpes velox)*	1.6–2.5 kg
Red fox *(Vulpes vulpes)*	3.6–7.6 kg
Fennec fox *(Vulpes zerda)*	1–1.9 kg

References

1 Kearns, K., Sleeman, J., Frank, L. et al. (2000). Zinc-responsive dermatosis in a red wolf (*Canis rufus*). *Journal of Zoo and Wildlife Medicine* 31 (2): 255–258.

2 Hurley-Sanders, J.L. and Sladky, K.K. (2015). Use of cortical bone fenestration, autogensous free skin graft, and thermography for wound treatment and monitoring in a red wolf (*Canis rufus gregoryi*). *Journal of Zoo and Wildlife Medicine* 46 (3): 617–620.

3 Anagnostou, T., Flouraki, E., Kostakis, C. et al. (2015). Anesthetic management of a 4-month-old red fox (*Vulpes vulpes*) for orthopedic surgery. *Journal of Zoo and Wildlife Medicine* 46 (1): 155–157.
4 Lee, S.Y., Jung, D.H., Park, S.J. et al. (2014). Unilateral laparoscopic ovariectomy in a red fox (*Vulpes vulpes*) with an ovarian cyst. *Journal of Zoo and Wildlife Medicine* 45 (3): 678–681.
5 Bicknese, B., Fagan, D.A., and Lamberski, N. (2008). Cyclic regimen of low-dose doxycycline to treat periodontal disease in a Chacoan peccary (*Catagonus wagneri*), Red pandas (*Ailurus fulgens*), and Bat-eared foxes (*Otocyon megalotis megalotis*). *Proceedings of the American Association of Zoo Veterinarians*. 167–168.
6 Crawshaw, G.J., Mills, K.J., Mosley, C. et al. (2007). Field implantation of intraperitoneal radiotransmitters in Eastern Wolf (*Canis lycaon*) pups using inhalation anesthesia with sevoflurane. *Journal of Wildlife Diseases* 43 (4): 711–718.
7 McKenzie, A.A. (1993). Capture, care, accommodation and transportation of wild African animals. In: *The Capture and Care Manual: Capture, Care, Accommodation, and Transportation of Wild African Animals* (ed. A.A. McKenzie), 161–164. Pretoria, SA: Wildlife Decision Support Services.
8 Padilla, L.R. and Hilton, C.D. (2014). Canidae. In: *Fowler's Zoo and Wild Animal Medicine*, vol. 8 (ed. R.E. Miller and M. Fowler), 457–465. St. Louis, MO: Elsevier Saunders.
9 Gutema, T.M., Atickem, A., and Lemma, A. (2018). Capture and immobilization of African wolves (*Canis lupaster*) in the Ethiopian highlands. *Journal of Wildlife Diseases* 54 (1): 175–179.
10 Langan, J.N. and Jankowski, G. (2019). Overview of African wild dog medicine. In: *Fowler's Zoo and Wild Animal Medicine Current Therapy*, vol. 9 (ed. R.E. Miller, N. Lamberski and P.P. Calle), 539–545. St. Louis, MO: Elsevier Saunders.
11 Aguirre, A.A., Principe, B., Tannerfeldt, M. et al. (2000). Field anesthesia of wild arctic fox (*Alopex lagopus*) cubs in the Swedish lapland using medetomidine-ketamine-atipamezole. *Journal of Zoo and Wildlife Medicine* 31 (2): 244–246.
12 King, R., Lapid, R., Epstein, A. et al. (2008). Field anesthesia of golden jackals (*Canis aureus*) with the use of medetomidine-ketamine or medetomidine-midazolam with atipamezole reversal. *Journal of Zoo and Wildlife Medicine* 39 (4): 576–581.
13 Holz, P., Holz, R.M., and Barnett, J.E.F. (1994). Effects of atropine on medetomidine/ketamine immobilization in the gray wolf (*Canis lupus*). *Journal of Zoo and Wildlife Medicine* 25: 209–213.
14 Kreeger, T.J., Arnemo, J.M., and Raath, J.P. (2002). *Handbook of Wildlife Chemical Immobilization*. Fort Collins, Colorado: Wildlife Pharmaceuticals Inc.
15 Sladky, K.K., Kelly, B.T., Loomis, M.R. et al. (2000). Cardiorespiratory effects of four alpha-2-adrenoceptor agonist-ketamine combinations in captive red wolves. *Journal of the American Veterinary Medical Association* 217 (9): 1366–1371.
16 Cirone, F., Gabriella, E., Marco, C. et al. (2004). Immunogenicity of an inactivated oil-emulsion canine distemper vaccine in African wild dogs. *Journal of Wildlife Diseases* 40: 343–346.
17 Van Heerden, J. (1993). Chemical capture of the wild dog. In: *The Capture and Care Manual: Capture, Care, Accommodation, and Transportation of Wild African Animals* (ed. A.A. McKenzie), 251–254. Pretoria, SA: Wildlife Decision Support Services.
18 Acosta-Jamett, G., Astorga-Arancibi, F., and Cunningham, A.A. (2010). Comparison of chemical immobilization methods in wild foxes (*Pseudalopex griseus* and *Pseudalopex culpaeus*) in Chile. *Journal of Wildlife Diseases* 46 (4): 1204–1213.
19 Bertelsen, M.F. and Villadsen, L. (2009). A comparison of the efficacy and cardiorespiratory effects of four medetomidine-based anesthetic protocols in the red fox (*Vulpes vulpes*). *Veterinary Anaesthesia and Analgesia* 36: 328–333.
20 Shilo, Y., Lapid, R., King, R. et al. (2010). Immobilization of red fox (*Vulpes vulpes*) with medetomidine-ketamine or medetomidine-midazolam and antagonism with atipamezole. *Journal of Zoo and Wildlife Medicine* 41 (1): 28–34.
21 DeMatteo, K., Silver, S., Porton, I. et al. (2006). Preliminary tests of a new reversible male contraceptive in bush dog, *Speothos venaticus*: open-ended vasectomy and microscopic reversal. *Journal of Zoo and Wildlife Medicine* 37 (3): 313–317.

22 Brash, M.G.I. Foxes. In: *BSAVA Management of Wildlife Casualties* (ed. E. Mullineaux, R. Best and J.E. Cooper), 154–160. Gloucester, UK: BSAVA.

23 Osofosky, S.A., McNutt, J.W., and Hirsch, K.J. (1996). Immobilization of free-ranging African wild dogs (*Lycaeon pictus*) using a ketamine/xylazine/atropine combination. *Journal of Zoo and Wildlife Medicine* 27: 528–532.

24 Pessutti, C., Bodini Santiago, M.E., and Fernandes Oliveira, L.T. (2001). Order carnivora, family canidae (dogs, foxes, maned wolves). In: *Biology, Medicine, and Surgery of South American Wild Animals* (ed. M.E. Fowler and Z.S. Cubas). Ames, IA: Iowa State University Press.

25 Larsen, R.S. and Kreeger, T.J. (2014). Canids. In: *Zoo Animal and Wildlife Immobilization and Anesthesia*, 2e (ed. G. West, D. Heard and N. Caulkett), 585–598. Ames, IA: Wiley Blackwell.

26 Telesco, R.L. and Sovada, M.A. (2002). Immobilization of swift foxes with ketamine hydrochloride-xylazine hydrochloride. *Journal of Wildlife Diseases* 38 (4): 764–768.

27 Travaini, A., Ferreras, P., Delibes, M. et al. (1992). Xylazine hydrochloride-ketamine hydrochloride immobilization of free-living red foxes (*Vulpes vulpes*) in Spain. *Journal of Wildlife Diseases* 28 (3): 507–509.

28 Larsen, R.S., Loomis, M.R., Kelly, B.T. et al. (2002). Cardiorespiratory effects of medetomidine-butorphanol, medetomidine-butorphanol-diazepam, and medetomidine-butorphanol-ketamine in captive red wolves (*Canis rufus*). *Journal of Zoo and Wildlife Medicine* 33 (2): 101–107.

29 Travaini, A. and Delibes, M. (1994). Immobilization of free-ranging red foxes (*Vulpes vulpes*) with tiletamine hydrochloride and zolazepam hydrochloride. *Journal of Wildlife Diseases* 30 (4): 589–591.

30 Dubey, J.P., Whitesell, L.E., Culp, W.E. et al. (2014). Diagnosis and treatment of *Neospora caninum* – associated dermatitis in a red fox (*Vulpes vulpes*) with concurrent *Toxoplasma gondii* infection. *Journal of Zoo and Wildlife Medicine* 45 (2): 454–457.

31 Leschnik, M., Kirtz, G., Viranyi, Z. et al. (2012). Acute granulocytic anaplasmosis in a captive timber wolf (*Canis lupus occidentalis*). *Journal of Zoo and Wildlife Medicine* 43 (3): 645–648.

32 Cypher, B.L., Rudd, J.L., Westall, T.L. et al. (2017). Sarcoptic mange in endangered kit foxes (*Vulpes macrotis mutica*): case histories, diagnoses, and implications for conservation. *Journal of Wildlife Diseases* 53 (1): 46–53.

33 Martony, M.E., Krause, K.J., Weldy, S.H. et al. (2016). Xenotransfusion in an island fox (*Urocyon littoralis clementae*) using blood from a domestic dog (*Canis lupus familiaris*). *Journal of Zoo and Wildlife Medicine* 47 (3): 923–926.

34 Anderson, K., Case, A., Woodie, K. et al. (2014). Duration of immunity in red wolves (*Canis rufus*) following vaccination with a modified live parvovirus and canine distemper vaccine. *Journal of Zoo and Wildlife Medicine* 45 (3): 550–554.

35 Coke, R.L., Backues, K.A., Hoover, J.P. et al. (2005). Serologic responses after vaccination of fennec foxes (*Vulpes zerda*) and meerkats (*Suricata suricatta*) with a live, canarypox-vectored canine distemper virus vaccine. *Journal of Zoo and Wildlife Medicine* 36 (2): 326–330.

36 Nevitt, B.N., Langan, J.N., Adkesson, M.J. et al. (2014). Diagnosis and treatment of chronic lymphocytic leukemia in a bat-eared fox (*Otocyon megalotis*). *Journal of the American Veterinary Medical Association* 245 (12): 1391–1395.

37 Acton, A.E., Beale, A.B., Gilger, B.C. et al. (2006). Sustained release cyclosporine therapy for bilateral keratoconjunctivitis sicca in a red wolf (*Canis rufus*). *Journal of Zoo and Wildlife Medicine* 37 (4): 562–564.

38 Anthony, A.L. (2018). Treatment of suspected exertional myopathy using dantrolene in a coyote (*Canis latrans*). *Journal of Zoo and Wildlife Medicine* 49 (2): 508–510.

39 Bertschinger, H.J., Trigg, T.E., Jochle, W., and Human, A. (2002). Induction of contraception in some African wild carnivores by down regulation of LH and FSH secretion using the GnRH analogue deslorelin. *Reproduction Supplement* 60: 41–52.

10

Bears

Drug name	Drug dose	Species	Comments
Antimicrobials and Antifungals			
Amoxicillin/ clavulanic acid	12 mg/kg PO BID [1]	Polar bears	n = 1 captive, post hernia repair, no reported side effects.
Ampicillin	4–5 g PO TID [2]	Polar bears	
	9 mg/kg IM [3]	Sun bears	n = 1 intraoperative antibiotics during rostral mandibulectomy.
Carbenicillin	2.5 g PO QID × 5d [2]	Polar bears	n = 1 captive, 86 kg bear.
Cefazolin sodium	10 mg/kg IV q2 hr [4]	Polar bears	n = 1 humeral condylar fracture, given every 2 hrs intraoperative.
Ceftiofur (Naxcel)	2.3 mg/kg IM [1]	Polar bears	n = 1 captive, post hernia repair, no reported side effects.
Ceftiofur (Excenel)	2 mg/kg IM [5]	American black bears	n = 1 juvenile female, treatment for poor body condition, traumatic wounds and mange.
Cephalexin	11 mg/kg PO BID [1]	Polar bears	n = 1 captive, post hernia repair, no reported side effects.
	15 mg/kg PO BID [4]	Polar bears	n = 1 humeral condylar fracture, given for 19 days with no reported side effects.
Chloramphenicol	3–4 g PO BID to TID for 6–10d in adult bear, 2.5 g/l topical spray q7d [2]	Polar bears	
Doxycycline	1 mg/kg PO SID × 12d [2]	Polar bears	
	10 mg/kg PO BID [6]	Sun bears	n = 2 cases of salmon poisoning, treated for 21 days, no adverse effects reported.
Enrofloxacin	2.5 mg/kg IV once or PO × 14d [3]	Sun bears	n = 1 postoperative treatment of rostral mandibulectomy due to squamous cell carcinoma of mandible.
	5 mg/kg IM or 6 mg/kg PO SID [1]	Polar bears	n = 1 captive, post hernia repair, no reported side effects.

(*Continued*)

Drug name	Drug dose	Species	Comments
Flumethasone	0.6–1.25 mg IM PO SID [2]	Polar bears	
Oxytetracycline (LA200)	10 mg/kg IM SID [6]	Sun bears	n = 2 cases of salmon poisoning, initially treated for 12 days via dart, then switched to oral doxycycline, no adverse affects reported.
	10 mg/kg IM BID [2]	Polar bears	
Penicillin (K)	15 000 IU/kg IM q3d [2]	Polar bears	Procaine and penicillin doses combined.
Piperazine	100 mg/kg PO [2]	Polar bears	
Procaine penicillin	15 000 IU/kg IM q3d [2]	Polar bears	Procaine and penicillin doses combined.
Procaine penicillin G with benzathine	30 000 IU/kg q3d [2]	Polar bears	
	44 000 IU/KG IM EOD [1]	Polar bears	n = 1 captive, post hernia repair, no reported side effects.
Tetracycline	5 mg/kg PO q7d [2]	Polar bears	For treatment of skin conditions.
Trimethoprim sulfadiazine	30 mg/kg PO SID [1]	Polar bears	n = 1 captive, post hernia repair, no reported side effects.
Trimethoprim sulfadimethoxazole	16 mg/kg PO BID [1]	Polar bears	n = 1 captive, post hernia repair, no reported side effects.
Trimethoprim sulfadimethoxazole	32 mg/kg PO BID × 7d [5]	Black bears	n = 1 juvenile female, treated for poor body condition, traumatic wounds, and mange.
Analgesia			
Bupivicaine	10–15 mg [7]	Polar bears	Given as a nerve block prior to removal of a premolar tooth for aging free-ranging bears.
Buprenorphine	0.01 mg/kg IM SID [1]	Polar bears	n = 1 captive, post hernia repair for pain control, no reported side effects.
Butorphanol	0.2–0.4 mg/kg IM BID [1]	Polar bears	n = 1 captive, post hernia repair for pain control, no reported side effects.
Carprofen	0.75 mg/kg IM, 0.85 mg/kg PO [1]	Polar bears	n = 1 captive post hernia repair, 1 dose of IM and 2 doses PO.
	5 mg/kg PO SID [3]	Sun bears	n = 1 case of chemotherapy to treat squamous cell carcinoma of mandible.
Meloxicam	0.1 mg/kg PO SID × 14d [1]	European brown bears	n = 1 female with femoral head and neck excision.
	0.1–0.2 mg/kg SC once [8]	Brown bears	n = 31 not a pharmacokinetic study, Given as analgesia during a study involving immobilization of free-ranging bears with minor surgical procedures.

Drug name	Drug dose	Species	Comments
	0.2 mg/kg loading dose followed by 0.1 mg/kg PO SID [9]	Asiatic black bears	n = 129 bears post bile collection confiscation with varying degrees of osteoarthritis. Combined with tramadol and gabapentin as needed.
Ketoprofen	2 mg/kg IM [3]	Sun bears	n = 1 case of chemotherapy for oral squamous cell carcinoma.
	2 mg/kg IM once followed by 1 mg/kg PO SID × 3d [4]	Polar bears	n = 1 humeral condylar fracture intra and postoperative care.
Morphine	0.5 mg/kg IV, with supplemental 0.1 mg/kg IV as needed perioperatively [3]	Sun bears	n = 1 case of chemotherapy for oral squamous cell carcinoma, morphine given as pain prevention.
Anesthetic and Sedation			
Butorphanol + azaperone + medetomidine	B: 0.3 mg/kg + A: 0.25 mg/kg + M: 0.1 mg/kg IM; antagonize with atipamezole at 5 mg/mg Medetomidine and naltrexone at 5 mg/mg of butorphanol administered [6].	Black bears	n = 16 captive and 5 free-ranging bears, all had reliable induction, no adverse effects, and recoveries were more rapid than with other combinations reported in the species.
Carfentanil	0.0054–0.0076 mg/kg IM or 0.0068–0.0188 mg/kg PO; antagonize with 100 mg naltrexone per 1 mg carfentanil [10]	Black, Brown, and Polar bears	Immobilization.
Carfentanil	0.001–0.038 mg/kg IM; antagonize with 2–3 mg diprenorphine SC + 30–50 mg IV and 30–40 mg IM naloxone [11]	Polar bears	n = 64 free-ranging bears, one death post procedure of an obese animal, 3 reversal strategies used and the one reported here, represents the least renarcotization observed, all experienced profound respiratory suppression, especially those receiving >0.01 mg/kg carfentanil.
Carfentanil + diazepam	C: 0.7–3.0 mg in 5–20 ml of honey, (0.0068–0.018 mg/kg) (0.008 mg/kg PO in Brown bears) D given later: 10–25 mg IV; antagonize with 100 mg naltrexone per mg of carfentanil [12]	Black and Brown bears	n = 10 experienced muscle rigidity (thus diazepam was given to alleviate), as well as bradypnea and oxygen desaturation. Bear at lowest dose of carfentanil was 6.8 μg/kg, and received 1.9 mg/kg Ketamin IV to fully induce.
Carfentanil + xylazine	C: 0.012 mg/kg + X: 0.3 mg/kg IM; antagonize with 100 mg naltrexone per 1 mg carfentanil used [10]	Black, Brown, and Polar bears	Immobilization.
	C: 0.01 mg/kg + X: 0.1 mg/kg IM; antagonize with 1 mg/kg naltrexone and 2 mg/kg tolazoline [13, 14]	Brown and Black bears	n = 7 Brown and 3 Black bears, wild caught in traps, all experienced respiratory suppression but had smooth and uneventful induction and recovery.

(*Continued*)

Drug name	Drug dose	Species	Comments
Detomidine + Telazol	D: 0.03 mg/kg + T: 1.5 mg/kg IM; antagonize with atipamezole 0.12 mg IV or 50% of this dose IV and 50% IM [15]	Asiatic black bears	n = 12 captive.
Dexmedetomidine + Telazol	Based on Age range: Yearling: 0.83 mg D + 83.3 mg T; 2 yr olds: 1.25 mg D + 125 mg T; Adults: 0.025 mg/kg D + 2.45 mg/kg T; antagonize with 10 mg atipamezole per mg dexmedetomidine used [8].	Brown bears	n = 31 free-ranging.
	Captive: D:6 μg/kg + T: 2.46 mg/kg (Hibernating bears use 50%), Free ranging: D: 10 μg/kg + T 4.12 mg/kg IM; antagonize with atipamezole IV 5–10 μg/μg of dexmedetomidine [16]	Brown bears	n = 10 captive, 21 free-ranging.
Diazepam	0.22 mg/kg PO [3]	Sun bears	n = 1 premedication.
Etorphine	0.02–0.06 mg/kg IM [10]	Black, Brown, and Polar bears	Immobilization.
	0.035 mg/kg IM; antagonize with 0.07 mg/kg diprenorphine [14]	Polar bears	Immobilization.
	0.011–0.132 mg/kg IM [17]	Brown bears	n = 17 bears, 27 procedures, higher doses resulted in significant respiratory suppression.
Gabapentin	3.5 mg/kg SID 6 mg/kg BID PO [9]	Asiatic black bears	n = 129 bears, post bile collection, confiscation with varying degrees of osteoarthritis. Combined with meloxicam as well as tramadol as needed.
Guaifenesin + ketamine + medetomidine CRI	Initial induction with ketamine 2 mg/kg + medetomidine 0.04 mg/kg IM, then maintenance with either isoflurane or guaifenesin/ketamine/medetomidine CRI at a rate of G: 50 mg/kg/hr + K: 1 mg/kg/hr + M: 0.01 mg/kg/hr [18]	Black bears	n = 7 regardless of constant rate infusion or isoflurane, all had mild hypertension and mild respiratory acidosis.
Hyaluronidase 150 IU + xylazine and Telazol	H: 150 IU + X: 2 mg/kg + T: 3 mg/kg [7]	Polar bears	n = 60 free-ranging bears; 16/34 control bears that did not include hyaluronidase in the dart required 2 or more injections of medication for full induction. So it was concluded that the addition of hyaluronidase decreased overall drug dose required and induction time.

Drug name	Drug dose	Species	Comments
Ketamine + diazepam	K: 5–7 mg/kg + D: 0.13 mg/kg IM; antagonize with flumazenil [10]	Not specified	
Ketamine + midazolam + medetomidine	K: 2.5–4 mg/kg + Mid: 0.05–0.09 mg/kg + Med: 0.035–0.075 mg/kg IM; antagonize with flumazenil [10]	Black, Sloth, Spectacled, and Polar bears	Immobilization.
Ketamine + midazolam	K: 2.5–4 mg/kg + M: 0.05–0.09 mg/kg IM; antagonize with flumazenil [10]	Not specified	Immobilization.
Ketamine + xylazine	K: 4–11 mg/kg + X: 0.06–0.11 mg/kg IM; antagonize with yohimbine 0.11 mg/kg IV or tolazoline 2–4 mg/kg split IV and IM [10]	Not specified	Xylazine may induce respiratory suppression.
	K: 4.4 mg/kg + X: 2 mg/kg,; antagonize with yohimbine 0.15 mg/kg IM [14, 19]	Black bears	Immobilization.
	K: 7.5 mg/kg + X: 2 mg/kg IM; antagonize with 0.125 mg/kg yohimbine [14]	Sloth bears	Immobilization.
	K: 5.8–9.75 mg/kg + X: 1.4–2.44 mg/kg IM; antagonize with yohimbine 0.125 mg/kg IV [20]	Sloth bears	n = 5 bears in 6 immobilizations, smooth induction and recovery.
Ketamine + xylazine	Created a suspension with 200 mg K + 200 mg X = 400 mg per ml: using 6.8–7 mg/kg of combined solution in adults and 2.8–3 mg/kg in yearlings [14, 21]	Polar bears	n = 45 bears, 21 adults, 18 subadults, and 6 yearlings, induction longer than other protocols and only lasted 30 min in most bears. 27 induced with one dart, 12 had partial or incomplete darting and required a 2nd injection and 6 required 3 or more injections. During summer, higher doses may be required.
	K: 4.8 mg/kg + X: 0.43 mg/kg IM [14]	Giant pandas	Supplemental 2.5 mg/kg ketamine.
Medetomidine + acepromazine	M: 0.09–0.22 mg/kg + A: 0.02–0.12 mg/kg IM; antagonize with tolazoline 100 mg and 15 mg atipamezole. 2nd study: M 0.11 mg/kg + A: 0.08 mg/kg IM, reversed with 5 mg atipamezole/mg medetomidine, or 0.4 mg/kg tolazoline + 2 mg atipamezole [22]	Black bears	2 studies: 1st involved 25 subadult bears in rehabilitation, 2nd involved adult free-range and nuisance bears. Overall only provided heavy sedation. In 2nd study 36% required additional dosing for safety and 6 procedures provided in appropriate sedation.

(Continued)

Drug name	Drug dose	Species	Comments
Medetomidine + ketamine	M: 0.06–0.08 + K: 2–3 mg/kg IM; antagonize with 0.35 mg/kg atipamezole with 50% IV and 50% IM [14, 19]	Sun bears	Immobilization, supplement with 2 mg/kg ketamine.
	M: 0.12–0.15 mg/kg + K: 3–4 mg/kg; antagonize at 1 hr with atipamezole at 4 × M dose, 50% IV and 50% IM, or 0.6 mg/kg [14, 23]	Polar bears	n = 12 Hypertension, bradycardia and decreased PaO2 seen, 2 bears had spontaneous arousal at 15 min post administration, 3 bears had spontaneous arousal during handling or at the conclusion of handling prior to reversal. 4 required top-up of induction medications.
	M: 0.02–0.04 mg/kg + K: 1.5–3 mg/kg IM; antagonize with 0.2 mg/kg atipamezole [10, 23]	Black bears	Immobilization; hypertension, bradycardia and decreased PaO2 seen; 2 bears had spontaneous arousal at 15 min post administration, 3 bears had spontaneous arousal during handling or at the conclusion of handling prior to reversal, 4 required top up of induction medications.
Medetomidine + ketamine + midazolam	Med: 0.035–0.075 mg/kg + K: 2.5–4 mg/kg + Mid: 0.05–0.09 mg/kg IM; antagonize with atipamezole 0.119–0.189 mg/kg half SC and half IM [24]	Sloth, Black, Polar, and Spectacled bears	n = 9 bears with 14 immobilizations, Induction in 9–15 min, recovery in 20–60 min.
Medetomidine + Telazol	M: 0.01–0.06 mg/kg T: 0.5–2 mg/kg IM; antagonize with atipamezole 0.2 mg/kg IV [10]	Not specified	
	M: 0.03–0.045 mg/kg + T: 1.54–2.3 mg/kg IM; antagonize with atipamezole 0.15–0.225 mg/kg IV or split into IV and IM [25]	Asiatic black bears	n = 60 captive and wild bears who underwent 373 immobilizations,.
Medetomidine + Telazol + ketamine	M: 0.02–0.06 mg/kg + T: 0.9–2.8 mg/kg IM + ketamine 1.5 mg/kg in 4 bears as supplement and 1.1–3 mg/kg added to original dart in 6 bears [26].	Brown bears	n = 13 free-ranging hibernating bears, 2/13 fled from den post darting and required higher doses, 11/13 abandoned den post recovery within 10 days and this resulted in increased energy costs and should be considered in hibernating bears.
Medetomidine + Telazol	M: 0.075 mg/kg + T: 1.8–2.5 mg/kg IM; antagonize with atipamezole 0.04 mg/kg IM [27]	Giant pandas	n = 7 free-range, 1 hr procedures, no adverse effects, 6/7 smooth recoveries, 1 rough.

Drug name	Drug dose	Species	Comments
	M: 0.01 mg/kg + T: 0.5 mg/kg IM; antagonize with atipamezole 0.05 mg/kg IV [28]	Himalayan black bears	n = 5 no adverse effects.
	M: 0.05 mg/kg + T: 2 mg/kg IM; antagonize with atipamezole 0.25 mg/kg IV [29]	Sun bears	n = 16 bears, 22 immobilizations, > 1 hr procedures, Temperature and heart rate decreased significantly within 10 min of induction.
	Based on Age range: Yearling: 1.66 mg D + 83.3 mg T; 2 yr olds: 2.5 mg D + 125 mg T; Adults: 0.05 mg/kg D + 2.45 mg/kg T; antagonize with 5 mg atipamezole per mg medetomidine used [30].	Brown bears	n = 31 free-ranging bears.
	M: 1.25–15 mg + T: 62–750 mg total; antagonize with atipamezole at 5 × the medetomidine dose [30]	Brown bears	n = 52 free-ranging and 6 captive bears, doses based on age range or size: Adult Females 5–10 mg M + 250–500 mg T; adult males 10–15 mg M + 500–750 mg T. Yearlings to juveniles: 1.25–5 mg M + 62–250 mg T. Capture-induced hyperthermia and lactic acidemia in free-ranging bears and hypoxemia seen in both captive and free-ranging bears.
	M: 0.05 mg/kg + T: 2.5 mg/kg IM; antagonize with 0.25 mg/kg atipamezole [14]	Brown bears	Immobilization.
	M: 0.05 mg/kg + T: 2 mg/kg IM; antagonize with 0.25 mg/kg atipamezole [19, 31]	Black bears	Immobilization.
	M: 0.052 mg/kg + T: 1.72 mg/kg IM; antagonize with 0.24 mg/kg IM [32]	Black bears	n = 4 recovery after 1 hr procedure within 2–10 min of administration of atipamezole.
	T: 3 mg/kg + M: 0.04 mg/kg IM [31]	Japanese black bears	n = 4 IV glucose tolerance study was affected by medetomidine and resulted in hyperglycemia and hypoinsulinemia. In the study, Telazol alone or combined with acepromazine or butorphanol did not affect the IV glucose tolerance test.
Medetomidine + Telazol	M: 0.052–0.06 mg/kg + T: 2–2.5 mg/kg IM; antagonize at 1 hr with atipamezole at 4 × M dose, 50% IV and 50% IM, or 0.24 mg/kg IM [14, 23, 33, 34]	Polar bears	n = 51 hypertension, bradycardia and decreased PaO2 seen, 9 animals required top-up of induction medications. 1 animal died post reversal in 3 hrs of hyperthermia after 8–10 min of convulsions.

(*Continued*)

Drug name	Drug dose	Species	Comments
Telazol	3–9 mg/kg; antagonize with flumazenil after 30 min of anesthesia time at 0.01 mg/kg IV [10]	All species of Ursids	Long recoveries are typical with this drug.
	3.2–11 mg/kg IM [19]	Spectacled bears	
	7 mg/kg IM [14]	Black bears	Immobilization, supplement with 3.5 mg/kg ketamine, as needed.
	8 mg/kg IM [14]	Brown bears	Immobilization, supplement with 4 mg/kg ketamine IM as needed.
	9 mg/kg [31]	Asiatic black bears	n = 4
	5–18 mg/kg [35]	Asiatic black bears	n = 75 43 wild and captive bears administered 9 mg/kg, 8 captive bears received 18 mg/kg, and 13 hibernating bears received 5 mg/kg. All bears induced and recovered successfully with minimal side effects.
	5.1 mg/kg [11]	Polar bears	n = 39 free-ranging bears, cubs <1 yr of age recovered more quickly than adults.
	8–9 mg/kg IM [36]	Polar bears	n = 319 bears, immobilization.
	2.8–4.4 or 8 mg/kg IM [19]	Asiatic black bears	Immobilization, supplement with 4 mg/kg ketamine IM, as needed.
	10 mg/kg IM [37]	Polar bears	Injected remotely and relocated. Tissue and blood levels of drugs were evaluated for up to 11 days to discuss safety of consumption post immobilization. Most metabolites, except zolazepam 2, were at trace or lower levels by 24 hrs, and this metabolite was detectable in muscle at fat at 11 days post immobilization.
	6.5 mg/kg IM (3.76–12 mg/kg) [23]	Polar bears	n = 30 recommended for short anesthesias that do not need analgesia. Animals in study were captive for at least 7 days but up to a year. Bears were ataxic during induction, and during procedure had rigid extremities, increased salivation, and occasional movements of jaw and palpebrae that intensified with stimulation. 8 required top-up of induction drugs.
	7–9 mg/kg [14, 38]	Polar bears	n = 9 captive animals, supplement with 2 mg/kg ketamine, as needed.

Drug name	Drug dose	Species	Comments
	6 mg/kg IM [14]	Sloth and Spectacled bears	Immobilization, supplement with 2 mg/kg ketamine, as needed.
	5.8–6.6 mg/kg IM [13]	Giant pandas	
Telazol + acepromazine	T: 6 mg/kg + A: 0.1 mg/kg IM [31]	Asiatic black bears	n = 4
Telazol + butorphanol	T: 6 mg/kg + B: 0.3 mg/kg IM [31]	Asiatic black bears	n = 4
Telazol + detomidine, antagonize with atipamezole	T: 1.5 mg/kg + D: 0.03 mg/kg; antagonize with A: 0.12 mg/kg [14]	Asiatic black bears	Immobilization.
Thiafentanil + xylazine	T: 0.03 mg/kg + X: 0.1 mg/kg IM, antagonize with 0.3 mg/kg naltrexone + 2 mg tolazoline IM [14]	Brown and Black bears	Immobilization.
Tramadol	2–4 mg/kg PO BID [10]	Asiatic black bears	n = 129 bears post bile collection and confiscation, with varying degrees of osteoarthritis. Combined with meloxicam as well as gabapentin as needed.
Xylazine + Telazol	X: 2 mg/kg + T: 3 mg/kg IM [38]	Polar bears	In a study comparing with 7–9 mg/kg Telazol,: 9 captive and 17 free-ranging polar bears were evaluated. The XTZ anesthesias were characterized by decreased pulse rate, higher arterial pressure, and when a claw was pinched as a stimulus better analgesia control. Free ranging bears were reversed with atipamezole 0.15 mg/kg or yohimbine 0.2 mg/kg. Captive bears were reversed with tolazoline at 2 × the xylazine dose.
	X: 2.2 mg/kg + T: 3 mg/kg IM, antagonize with 0.11 mg/kg yohimbine [31]	Black bears	Immobilization.
	X: 3 mg/kg + T: 4 mg/kg IM, antagonize with 0.11 mg/kg yohimbine IM [14]	Brown bears	Immobilization.
Antiparasitic			
Fenbendazole	10 mg/kg PO SID × 2d [2]	Polar bears	Cleared ascarid and hookworm infestation.
Ivermectin	0.3 mg/kg SC q7d × 4 treatments [5]	Black bears	n = 1 female juvenile treated for audycoptid mange, *Ursicoptes americanus*, first successful treatment, at 6 wks only dead mites and hair regrowth, and at 4 months no reoccurrence.

(*Continued*)

Drug name	Drug dose	Species	Comments
	0.1 mg/kg IM q7d × 2 doses [2]	Polar bears	
Mebendazole	20 mg/kg PO SID [2]	Polar bears	
Milbemycin oxime	1 mg/kg PO q30d [2, 39]	Polar and Kodiak brown bears	n = 3 of each species, infested with *Baylisascaris transfuga*, all cleared after 12 mo of treatment.
Praziquantel	4 mg/kg IM SID × 3d, followed by 12 mg/kg PO once [6]	Sun bears	n = 2 cases of salmon poisoning, initially treated IM, but based on recommendations from successfully treated dogs increased to one higher oral dose. Both bears cleared the infestation within 9 days and recovered.
Niclosamide	80 mg/kg PO [2]	Polar bears	
Other			
Ascorbic acid	2–4 g PO SID [2]	Polar bears	
Canary pox vectored canine distemper virus vaccine	1 ml given every 3 weeks for 3 treatments IM, then boostered 1 yr later SC [40]	Giant pandas	n = 2 appeared safe without adverse effects and serum titers appeared protective based on other species from both routes.
Cimetidine	3.5 mg/kg IM SID [1]	Polar bears	n = 1 captive, post hernia repair, one dose.
Cisplatin gel	3 mg topically × 2 treatments [3]	Sun bear	n = 1 for treatment of squamous cell carcinoma of the mandible, 2 yrs post treatment no cancer is detectable.
Cyclosporin	5 mg/kg PO SID [41]	Andean bears	n = 1 case of alopecia syndrome with partial resolution.
Dexamethasone	0.1 mg/kg IM [2]	Polar bears	
Dichlorvos	20 mg/kg PO SID [2]	Polar bears	
Diphenhydramine	2 mg/kg IM [3]	Sun bears	n = 1 to decrease possible reaction to topical chemotherapy in a sun bear with squamous cell carcinoma of the mandible.
Famotidine	0.5 mg/kg IM or PO BID [1]	Polar bears	n = 1 captive, post hernia repair, one dose.
	0.5 mg/kg PO BID [6]	Sun bears	n = 2 cases of salmon poisoning.
Fluoxetine	1 mg/kg PO SID [10]	Polar bears	n = 1 for treatment of stereotypical pacing behavior in a captive bear.

Drug name	Drug dose	Species	Comments
	0.62 mg/kg PO SID [10]	Brown bears	Treatment of stereotypical pacing.
J956 antiprogestin contraception	10 mg/kg PO or IM [42]	Black, Brown, Polar, Asiatic black and Spectacled bears	Led to sustained plasma levels of almost 2 months in 1 black bear and 5 brown bears, and prevented embryo implantation in 8 female bears. In a 2nd study with 11 polar bears, 1 Asiatic black bear and 1 spectacled bear, oral was successful if given prior to implantation or up to 30 days post implantation, but not after. Parenteral administration was successful in 100% of bears. Study monitored bears with fecal and serum progesterone and via abdominal ultrasonography.
Levothyroxine	0.018–0.022 mg/kg PO BID [43]	Black bears	n = 1 case of hypothyroidism successfully treated and responded within 30 days to oral medication, decreased to lower dose at 6 mo recheck based on thyroid analyte testing results.
Nitrofurantoin	4–6 mg/kg PO TID [2]	Polar bears	
Oclacitinib maleate (Apoquel)	0.46–0.5 mg/kg PO BID [41]	Andean bears	n = 3 cases, rapid and complete resolution of pruritis and improvement in demeanor and hair regrowth.
Peptobismol	1 ml/kg PO QID [2]	Polar bears	For use in an 86 kg bear.
Prednisolone	20 mg PO SID or 1–5 mg/kg IV IM or SID [2]	Polar bears	For treatment of allergies, and respiratory distress respectively.
Thiamin	Either 1 mg/kg IM SID followed by 2–4 mg/kcal/feed PO SID given initially IM then following up 2 h prior to feeding with PO dose. Or to give 25–35 mg/kg fish PO at feeding [2]	Polar bears	
Thyroxine	3 mg PO BID [2]	Polar bears	
TSH	30 IU IM [2]	Polar bears	For thyroid supplementation test.
Vitamin A	1 million IU/day PO SID [2]	Polar bears	As a dietary supplement.
Vitamin E	600–2400 IU PO 30d [2]	Polar bears	

Species	Weight [14]
Asiatic black bear *(Ursus thibetanus)*	Female: 65–90 kg, Male: 110–150 kg
Black bear *(Ursus americanus)*	Female: 92–140 kg, Male: 115–270 kg
Brown bear *(Ursus arctos)*	100–325 kg
Polar bear *(Ursus maritimus)*	Female: 150–300 kg, Male: 300–800 kg
Sloth bear *(Melurus ursinus)*	55–145 kg
Spectacled bear *(Tremarctos ornatus)*	60–140 kg
Sun bear *(Ursus malayanus)*	50–73 mg
Giant panda *(Ailuropoda melanoleuca)*	75–160 kg

References

1 Velguth, K.E., Rochat, M.C., Langan, J.N. et al. (2009). Acquired umbilical hernias in four captive polar bears (*Ursus maritimus*). *Journal of Zoo and Wildlife Medicine* 40 (4): 767–772.

2 Dierauf, L.A. and Gulland, F.D. (2001). *CRC Handbook of Marine Mammal Medicine*. Florida: CRC Press.

3 Mylniczenko, N.D., Manharth, A.L., Clayton, L.A. et al. (2005). Successful treatment of mandibular squamous cell carcinoma in a Malayan sun bear (*Helarctos malayanus*). *Journal of Zoo and Wildlife Medicine* 36 (2): 346–348.

4 Tremblay, J., Mulon, P.Y., and Desrochers, A. (2005). Management of a lateral humeral condylar fracture in a polar bear. *Proceedings of the American Association of Zoo Veterinarians*. 308–310.

5 Joyner, P.H., Shreve, A.A., Snead, S.E. et al. (2004). Successful treatment of ursicoptic mange in a black bear (*Ursus americanus*) using Ivermectin. *Proceedings of the American Association of Zoo Veterinarians*. 584–586.

6 Wolfe, L.L., Goshorn, C.T., and Baruch-Mordo, S. (2008). Immobilization of black bears (*Ursus americanus*) with a combination of butorphanol, azaperone, and medetomidine. *Journal of Wildlife Diseases* 44 (3): 748–752.

7 Cattet, M.R. and Obbard, M.E. (2010). Use of hyaluronidase to improve chemical immobilization of free-ranging polar bears (*Ursus maritimus*). *Journal of Wildlife Diseases* 46 (1): 246–250.

8 Fandos, E.N., Cattet, Zedrosser, M., A. et al. (2017). A double-blinded, randomized comparison of Medetomidine-Tiletamine-Zolazepam and Dexmedetomidine-Tiletamine-Zolazepam anesthesia in free-ranging brown bears (*Ursus Arctos*). *PLoS One* 12 (1).

9 Monica, K.H., Bando, B.S., Webster, N. et al. (2012). Prevalence and management of osteoarthritis in Asiatic Black bears (*Ursus thibetanus*) rescued from bile farms in China. *Proceedings of the American Association of Zoo Veterinarians*. 219.

10 Miller, R.E. and Fowler, M.E. (2015). Ursidae. In: *Fowler's Zoo and Wild Animal Medicine*, vol. 8 (ed. R.E. Miller and M. Fowler), 498–508. St. Louis, MO: Elsevier Saunders.

11 Haigh, J.C., Lee, L.J., and Schweinsburg, R.E. (1983). Immobilization of polar bears with carfentanil. *Journal of Wildlife Diseases* 19 (2): 140–144.

12 Ramsay, E.C., Sleeman, J.M., and Clyde, V.L. (1995). Immobilization of black bears (*Ursus americanus*) with orally administered carfentanil citrate. *Journal of Wildlife Diseases* 31 (3): 391–393.

13 Kreeger, T.J., Bjornlie, D., Thompson, D. et al. (2013). Immobilization of Wyoming bears using carfentanil and Xylazine. *Journal of Wildlife Diseases* 49 (3): 674–678.

14 Kreeger, T.J., Arnemo, J.M., and Raath, J.P. (2012). *Handbook of Wildlife Chemical Immobilization*. Fort Collins, Colorado, U.S.A.: Wildlife Pharmaceuticals Inc.
15 Laricchiuta, P., Gelli, D., Campolo, M. et al. (2008). Reversible immobilization of Asiatic black bear (*Ursus thibetanus*) with Detomidine-Tiletamine-Zolazepam and atipamezole. *Journal of Zoo and Wildlife Medicine* 39 (4): 558–561.
16 Teisberg, J.E., Farley, S.D., Nelson, O.L. et al. (2014). Immobilization of grizzly bears (*Ursus arctos*) with dexmedetomidine, tiletamine, and zolazepam. *Journal of Wildlife Diseases* 50 (1): 74–83.
17 Herbert, D.M., Lay, D.W., and Turnbull, W.G. (1980). Immobilization of coastal grizzly bears with etorphine hydrochloride. *Journal of Wildlife Diseases* 16 (3): 339–342.
18 Bauer, K.L., Siegal-Willet, J., Hayek, L.S.C. et al. (2017). Comparison of a Guifenesin, Ketamine, and Medetomidine constant-rate-infusion with isoflurane gas for anesthesia maintenance in American Black bears (*Ursus americanus*). *Annual Proceedings of the American Association of Zoo Veterinarians*. 3.
19 West, G., Heard, D., and Caulkett, N. (2014). Ursids. In: *Zoo Animal and Wildlife Immobilization and Anesthesia*, 2e (ed. G. West, D. Heard and N. Caulkett), 599–606. Ames, IA: Wiley Blackwell.
20 Page, C.D. (1986). Sloth bear immobilization with a ketamine-Xylazine combination: reversal with yohimbine. *Journal of the American Veterinary Medical Association* 189 (9): 1050–1051.
21 Lee, J., Schweinsburg, R., Kernan, F. et al. (1981). Immobilization of polar bears (*Ursus maritimus*, Phipps) with ketamine hydrochloride and Xylazine hydrochloride. *Journal of Wildlife Diseases* 17 (3): 331–336.
22 Wolfe, L.L., Johnson, H.E., Fisher, M.C. et al. (2014). Use of acepromazine and medetomidine in combination for sedation and handling of Rocky Mountain elk (*Cervus elaphus nelsoni*) and black bears (*Ursus americanus*). *Journal of Wildlife Diseases* 50 (4): 979–981.
23 Caulkett, N.A., Cattet, M.R., Caulkett, J.M. et al. (1999). Reversible immobilization of free-ranging polar bears with Medetomidine-Zolazepam-Tiletamine and atipamezole. *Journal of Zoo and Wildlife Medicine* 30 (4): 504–509.
24 Curro, T.G., Okeson, D., Zimmerman, D. et al. (2004). Xylazine-midazolam-ketamine versus Medetomidine-midazolam-ketamine anesthesia in captive Siberian tigers (*Panthera tigris altaica*). *Journal of Zoo and Wildlife Medicine* 35 (3): 320–327.
25 Jeong, D.H., Yang, J.J., Seok, S.H. et al. (2017). Immobilization of Asiatic black bears (*Ursus thibetanus*) with medetomidine-zolazepam-tiletamine in South Korea. *Journal of Wildlife Diseases* 53 (3): 636–641.
26 Evans, A.L., Sahlen, V., Stoen, O.G. et al. (2012). Capture, anesthesia, and disturbance of free-ranging brown bears (*Ursus arctos*) during hibernation. *PLoS One* 7 (7): Epub 2012.
27 Jin, Y., Qiao, Y., Liu, X. et al. (2016). Immobilization of wild giant panda (*Ailuropoda melanoleuca*) with dexmedetomidine-tiletamine-zolazepam. *Veterinary Anaesthesia and Analgesia* 43 (3): 333–337.
28 Arun, A.S., Krishna, S., Antony, L. et al. (2016). Effective reversible immobilization of captive Himalayan black bears (*Selenarctos thibetanus laniger*) with Medetomidine-Tiletamine-Zolazepam and atipamezole. *Journal of Wildlife Diseases* 52 (2): 400–402.
29 Onuma, M. (2003). Immobilization of sun bears (*Helarctos malayanus*) with Medetomidine-Zolazepam-Tiletamine. *Journal of Zoo and Wildlife Medicine* 34 (2): 202–205.
30 Fahlman, A., Arnemo, J.M., Swenson, J.E. et al. (2011). Physiologic evaluation of capture and anesthesia with Medetomidine-Zolazepam-tiletamine in brown bears (*Ursus arctos*). *Journal of Zoo and Wildlife Medicine* 42 (1): 1–11.
31 Kamine, A., Shimozuru, M., Shibata, H. et al. (2012). Effects of intramuscular administration of Tiletamine-Zolazepam with and without sedative pretreatment on plasma and serum

biochemical values and glucose tolerance test results in Japanese black bears (*Ursus thibetanus japonicus*). *American Journal of Veterinary Research* 73 (8): 1282–1289.

32 Caulkett, N.A. and Cattet, M.R. (1997). Physiological effects of medetomidine-zolazepam-tiletamine immobilization in black bears. *Journal of Wildlife Diseases* 33 (3): 618–622.

33 Cattet, M.R., Caulkett, N.A., Polischuk, S.C. et al. (1997). Comparative physiologic effects of Telazol, medetomidine-ketamine, and medetomidine-Telazol in captive polar bears (*Ursus maritimus*). *Journal of Wildlife Diseases* 33 (3): 611–617.

34 Curry, E., Wyatt, J., Sorel, L.J. et al. (2014). Ovulation induction and artificial insemination of a captive polar bear (*Ursus maritimus*) using fresh semen. *Journal of Zoo and Wildlife Medicine* 45 (3): 645–649.

35 Asano, M., Tsubota, T., Komatsu, T. et al. (2007). Immobilization of Japanese black bears (*Ursus thibetanus japonicus*) with tiletamine hydrochloride and Zolazepam hydrochloride. *The Journal of Veterinary Medical Science* 69 (4): 433–435.

36 Stirling, I., Spencer, C., and Andriashek, D. (1989). Immobilization of polar bears (*Ursus maritimus*) with Telazol in the Canadian Arctic. *Journal of Wildlife Diseases* 25 (2): 159–168.

37 Semple, H.A., Gorecki, D.K., Farley, S.D. et al. (2000). Pharmacokinetics and tissue residues of Telazol in free-ranging polar bears. *Journal of Wildlife Diseases* 36 (4): 653–662.

38 Cattet, M.R., Caulkett, N.A., and Lunn, N.J. (2003). Anesthesia of polar bears using xylazine-zolazepam-tiletamine or zolazepam-tiletamine. *Journal of Wildlife Diseases* 39 (3): 655–664.

39 Hedberg, G.E., Hedberg, A.H.T., and Bennett, R.A. (1995). Preliminary studies on the use of Milbemycin oxime for treatment of polar bears (*Ursus maritimus*) with chronic *Baylisascaris transfuga* infection. *Annual Proceedings of the American Association of Zoo Veterinarians*. 299–303.

40 Bronson, E., Deem, S.L., Sanchez, C. et al. (2007). Serologic response to a canarypox-vectored canine distemper virus vaccine in the giant panda (*Ailuropoda melanoleuca*). *Journal of Zoo and Wildlife Medicine* 38 (2): 363–366.

41 Drake, G.J., Nuttall, T., Lopez, J. et al. (2017). Treatment success in three Andean bears (*Tremarctos ornatus*) with alopecia syndrome using Oclacitinib maleate (Apoquel). *Journal of Zoo and Wildlife Medicine* 48 (3): 818–828.

42 Jewgenow, K., Quest, M., Elger, W. et al. (2001). Administration of antiprogestin J956 for contraception in bears: a pharmacological study. *Theriogenology* 56 (4): 601–611.

43 Storms, T.N., Graham, P.A., and Ramsay, E.C. (2002). Hypothyroidism in an American black bear (*Ursus americanus*) and thyroid testing in bears. *Proceedings of the American Association of Zoo Veterinarians*. 28–30.

11

Small Omnivores and Carnivores: Red Pandas, Fossa, Skunks, Meerkats, Mustelids, Procyonids, and Viverrids

Drug name	Drug dose	Species	Comments
Antimicrobials and Antifungals			
Ailurid: Red Pandas			
Amoxicillin long-acting (Bivamox) [1]	15 mg/kg IM q48 hr × 7 d	Red pandas	n = 1 animal postoperative for surgical repair of avascular necrosis of femoral head (bilateral).
Amoxicillin-clavulanic acid	No dosage [2]	Red pandas	n = 1, 4-week old red panda cub with dermatophytosis.
Doxycycline	0.3 mg/kg PO BID (on 30d, off 30d, in 5–7 cycles) [3]	Red pandas	n = 3 animals, to treat peridontitis not responsive to standard cleanings.
	13–25 mg PO BID [4]	Red pandas	n = 2 animals, treated for keratomycosis.
Enrofloxacin	5 mg/kg IM SID × 7d [1]	Red pandas	n = 1 animal postoperative repair of avascular necrosis of femoral head (bilateral).
Fluconazole	50 mg PO SID × 20d [4]	Red pandas	n = 2 animals, treated for keratomycosis.
Itraconazole	5–10 mg/kg PO SID to BID [5, 6]	Red pandas	For dermatophytosis, areas on chest or tail may rapidly progress in young cubs and require oral treatment in addition to topical.
Euplerid: Fossas			
Ampicillin	10 mg/kg IM [7]	Fossas	n = 1 for dermatopathy of unknown cause.
Amoxicillin	30 mg/kg PO BID × 10d [7]	Fossas	n = 1 for dermatopathy of unknown cause.
Amoxicillin-clavulanate	15 mg/kg PO BID × 10d [7]	Fossas	n = 1 for dermatopathy of unknown cause.
Ceftiofur crystalline-free acid	6 mg/kg SC [7]	Fossas	n = 1 for dermatopathy of unknown cause.

(*Continued*)

Zoo and Wild Mammal Formulary, First Edition. Alicia Hahn.

Drug name	Drug dose	Species	Comments
Fluconazole	2.5 mg/kg PO SID × 21d [7]	Fossas	n = 1 for dermatopathy of unknown cause.
Herpestids			
Cefadroxil	30 mg/kg PO BID × 14d [8]	Meerkats	n = 4 animals, captive, diagnosed with persimmon phytobezoars and treated post removal with famotidine, cefadroxil and buprenorphine.
Cefazolin	25 mg/kg IV [9]	Meerkats	n = 1 treatment of clinical toxoplasmosis.
Enrofloxacin	5 mg/kg SC × 14d [10]	Meerkats	n = 4 full siblings, captive, with presumptive pancreatitis. One animal survived ultimately.
Metronidazole	15 mg/kg IV [9]	Meerkats	n = 1 treatment of clinical toxoplasmosis.
Mephitids: Skunks			
Amoxicillin/ clavulanic acid	12.5 mg/kg IM BID [11]	Skunks	n = 1 adjunctive treatment for mediastinal lymphoma and chylothorax.
	12.5 mg/kg PO BID × 7d [12]	Skunks	n = 1 induction of anesthesia.
Cefazolin	20 mg/kg IV q2h (perioperatively), 20 mg/kg IV q12h (postoperatively) [13]	Skunks	n = 1 perioperative analgesia.
Mustelids			
Amikacin	5 mg/kg IM BID or 10 mg/kg SID [14]	sea otters	Nephrotoxicity reported.
Amoxicillin	10–20 mg/kg PO QID [14]	Sea otters	
Cefazolin	10–30 mg/kg IM QID [14]	Sea otters	
	22 mg/kg IV [15]	Cape clawless otters	n = 1 Perioperative antibiotic therapy for orthopedic surgery.
Cefovecin	8 mg/kg SC once [16]	Sea otters	n = 7 adult otters, pharmacokinetics based on Isolate, drug may be efficacious for 2.5–10 days.
Cephalexin	20 mg/kg PO BID [14]	Sea otter pups	
Enrofloxacin	2.5 mg/kg PO BID × 10–14d [17]	Marine otters	n = 5 marine otters captured and treated for 14 days prior to placement of intra-abdominal radiotransmitters.
	5–20 mg/kg SID [14]	Sea otters	

Drug name	Drug dose	Species	Comments
Flucloxacilin	25 mg/kg PO QID × 14d [17]	Marine otters	n = 1 marine otter that sustained a digit fracture and was treated for 14 days prior to placement of intra-abdominal radiotransmitters.
Gentamicin	Adults 2 mg/kg IM TID, Pups: 2 mg/kg BID × 5d [14]	Sea otters	4.4 mg/kg IM BID has been associated with nephrotoxicity.
Griseofulvin	30 mg/kg PO BID × 45d [14]	Sea otters	
Hetacillin	20 mg/kg PO BID [14]	Sea otters	
Ketoconazole	10 mg/kg PO TID [14]	Sea otters	
Lincomycin	20 mg/kg IM BID [14]	Sea otters	
Metronidazole	25–30 mg/kg PO BID × 5d [14]	Sea otters	
Neomycin	10–14 mg/kg PO SID [14]	Sea otters	
Oxacillin	20 mg/kg IM TID [14]	Sea otters	
Penicillin G	20–22 000 IU/kg IM SID to BID [14]	Sea otters	
Procaine penicillin G with benzathine	30 000 IU/kg IM once [17]	Marine otters	n = 6 marine otters captured for placement of intra-abdominal radio transmitters – given intraoperative.
Tetracycline	20 mg/kg IM SID [14]	Sea otters	Can cause muscle necrosis.
Trimethoprim sulfadiazine	33.6 mg/kg PO BID or 20 mg/kg IM BID [14]	Sea otters	Lower dose for hemorrhagic diarrhea in pups.
Procyonids			
Amoxicillin-clavulanate	15 mg/kg PO BID × 14d [18]	Coatis	n = 1 antimicrobial treatment for pyometra.
Enrofloxacin	2.5 mg/kg SC once, 5 mg/kg SID × 10d [19]	Raccoons	n = 2 analgesia for thyroidectomy.
Procaine benzyl penicillin	20 000 IU/kg IM [20]	Coatis	n = 1 perioperative antibiotic for ectopic testicle orchidectomy.
Viverrids			
Azithromycin	10 mg/kg PO SID × 30d [21]	Binturongs	n = 1; antimicrobial treatment of pyoderma.
Marbofloxacin	2.5 mg/kg PO SID × 14d [22]	Masked palm civets	n = 1 treatment for bacterial dermatitis secondary to Notoedres, Sarcoptes and Demodex mites.
	5 mg/kg PO SID × 30d [21]	Binturongs	n = 1; antimicrobial treatment of pyoderma.

(Continued)

Drug name	Drug dose	Species	Comments
Analgesia:			
Ailurid: Red Pandas			
Buprenorphine	0.045 mg IM once [4]	Red pandas	n = 1 treated for keratomycosis.
Carprofen	10 mg SC, 10 mg PO, 5 mg PO SID × 5d [4]	Red pandas	n = 1 treated for keratomycosis.
Meloxicam	1 mg IM once; 0.45 mg PO SID [4]	Red pandas	n = 1 treated for keratomycosis.
Tramadol	5 mg PO TID × 5d [4]	Red pandas	n = 1 treated for keratomycosis.
Euplerid: Fossas			
Meloxicam	0.1 mg/kg SC [7]	Fossas	n = 1 treated for dermatopathy of unknown cause.
Herpestids:			
Buprenorphine	0.02 mg/kg SC × 14d [10]	Meerkats	n = 4 full siblings, captive, with presumptive pancreatitis. One animal survived.
	0.03 mg/kg PO BID × 3d [8]	Meerkats	n = 4 animals, captive, diagnosed with persimmon phytobezoars and treated post removal with famotidine, cefadroxil and buprenorphine.
Flunixin meglumine	1 mg/kg IV [10]	Meerkats	n = 1 captive, with presumptive pancreatitis, treated intraoperatively.
Meloxicam	0.2 mg/kg SC [9]	Meerkats	n = 1 treatment of clinical toxoplasmosis.
Mephitids:			
Buprenorphine	0.3 mg/kg IV q8 h [13]	Skunks	n = 1 perioperative analgesia.
	0.03 mg/kg IM [23]	Skunks	n = 20 perioperative analgesia.
Carprofen	2 mg/kg PO BID × 10d [12]	Skunks	n = 1 postoperative analgesia for hemilaminectomy.
Fentanyl	2 μcg/kg IV bolus followed by 2 μcg/kg/h IV CRI [13]	Skunks	n = 1 perioperative analgesia.
	5 μ/kg/h IV [12]	Skunks	n = 1 perioperative analgesia.
Meloxicam	0.1 mg/kg SC [13]	Skunks	n = 1 perioperative analgesia.
	0.2 mg/kg SC [23]	Skunks	n = 20 perioperative analgesia.
Tramadol	4 mg/kg PO q8–12 h × 7d [13]	Skunks	n = 1 perioperative analgesia.

Drug name	Drug dose	Species	Comments
Mustelids			
Aspirin (acetylsalicylic acid)	10 mg/kg PO Q 36 hrs [14]	Sea otters	
Carprofen	1.5–2 mg/kg PO BID for 5–10d [14]	Sea otters	For injection site pain.
Ketoprofen	0.5 mg/kg PO SID × 3–5d (superficial skin wounds); 1 mg/kg PO SID × 5d postoperative [17]	Marine otters	n = 6 marine otters captured and treated for skin wounds/ fractured digit and post placement of intra-abdominal radiotransmitters.
Lidocaine	2 mg/kg bolus, repeat in 20 min [14]	Sea otters	
Meloxicam	0.2 mg/kg IM [15]	Cape clawless otters	n = 1 perioperative analgesic therapy for orthopedic surgery.
Procyonids			
Buprenorphine	0.006–0.01 mg/kg SC [19]	Raccoons	n = 2 analgesia for thyroidectomy.
Meloxicam	0.2 mg/kg IV [24]	Coatis	n = 1 perioperative analgesia for hysterectomy.
	0.2 mg/kg IM [20]	Coatis	n = 1 perioperative analgesia for ectopic testicle orchidectomy.
	0.1–0.2 mg/kg SC [19]	Raccoons	n = 2 analgesia for thyroidectomy.
Viverrids			
Hydromorphone	1 mg IV [25]	Binturongs	n = 1 Perioperative analgesia for hemilaminectomy.
Fentanyl	75 mg IV [25]	Binturongs	n = 1 Perioperative analgesia for hemilaminectomy.
Anethesia and Sedation			
Ailurid: Red Pandas			
Ketamine + medetomidine	K: 4 mg/kg + M: 0.1 mg/kg IM; antagonize with atipamezole 0.5 mg/kg [26]	Red pandas	
	K: 6.6 mg/kg + M: 0.08 mg/kg IM; antagonize with atipamezole 0.4 mg/kg [6]	Red pandas	
Ketamine + xylazine	K: 10 mg/kg + X: 2 mg/kg IM [26]	Red pandas	
Telazol	T: 5 mg/kg IM [26]	Red pandas	Supplement with ketamine 5 mg/kg as needed.
Euplerid: Fossas			
Ketamine + medetomidine	K: 5 mg/kg + M: 0.1 mg/kg; antagonize with atipamezole 0.5 mg/kg [6]	Fossas	

(*Continued*)

Drug name	Drug dose	Species	Comments
Ketamine + xylazine	K: 10.5–20 mg/kg + X: 2.5–5 mg/kg IM [6]	Fossas	Antagonize with yohimbine 0.125 mg/kg.
Telazol	T: 6 mg/kg IM [26]	Fossas	Supplement with ketamine 6 mg/kg as needed.
Herpestids			
Ketamine	K: 45 mg/kg IM [26]	African water mongooses, Mongooses (Herpestes spp.)	
Ketamine + acepromazine	K: 30 mg/kg + A: 0.75 mg/kg IM [26]	Mongooses (Herpestes spp.)	
Ketamine + xylazine	K: 6 mg/kg + X: 6 mg/kg IM [6, 26]	Mongooses (Herpestes spp.)	
Sevoflurane	6.5% induction and 4% maintenance [27]	Meerkats	n = 20 animals, captive, induced via facemask.
Telazol	T: 4.4 mg/kg IM [6, 26]	Black-legged mongooses	Supplement with ketamine 4.4 mg/kg as needed.
	T: 5 mg/kg IM [6, 26]	Mongooses (Herpestes spp.), Malagasy ring-tailed mongooses	Supplement with ketamine 5 mg/kg as needed.
	T: 5.5 mg/kg IM [6, 26]	African water mongooses	Supplement with ketamine 5.5 mg/kg as needed.
Mustelids and Mephitids			
Butorphanol + midazolam	B: 0.25 mg/kg + M: 0.25 mg/kg IM [13]	Skunks	n = 1 sedation for exam.
Butorphanol or Oxymorphone	B: 0.5 mg/kg or O: 0.3 mg/kg [28, 29]	Sea otters	Sedation. Antagonize with naltrexone 0.04 mg/kg IV or IM.
Butorphanol + dexmedetomidine + midazolam	B:0.2 mg/kg + D: 0.015 mg/kg + Mid: 0.15 mg/kg [26];	Asian small clawed otters	Antagonize with naloxone 0.1 mg/kg + atipamezole 0.2 mg/kg + flumazenil 0.06 mg/kg.
Diazepam + Oxymorphone	D: 0.5 mg/kg + O: 0.3 mg/kg IM [29]	Sea otters	
Isoflurane	Chamber induction [26]	Pine martens	Wild animals have been immobilized successfully in the field, avoid animal overheating.
Etorphine + xylazine	E: 0.1 mg/kg + X: 1 mg/kg; antagonize with diprenorphine 0.2 mg/kg and yohimbine 0.15 mg/kg [26]	Wolverines	
Fentanyl + acepromazine + diazepam	F: 0.1 mg/kg + Ace: 0.14 mg/kg + D: 0.2 mg/kg IM [29]	Sea otters	n = 32 animals.

Drug name	Drug dose	Species	Comments
Fentanyl + azaperone	F: 0.3 mg/kg + A: 0.25 mg/kg IM [26]	Sea otters	
Fentanyl + azaperone + diazepam	F: 0.1 mg/kg + A: 0.5 mg/kg + D: 0.1 mg/kg IM [29]	Sea otters	n = 61 animals, deeper sedation than F + D and duration up to 2.5 hrs.
Fentanyl + diazepam	F: 0.1–0.3 mg/kg + D: 0.1 mg/kg; antagonize with naltrexone 0.6 mg/kg [26, 29]	Sea otters	n = 597 free-ranging otters, supplement with 0.15 mg/kg fentanyl as needed. Higher end of F dose range for surgical procedures.
Fentanyl + xylazine	F: 0.2 mg/kg + X: 1 mg/kg IM; antagonize with naloxone 0.2 mg/kg + yohimbine 0.15 mg/kg [26]	Sea otters	
Ketamine	K: 10 mg/kg IM [26, 29]	Asian small clawed otters, American river otters	
	K: 10–40 mg/kg [29]	Mustelids	
	K: 15 mg/kg IM [26]	Tayras	
Ketamine	K: 20 mg/kg IM [26, 29]	European badgers, Fishers	Prolonged recovery.
	K: 33–70 mg/kg IM [29]	Striped skunks	n = 121 kits/offspring, field immobilization, scent gland removal, one mortality due to aspiration.
Ketamine + acepromazine	K: 15 mg/kg + A: 0.2 mg/kg [26, 28, 29]	Hog-nosed, Hooded, Spotted and Striped skunks	
	K: 15 mg/kg + A: 0.4 mg/kg [26, 29]	European badgers	
	K: 20 mg/kg + A: 0.1 mg/kg [29]	Fishers	
	K: 20 mg/kg + A: 0.2 mg/kg [26, 28]	Wolverines	
	K: 25 mg/kg + A: 1.1 mg/kg IM [26]	Ferrets	
Ketamine + diazepam	K: 10–12 mg/kg + D: 0.3–5 mg/kg IM [28]	American river otters	
	K: 15–18 mg/kg + D: 0.4–0.5 mg/kg IM [26, 29]	European otters	
	K: 22 mg/kg + D: 0.4 mg/kg IM [29]	Mustelids	
	K: 15–35 mg/kg + D: 0.1–0.2 mg/kg IM [26, 28, 29]	Black-footed ferrets	

(*Continued*)

Drug name	Drug dose	Species	Comments
Ketamine + medetomidine	K: 2.5–3 mg/kg + M: 0.025–0.03 mg/kg IM; antagonize with atipamezole 0.125 mg/kg [28, 29]	American river otters	
	K: 3 mg/kg + M: 0.075 mg/kg IM; antagonize with atipamezole 0.45 mg/kg [26, 28, 29]	Black-footed ferrets	Supplement with ketamine 1.5 mg/kg IM as needed.
	K: 4 mg/kg + M: 0.03 mg/kg IM; antagonize with atipamezole 0.15 mg/kg [26]	Giant otters	Supplement with ketamine 2 mg/kg IM as needed.
	K: 4 mg/kg + M: 0.04 mg/kg IM; antagonize with atipamezole 0.2 mg/kg [26]	American river otters	Supplement with ketamine 2 mg/kg IM as needed.
	K: 4 mg/kg + M: 0.08 mg/kg IM; antagonize with atipamezole 0.4 mg/kg [26, 29]	Fishers	Supplement with ketamine 2 mg/kg IM as needed.
	K: 5 mg/kg + M: 0.05 mg/kg IM; antagonize with atipamezole 0.25 mg/kg [26, 29]	European otters, Marine otters	Supplement with ketamine 2.5 mg/kg as needed, In 38 free-ranging animals used: K: 4.3–5.9 mg/kg + M: 0.04–0.06 mg/kg.
	K: 5–10 mg/kg + M: 0.05–0.1 mg/kg IM; antagonize with atipamezole 0.25–0.5 mg/kg [29]	European badgers	Preferred combination.
	K: 5 mg/kg + M: 0.1 mg/kg IM [26, 28, 29]	Ferrets, Yellow-throated marten, Ermine, Mink	
Ketamine + medetomidine	K: 5 mg/kg + M: 0.12 mg/kg IM; antagonize with atipamezole 0.6 mg/kg [26, 28, 29]	Asian small clawed otters	Supplement with ketamine 2.5 mg/kg as needed.
	K: 7 mg/kg + M: 0.3 mg/kg; antagonize with atipamezole 1.5 mg/kg IM [26].	Wolverines	If not down in 15 min, repeat full dose. In captive animals, may be able to decrease dose by 50%.
	K: 10 mg/kg + M: 0.1 mg/kg; antagonize with atipamezole 0.4 mg/kg IM [26].	European badgers	
	K: 10 mg/kg + M: 0.2 mg/kg; antagonize with atipamezole 1 mg/kg IM [26, 28, 29].	Pine martens, European minks	Supplement with ketamine 5 mg/kg IM as needed. Monitor for hypothermia.

Drug name	Drug dose	Species	Comments
	K: 20 mg/kg + M: 0.04 mg/kg; antagonize with atipamezole 0.02 mg/kg IM [29].	Fishers	
Ketamine + medetomidine + butorphanol	K: 0.04–0.06 mg/kg + M: 0.02 mg/kg + B: 0.04–0.08 mg/kg IM [29]	European badgers	
Ketamine + midazolam	K: 10 mg/kg + Mid: 0.25 mg/kg IM [29]	American river otters	
	K: 10 mg/kg + Mid: 0.3 mg/kg IM [26, 29]	Asian small clawed otters	
	K: 15–18 mg/kg + Mid: 0.75–1 mg/kg	Asian small clawed otters	
Ketamine + midazolam	K: 10–15 mg/kg + Mid: 0.4–1 mg/kg IM [29]	European badgers	Minimal advantage over ketamine alone.
	K: 15 mg/kg + Mid: 0.5 mg/kg IM [26, 28, 30]	American river otters	n = 14 American river otters, with wide safety margin.
	K 15–18 mg/kg + Mid: 0.75–1 mg/kg IM [26, 28, 30]	Asian small clawed otters	
Ketamine + xylazine	K: 5–10 mg/kg + X: 1–2 mg/kg IM; antagonize with yohimbine 0.125 mg/kg [29]	American river otters	
Ketamine + xylazine	K: 6 mg/kg + X: 0.5 mg/kg IM [26, 28, 29]	Honey badgers	Approach animals with care.
	K: 7.5 mg/kg + X: 1.5 mg/kg IM [26]	American river otters	
	K: 8 mg/kg + X: 1 mg/kg IM [26, 29]	Clawless otters, Spotted-necked otters	
	K: 8.5–10.6 mg/kg + X: 1.5–2 mg/kg IM [28]	Giant otters	
Ketamine + xylazine	K: 10 mg/kg + X: 1–2 mg/kg; antagonize with yohimbine 0.125 mg/kg or atipamezole 0.02–0.06 mg/kg [29]	Mustelids	
	K: 15 mg/kg + X: 1 mg/kg IM [26, 28, 29]	Badgers	
	K: 16 mg/kg + X: 6 mg/kg IM [26, 29]	European badgers	
	K: 16 mg/kg + X: 8 mg/kg IM [26]	Spotted skunks	
	K: 18 mg/kg + X: 1.6 mg/kg IM [26, 29]	Pine martens	
	K: 20 mg/kg + X: 2 mg/kg [26, 29]	European otters, Mustelids in general	

(Continued)

Drug name	Drug dose	Species	Comments
	K: 25 mg/kg + X: 2 mg/kg [26]	Ferrets	Supplement with ketamine 12 mg/kg IM as needed.
	K: 30–40 mg/kg + X: 1 mg/kg IM [26]	Yellow-throated martens	Supplement with ketamine 15 mg/kg IM as needed.
	K: 40 mg/kg + X: 1 mg/kg IM [28, 29]	Minks	
Morphine + lidocaine epidural block	Morphine 0.1 mg/kg + lidocaine 0.2 mg/kg epidural [13]	Skunks	n = 1 perioperative analgesia.
Propofol	To effect, 4 mg IV total [13]	Skunks	n = 1 anesthetic induction after sedation.
	1.4 mg/kg IV [12]	Skunks	n = 1; induction of anesthesia.
Telazol	T: 1.5–22 mg/kg IM [29]	Mustelids	Antagonize with flumazenil 0.05–0.1 mg/kg IM.
	T: 2.2 mg/kg IM [26, 28, 29]	Honey badgers	Supplement with ketamine 2.2 mg/kg IM as needed.
	T: 3 mg/kg IM [26]	Sea otters	Avoid overheating by monitoring rectal temperature.
	T: 4–8 mg/kg IM; antagonize with flumazenil 0.08 mg/kg [26, 28, 29]	American river otters	
	T: 3.3 mg/kg IM [26, 28, 29]	Tayras	Supplement with ketamine 3.3 mg/kg IM as needed.
	T: 3–6 mg/kg IM [29]	Mustelids	
	T: 4.4 mg/kg IM [26, 28, 29]	Hog badgers, Badgers	Supplement with ketamine 2.2 mg/kg IM as needed. (Badger-4.4 mg/kg ketamine as needed.).
	T: 5 mg/kg IM [26, 29]	Ferret badgers, Clawless otters, Spotted-necked otters, Chinese ferret badgers	Supplement with ketamine 2.5–5 mg/kg IM as needed.
	T: 6–9 mg/kg IM [26, 29]	Asian small clawed otters	
Telazol	T: 10 mg/kg IM [26, 29]	European badgers	Supplement with ketamine 5 mg/kg IM as needed.
	T: 10 mg/kg IM [26, 28, 29]	Hog-nosed, Hooded, Spotted, and Striped skunks	Supplement with ketamine 10 mg/kg as needed.
	T: 11 mg/kg IM [26]	Fishers	
	T: 11–22 mg/kg [28, 29]	Ermines	
	T: 15 mg/kg IM [26, 28, 29]	Ferrets, Yellow-throated martens, Wolverines, Mink	Supplement with ketamine 15 mg/kg IM as needed. Wolverine: In captive animals may be able to decrease dose by 50%.

Drug name	Drug dose	Species	Comments
Telazol + medetomidine	T: 2.5 mg/kg + M: 0.04 mg/kg IM; antagonize with atipamezole 0.2 mg/kg [29]	European badgers	
Telazol + xylazine	T: 3 mg/kg + X: 2 mg/kg [26]	Fishers, Pine martens	
Procyonids			
Ketamine	K: 10 mg/kg IM [26]	Cuscuses	Supplement with ketamine 5 mg/kg IM as needed.
	K: 10–30 mg/kg [29]	Procyonids	Higher end of dose range only for smaller species.
	K: 25 mg/kg IM [26, 29]	Kinkajous	
Ketamine + acepromazine	K: 10 mg/kg + A: 0.2 mg/kg [29]	Ringtails	
	K: 15 mg/kg + A: 0.1 mg/kg [26]	Coatimundis	Keep separate from conspecifics for at least 24 hrs if possible.
	K: 20 mg/kg + A: 0.1 mg/kg [26, 29]	Raccoons	
Ketamine + diazepam	K: 10 mg/kg + D: 0.5 mg/kg [29]	Procyonids	
Ketamine + medetomidine	K: 2–5 mg/kg + M: 0.025–0.05 mg/kg; antagonize with atipamezole 0.1 mg/kg [29]	Procyonids	
	K: 5.5 mg/kg + M: 0.1 mg/kg; antagonize with atipamezole 0.5 mg/kg [26, 28, 29, 31]	Kinkajous	Supplement with ketamine 3 mg/kg IM as needed.
Ketamine + medetomidine + butorphanol	K: 2.5–7.7 mg/kg + M: 0.05–0.064 mg/kg + B: 0.34–0.36 mg/kg IM; antagonize with atipamezole 0.25 mg/kg, half IV and half IM [29]	Coatimundis	
Ketamine + midazolam	K: 10 mg/kg + Mid: 0.25–0.5 mg/kg IM [29]	Procyonids	
Ketamine + xylazine	K: 10 mg/kg + X: 1–2 mg/kg [29]	Procyonids	Good muscle relaxation.
	K: 20 mg/kg + X: 1 mg/kg [6, 26]	Coatimundis	Supplement with ketamine 10 mg/kg IM as needed. Keep separate from conspecifics for at least 24 hrs if possible.
Ketamine + xylazine + atropine	K: 20 mg/kg + X: 4 mg/kg; antagonize with yohimbine 0.15 mg/kg [26, 28, 29]	Raccoons	Supplement with ketamine 10 mg/kg IM as needed.

(*Continued*)

Drug name	Drug dose	Species	Comments
	K: 5–15 mg/kg + X: 1–2 mg/kg + At: 0.04 mg/kg IM [29]	Procyonids	Induction 3–5 min, Anesthesia 15–20 min, Recovery 60–90 min.
Telazol	T: 3 mg/kg IM [26]	Raccoons	Adequate immobilization with full recovery <1 hr.
	T: 3–5 mg/kg IM [29]	Procyonids	
	T: 4.76–11.6 mg/kg [32]	Coatimundis	n = 53 free-ranging animals immobilized, appeared safe overall. Older/larger animals should require smaller doses.
	T: 5 mg/kg IM [26, 28, 29]	Olingos	Supplement with ketamine 5 mg/kg IM as needed.
	T: 10 mg/kg IM [26, 29]	Kinkajous, Ringtails	
	T: 12 mg/kg IM [29]	Raccoons	
	T: 10–25 mg/kg IM [29]	Procyonids	Capture and minor surgery.
Telazol + xylazine	T: 3 mg/kg + X: 2 mg/kg IM [26, 28, 29]	Raccoons	
Viverrids:			
Ketamine	K: 10–15 mg/kg IM [33]	Viverrids	Induction in 3–5 min.
Ketamine + acepromazine	K: 30 mg/kg + A: 0.3 mg/kg IM [26]	Genets	
Ketamine + acepromazine + atropine	K: 17 mg/kg + Ace: 0.73 mg/kg + At: 0.04 mg/kg IM [33]	Owston's palm civets	Induction 9 min, no vomiting, decreased temp.
	K: 17 mg/kg + Ace: 0.73 mg/kg + At: 0.04 mg/kg IM [33]	Large Indian civets	Induction 11 min, no vomiting.
Ketamine + diazepam	K: 10 mg/kg + D: 0.5 mg/kg IM [33]	Viverrids	
Ketamine + medetomidine + butorphanol	K: 2 mg/kg + M: 0.04 mg/kg + B: 0.2 mg/kg IM [6, 26]	Binturongs	
Ketamine + medetomidine + butorphanol	K: 308 mg/kg + M: 0.02–0.06 mg/kg + B: 0.2–0.5 mg/kg IM [33]	Binturongs	Lower K and higher M doses provide a shorter recovery.
Ketamine + midazolam	K: 10 mg/kg + Mid: 0.25–0.5 mg/kg IM [33]	Viverrids	
Ketamine + xylazine	K: 5.7 mg/kg + X: 9.8 mg/kg IM [6]	Genets	
	K: 10 mg/kg + X: 0.5 mg/kg IM [26]	African civets	Do not dart free-range animals as they can become lost before drug takes effect.
	K: 15 mg/kg + X: 1.5 mg/kg IM [26]	Brown palm civets	Supplement with one half of original dose as needed.
Ketamine + xylazine	K: 20 mg/kg + X: 1.5 mg/kg IM [6, 26]	Binturongs	Antagonize with yohimbine 0.125 mg/kg.

Drug name	Drug dose	Species	Comments
	K: 30 mg/kg + X: 0.5 mg/kg IM [26]	Genets	
Telazol	T: 2 mg/kg IM [6, 26]	Binturongs	Supplement with ketamine 2 mg/kg as needed.
	T: 3–5 mg/kg IM [33]	Viverrids	Induction 15–20 min, best if silent during induction. Recovery 60–120 min.
	T: 4 mg/kg IM [26]	Palm masked civets	Supplement with ketamine 4 mg/kg as needed.
	T: 4.4 mg/kg IM [26]	African civets, Lesser Oriental civets, Oriental civets, Banded linsangs	Supplement with ketamine 4.4 mg/kg as needed.
	T: 5 mg/kg IM [26, 33]	Palm civets, Genets, Malay civets	Supplement with ketamine 5 mg/kg as needed.
	T: 6.6 mg/kg IM [26]	Banded palm civets	Supplement with ketamine 6.6 mg/kg as needed.
	T: 8.8 mg/kg IM [26]	African palm civets	Supplement with ketamine 8.8 mg/kg as needed.
	T: 15 mg/kg [33]	Madagascar carnivores	
Xylazine	X: 1–2 mg/kg IM [33]	Brown palm civets	
Antiparasitic			
Ailurid: Red panda			
Ivermectin	0.5 mg/kg PO q30d [6]	Red pandas	Heartworm prevention.
Melarsomine	FATAL [6, 34]	Red pandas, North American river otters	Treatment at canine doses has been fatal. 2.5–2.7 mg/kg – died within 22 hrs of receiving.
Euplerid: Fossa			
Ivermectin	0.2 mg/kg SC once, 0.4 mg/kg SC twice 14d apart [7]	Fossas	n = 2 for dermatopathy of unknown cause.
Mustelids			
Amprolium	19 mg/kg PO SID [28]	Mustelids	For coccidisis.
Carbaryl 5% shampoo	Topical bath [28]	Mustelids	Weekly for 3 treatments for mange.
Fenbendazole	20 mg/kg × 5d or 50 mg/kg for 3–5d, PO [28]	Mustelids	
Fipronil	1 pump of spray, or 1/5–1/2 cat dose q60d Topical [28]	Mustelids	Flea adulticide.
Ivermectin	0.006 mg/kg PO q30d [28]	Mustelids	For heartworm prevention.

(*Continued*)

Drug name	Drug dose	Species	Comments
Ivermectin	0.2–0.5 mg/kg SC or PO, repeat q14d as needed [28]	Mustelids	Ecto and endoparasites.
	0.05–0.3 mg/kg PO once [14]	Sea otters	
Levamisole	10 mg/kg PO or SC [28]	Mustelids	May be toxic at higher doses.
	15 mg/kg 7–10d PO SID [14]	Sea otters	
Mebendazole	50 mg/kg PO BID × 2d [28]	Mustelids	Nematodes
Melarsomine	FATAL [6, 34]	Red pandas, North American river otters	Treatment at canine doses has been fatal. 2.5–2.7 mg/kg – died within 22 hrs of receiving.
Metronidazole	15–20 mg/kg PO BID × 14d [28]	Mustelids	Clostridium spp and protozoal infections.
Praziquantel	5–25 mg/kg PO SC, repeat in 14d [28]	Mustelids	Cestodes and trematodes.
	6 mg/kg IM [14]	Sea otters	
Pyrantel pamoate	5–60 mg/kg PO q14d or 4.4 mg/kg q2 weeks [28]	Mustelids	Nematodes
Sulfadimethoxine	20–50 mg/kg PO Sid to BID [28]	Mustelids	Anticoccidian, antibacterial.
Thiacetarsemide	2.2 mg/kg IV BID × 2d [28]	Mustelids	Heartworm adulticide, Follow 3–4 wks later with Ivermectin. Caution must be used due to side effects of dying worms.
Procyonids:			
Sentinel	Used routinely/monthly at domestic animal doses [35]	Coatis	
Viverrids:			
Selamectin	15 mg/kg topical q2wk × 3 treatments [22]	Masked palm civets	n = 1 treatment for Notoedres, Sarcoptes and Demodex mites.
Other			
Activated charcoal	100 ml tube fed [14]	Sea otters	
Busipirone	10 mg/kg PO BID for 18 mo [28]	American badgers	For treatment of self-mutilation.
Cimetidine	5–10 mg/kg IV IM SC PO BID (Or 5 mg/kg IM TID) [14]	Sea otters	Results in reversible increases in liver enzymes. Latter dose is for pups with hemorrhagic diarrhea.
Deslorelin	0.18–0.23 mg/kg SC [14]	Sea otters	
Dexamethasone	2 mg/kg IV IM [14]	Sea otters	Repeat doses with caution.
Diphenhydramine	0.5–2 mg/kg PO BID [14]	Sea otters	

Drug name	Drug dose	Species	Comments
Famotidine	1 mg/kg PO SID × 7d [8]	Meerkats	n = 4 animals, diagnosed with gastric persimmon phytobezoars with ulcerative lesion and treated post removal with famotidine, cefadroxil and buprenorphine.
	5 mg/kg SC [10]	Meerkats	n = 4 full siblings, captive, with presumptive pancreatitis, treated with supportive care. One animals survived ultimately.
Folic acid	2.5 mg/kg PO [14]	Sea otters	
Furosemide	2 mg/kg IM [14]	Sea otters	
Hydrocortisone	50 mg/kg IV, 5–150 mg/kg [14]	Sea otters	For shock
Insulin	2 IU/kg (Adjustable) SC BID [14]	Sea otters	
Kaopectate	2 mg/kg PO q6 hrs [14]	Sea otters	
Lactulose	0.36 ml/kg [10]	Meerkats	n = 1 animal with presumptive pancreatitis and encephalitis, treated supportively. Did not survive.
Leuprolide acetate	3.75 mg (0.11–0.19 mg/kg) IM via hand injection in pelvic limb dorsally, reconstituted in 0.5–1.5 ml diluent, given monthly for 6 months of breeding season [36]	Sea otters	n = 4 males from 3.5–6 yrs. of age to control male associated aggression, 2 animals experienced anorexia, depression and injection site swelling, pain and lameness that was not responsive to flunixin or diphenhydramine therapy.
Metoclopramide	0.2 mg/kg IM BID [14]	Sea otters	For pups with hemorrhagic diarrhea.
Milk Thistle and S-adenosylmethionine (Denosyl)	M: 10.7–14.3 mg/kg PO SID + 31 mg/kg PO SID [10]	Meerkats	n = 1 animal with presumptive hepatitis diagnosed at age 8 mo, treated for 2 years and was stable until diagnosed with pancreatitis with 3 littermates.
Oxytocin	10–20 USP IV or IM [14]	Sea otters	For milk let down.
Prednisolone	2 mg/kg PO SID [11]	Skunks	n = 1; adjunctive treatment for mediastinal lymphoma and chylothorax.
Ranitidine	1–4 mg/kg PO TID [14]	Sea otters	
Vitamin B complex	2 ml/1 L LRS SC pups; 1 ml/10 kg SC Adults [14]	Sea otters	
Vitamin C (Ascorbic acid)	50–100 mg PO IM SC SID [14]	Sea otters	
Vitamin E	100 IU/kg fish SID; 400 IU/days [14].	Sea otters	

Species	Weight [6, 26, 28, 29, 33]
Ailurid:	
Red/Lesser Panda *(Ailurus fulgens)*	3–6 kg
Euplerid:	
Fossa *(Fossa fossa)*	1.5–2 kg
Herpestids:	
Meerkat *(Suricata suricatta)*	0.7–0.8 kg
Mongoose, African water *(Atilax paludinosus)*	3.5–4.1 kg
Mongoose, Black-legged *(Bdeogale spp.)*	0.9–3 kg
Mongoose *(Herpestes spp.)*	0.4–4 kg
Mongoose, Malagasy Ring-tailed *(Galidia elegans)*	0.7–0.9 kg
Mephitids:	
Skunk, Hog-nosed *(Conepatus leuconotus)*	2.3–4.5 kg
Skunk, Hooded *(Mephitis macroura)*	0.7–2.5 kg
Skunk, Spotted *(Spilogale spp.)*	0.2–1 kg
Skunk, Striped *(Mephitis mephitis)*	2–3 kg
Mustelids:	
Badger, European *(Meles meles)*	10–16 kg
Badger, Ferret *(Melogale moschata)*	1–3 kg
Badger, Hog *(Arctonyx collaris)*	7–14 kg
Badger, Honey *(Mellivora capensis)*	7–13 kg
Badger *(Taxidea taxus)*	4–12 kg
Ferret, Black-footed *(Mustela nigripes)*	0.7–1.5 kg
Ferret *(Mustela putorius furo)*	0.6–1.2 kg
Fisher *(Martes pennanti)*	2.6–5.5 kg
Marten, Pine *(Martes americana)*	0.5–1.5 kg
Marten, Yellow-throated *(Martes flavigula)*	2–3 kg
Mink *(Mustela vison)*	0.8–1.1 kg
Mink, European *(Mustela lutreola)*	0.4–1 mg/kg
Otter, American River *(Lontra canadensis)*	7–9 kg
Otter, Asian Small clawed *(Aonyx cinerea)*	1–5 kg
Otter, Clawless *(Aonyx capensis)*	13–34 kg
Otter, European *(Lutra lutra)*	3–14 kg
Otter, Giant *(Pteronura brasiiensis)*	22–30 kg
Otter, Marine *(Lontra feline)*	3–4 kg
Otter, Sea *(Enhydra lutris)*	Female 15–32 kg, Male: 22–45 kg
Otter, Spotted-necked *(Lutra maculicollis)*	3–14 kg
Tayra *(Eira barbara)*	4–5 kg
Wolverine *(Gulo gulo)*	7–32 kg
Procyonids:	
Cuscus *(Phalanger spp)*	1–5 kg

Species	Weight [6, 26, 28, 29, 33]
Coatimundi *(Nasua spp.)*	3–6 kg
Kinkajou *(Potus flavus)*	1.4–4.6 kg
Olingo *(Bassaricyon gabbi)*	0.9–1.5 kg
Ringtail *(Bassariscus astutus)*	0.8–1.3 kg
Raccoon *(Procyon lotor)*	2–12 kg
Viverrids:	
Binturong *(Arctictus binturong)*	16–28 kg
Civet, African palm *(Nandinia binotata)*	1.7–2.1 kg
Civet, African *(Civettictus civetta)*	7020 kg
Civet, Banded Palm *(Hemigalus derbyanus)*	1.75–3 kg
Civet, Brown Palm *(Paradoxurus jerdoni)*	1.2–3.5 kg
Civet, lesser oriental *(Viverricula indica)*	2–4 kg
Civet, Masked palm *(Paguma larvata)*	3.6–5 kg
Civet, Oriental *(Viverra zibetha)*	5–11 kg
Civet, Palm *(Paradoxurus hermaphroditus)*	1.5–4.5 kg
Genet *(Genetta spp.)*	1–3 kg
Linsang, Banded *(Prionodon linsang)*	0.6–0.8 kg

References

1 Delclaux, M., Talavera, C., Lopez, M. et al. (2002). Avascular necrosis of the femoral heads in a red panda (*Ailurus fulgens fulgens*): possible Legg-Calve-Perthes disease. *Journal of Zoo and Wildlife Medicine* 33 (3): 283–285.

2 Ilha, M.R.S. and Newman, S.J. (2012). Pathology in practice. *Journal of the American Veterinary Medical Association* 240 (8): 953–955.

3 Bicknese, E.J., Fagan, D.A., and Lamberski, N. (2008). Cyclic regimen of low-dose doxycycline to treat periodontal disease in a chacoan peccary (*C. wagneri*), Red pandas (*A. fulgens*), and Bat-eared foxes (*O. megalotis*). *Annual Proceedings of the American Association of Zoo Veterinarians*. 167–168.

4 Volk, H.A., O'Reilly, A., Bodley, K. et al. (2018). Keratomycosis in captive red pandas (*Ailurus fulgens*): 2 cases. *Open Veterinary Journal* 8 (2): 200–203.

5 Kearns, K.S., Pollock, C.G., and Ramsay, E.C. (1999). Dermatophytosis in red pandas (*Ailurus fulgens fulgens*): a review of 14 cases. *Journal of Zoo and Wildlife Medicine* 30 (4): 561–563.

6 Ramsay, E. (2015). Procyonids and viverrids. In: *Fowler's Zoo and Wild Animals*, 8e (ed. R.E. Miller and M. Fowler), 491–497. St. Louis, MO: Elsevier.

7 Ratliff, C. and Sutherland-Smith, M. (2017). Seasonal dermatopathy and concurrent reproductive findings in a captive fossa (*Cryptoprocta ferox*). *Journal of Zoo and Wildlife Medicine* 48 (4): 1181–1187.

8 Hahn, A., D'Agostino, J., Cole, G. et al. (2013). Persimmon phytobezoars in meerkats (*Suricata suricatta*). *Journal of Zoo and Wildlife Medicine* 44 (2): 505–508.

9 Levi, M.M., Horowitz, I., Fleiderovitz, O. et al. (2017). Clinical toxoplasmosis in two meerkats (*Suricata suricatta*) in Israel. *Israel Journal of Veterinary Medicine* 72 (1): 49–54.

10 Naples, L.M., Lacasse, C., Landolfi, J.A. et al. (2010). Acute pancreatitis in slender-tailed meerkats (*Suricata suricatta*). *Journal of Zoo and Wildlife Medicine* 41 (2): 275–286.

11 Liptovszky, M., Kerekes, Z., Perge, E. et al. (2017). Mediastinal lymphoma and chylothorax in a striped skunk (*Mephitis mephitis*). *Journal of Zoo and Wildlife Medicine* 48 (2): 598–601.

12 Krauss, M.W., Benato, L., Wack, A. et al. (2014). Intervertebral disk disease in 3 striped skunks (*Mephitis mephitis*). *Veterinary Surgery* 43: 589–592.

13 Summa, N., Eshar, D., Reynolds, D. et al. (2015). Successful diagnosis and treatment of bilateral perineal hernias in a skunk (*Mephitis mephitis*). *Journal of Zoo and Wildlife Medicine* 46 (3): 575–579.

14 Dierauf, L. and Gulland, F.M.D. (2001). *CRC Handbook of Marine Mammal Medicine*, 719–721. CRC Press.

15 Molter, C.M., Jackson, J., Clippinger, T.L. et al. (2015). Tibial plateau leveling osteotomy in a cape clawless otter (*Aonyx capensis*) with cranial cruciate ligament ruptures. *Journal of Zoo and Wildlife Medicine* 46 (1): 179–183.

16 Lee, E.A., Byrne, B.A., Young, M.A. et al. (2016). Pharmacokinetic indices for cefovecin after single-dose administration to adult sea otters (*Enhydra lutris*). *Journal of Veterinary Pharmacologic Therapy* 39 (6): 625–628.

17 Soto-Azat, C., Boher, F., Fabry, M. et al. (2008). Surgical implantation of intra-abdominal radiotransmitters in marine otters (*Lontra felina*) in Central Chile. *Journal of Wildlife Diseases* 44 (4): 979–982.

18 Chittick, E., Rotstein, D., Brown, T. et al. (2001). Pyometra and uterine adenocarcinoma in a melengesterol acetate-implanted captive coati (*Nasua nasua*). *Journal of Zoo and Wildlife Medicine* 32 (2): 245–251.

19 McCain, S.L., Allender, M.C., Bohling, M. et al. (2010). Thyroid neoplasia in captive raccoons (*Procyon lotor*). *Journal of Zoo and Wildlife Medicine* 41 (1): 121–127.

20 Lima, D.C.V., Siqueira, D.B., Valdemiro, A. et al. (2016). Ectopic testis in coati (*Nasua nasua*). *Pesquisa Veterinaria Brasileira* 36 (10): 999–1004.

21 Adamovicz, L., Kennedy-Stoskopf, S., Talley, A. et al. (2017). Mycobacterium intracellulare infection causing a retro-peritoneal mass in a binturong (*Arctictis binturong*). *Journal of Zoo and Wildlife Medicine* 48 (2): 544–548.

22 Olivier, L., Nardini, G., Leopardi, S. et al. (2015). Mite infection in a masked palm civet (*Paguma larvata*) treated by selamectin (Stronghold®, PFIZER LTD.). *Journal of Zoo and Wildlife Medicine* 46 (3): 592–595.

23 Hwang, Y.T., Gentes, M.L., Parker, D.L. et al. (2004). Effects of surgical implantation of temperature data loggers on reproduction of captive striped skunks (*Mephitis mephitis*). *Journal of Zoo and Wildlife Medicine* 35 (4): 515–519.

24 Minto, B.W., Nagatsuyu, C.E., Teixeira, C.R. et al. (2017). Minimally invasive hysterectomy in coatis (*Nasua nasua*). *Pesquisa Veterinária Brasileira* 37 (6): 627–629.

25 Spriggs, M., Arble, J., and Myers, G. (2007). Intervertebral disc extrusion and spinal decompression in a binturong (*Arctictis binturong*). *Journal of Zoo and Wildlife Medicine* 38 (1): 135–138.

26 Kreeger, T.J. and Arnemo, J.M. (2012). *Handbook of Wildlife Chemical Immobilization*. China: Kreeger.

27 Strike, T.B., Bielby, J., Feltrer, Y. et al. (2017). Comparison of isoflurane and sevoflurane for short-term anesthesia in meerkats (*Suricata suricatta*)-are there benefits that outweigh costs? *Journal of Zoo and Wildlife Medicine* 48 (2): 371–379.

28 Kollias, G.V. and Fernández-Morán, J. (2015). Mustelids. In: *Fowler's Zoo and Wild Animals*, 8e (ed. R.E. Miller and M. Fowler), 477–491. St. Louis, MO: Elsevier.

29 Kollias, G.V. and Abou-Madi, N. (2014). Procyonids and mustelids. In: *Zoo Animal and Wildlife Immobilization and Anesthesia*, 2e (ed. G. West, D. Heard and N. Caulkett), 607–617. Ames, IA: Wiley Blackwell.

30 Belfiore, N.M. (2008). Trapping and handling of North American river otters (*Lontra canadensis*) in a managed marsh. *Journal of Zoo and Wildlife Medicine* 39 (1): 13–20.

31 Fournier, P., Fournier-Chambrillon, C., and ViÈ, J.C. (1998). Immobilization of wild kinkajous (*Potos flavus*) with medetomidine-ketamine and reversal by atipamezole. *Journal of Zoo and Wildlife Medicine* 29 (2): 190–194.

32 Conforti, V.A., Cascelli de Azevedo, F.C., Paulo, O.L.O.H. et al. (2017). Chemical restraint of free-ranging south American coatis (*Nasua nasua*) with a combination of tiletamine and zolazepam. *Journal of Wildlife Diseases* 53 (1): 140–143.

33 Moresco, A. and Larsen, R.S. (2014). Viverrids. In: *Zoo Animal and Wildlife Immobilization and Anesthesia*, 2e (ed. G. West, D. Heard and N. Caulkett), 619–625. Ames, IA: Wiley Blackwell.

34 Neiffer, D.L., Klein, E.C., Calle, P.P. et al. (2002). Mortality associated with melarsomine dihydrochloride administration in two North American river otters (*Lontra canadensis*) and a red panda (*Ailurus fulgens fulgens*). *Journal of Zoo and Wildlife Medicine* 33 (3): 242–248.

35 Dumonceaux, G. (2018). Personal communication.

36 Calle, P.P., Stetter, M.D., and Raphael, B.L. (1997). Use of Depot Leuprolide Acetate to control undesirable male associated behaviors in the California Sea Lion (*Zalophus californianus*) and California Sea otter (*Enhydra lutris*). *Annual Proceedings of the International Association of Aquatic Animal Medicine.*

12

Hyenas

Drug name	Drug dose	Species	Comments
Antimicrobials and Antifungals			
Azithromycin	5 mg/kg IV over 60 min, then 5 mg/kg PO SID [1]	Spotted hyenas	n = 1 case of erythema multiforme in a spotted hyena likely due to either canine distemper vaccination or amoxicillin.
Clavamox	14 mg/kg PO BID [2]	Spotted hyenas	n = 1 case of rear limb lameness ultimately diagnosed as anal sac squamous cell carcinoma that was treated with Clavamox for 21 days.
Enrofloxacin	2.5–5.2 mg/kg PO BID × 10d [1]	Spotted hyenas	n = 2 One case of erythema multiforme in a spotted hyena likely due to either canine distemper vaccination or amoxicillin, given IV during procedure and then for 18 days orally. A second case for adjunct treatment of squamous cell carcinoma of anal sac.
Analgesic			
Buprenorphine	0.01 mg/kg IM or SC [3]	Not specified	For analgesia.
Etodolac	9–10 mg/kg PO SID [3]	Not specified	n = 1 for 30 day treatment at lower dose. Multiple animals given higher dose on multiple days, no adverse effects noted.
Gabapentin	2.5–5 mg/kg PO BID [2]	Spotted hyenas	n = 1 case of an animal with right rear limb lameness that was minimally responsive to NSAIDS and antibiotics, and was ultimately diagnosed with anal sac squamous cell sarcoma. While on gabapentin, animal became somnolent and the medication was discontinued. In the author's experience with another Spotted hyena in similar dosing, severe sedation was noted.

(Continued)

Zoo and Wild Mammal Formulary, First Edition. Alicia Hahn.

Drug name	Drug dose	Species	Comments
Meloxicam	0.1–0.2 mg/kg SC [2, 3]	Not specified	Higher dose given once for endodontic procedures.
Methocarbamol	9.6 mg/kg PO BID [2]	Spotted hyenas	n = 1 case of an animal with right rear limb lameness that was minimally responsive to NSAIDS and antibiotics, and was ultimately diagnosed with anal sac squamous cell sarcoma.
Anesthetic			
Etorphine + xylazine	E: 0.05 + X: 0.63 mg/kg [4]	Spotted hyenas	Antagonize with 100 mg naltrexone per mg etorphine, and 0.125 mg/kg yohimbine.
	E: 0.05 mg/kg + X: 0.6 mg/kg IM; antagonize with 0.1 mg/kg diprenorphine + 0.15 mg/kg yohimbine [5]	Spotted hyenas	Respiratory suppression can occur.
Ketamine	15 mg/kg IM [4]	Brown hyenas	
Ketamine + acepromazine	K: 15 mg/kg + A: 0.3 mg/kg IM [4]	Aardwolves	
Ketamine + medetomidine	K: 2–3 mg/kg + M: 0.035–0.045 mg/kg IM; antagonize with atipamezole at 5 × mg of medetomidine used [1, 4]	Brown hyenas, spotted hyenas	n = 1 Spotted hyena on 2 occasions, Wild hyenas, recumbency within 7 minutes, IM injection in neck or shoulder was consistently successful. Recommend to cover eyes and plug ears, and for supplement can consider 30–40 mg ketamine IM. Reversal in 5–10 minutes.
Ketamine + xylazine + atropine	K 4–6 mg/kg + X: 1 mg/kg + A: 0.045 mg/kg IM [3]	Cubs generally require 80% of the adult calculated dose. Recommend muzzling during procedure as the bite response is not as readily abolished as in domestic animals.	Dart hind end, as anxious animals will whip neck back and forth, making this area less desirable. Heavier animals may require an additional 1–2 mg/kg ketamine IM for full sedation, whereas lighter animals may experience rigidity and twitching. Diazepam 0.5 mg/kg IV will assist with this, but may lead to periods of apnea. Some reports in males that are inherently lower in body weight experience seizures at or close to 6 mg/kg K. Again diazepam assists with this.
Ketamine + xylazine	K: 8–10 mg/kg + X: 0.5–1.0 mg/kg IM; antagonize with yohimbine 0.11–0.125 mg/kg IM [4]	Brown, Striped, and Spotted hyenas	

Drug name	Drug dose	Species	Comments
	K: 13.2 + X: 6.3 mg/kg IM; antagonize with 0.125 mg/kg yohimbine or 3.7 mg/kg tolazoline [4]	Spotted hyenas	
	K: 10 mg/kg + X: 1 mg/kg; antagonize with 0.11 mg/kg yohimbine [5]	Brown, Striped, and Spotted hyenas	The long hair coat in brown hyena may lead to overestimation of body weight in this species.
Ketamine + xylazine + midazolam	Pre-sedation with M: 0.055 mg/kg + X: 0.57 mg/kg IM, then induced with K: 3.8 mg/kg IM [2]	Spotted hyenas	n = 1 case of an animal with right rear limb lameness that was minimally responsive to NSAIDS and antibiotics, and was ultimately diagnosed with anal sac squamous cell sarcoma.
Ketamine + Telazol	K: 5.5 mg/kg + T: 1.83 mg/kg IM [1]	Spotted hyenas	n = 2 immobilizations of one animal that developed erythema multiforme.
Medetomidine + butorphanol + midazolam	Med: 0.0192 mg/kg + B: 0.15 mg/kg + Mid: 0.2 mg/kg IM [2]	Spotted hyenas	n = 1 case, 25 yr old with rear leg lameness and eventually diagnosed with anal sac squamous cell carcinoma.
Telazol	5 mg/kg IM [4]	Brown, Striped, and Spotted hyenas	
	6.5 mg/kg IM free-ranging, 5 mg/kg captive, supplemental 3 mg/kg ketamine IM [5]	Brown, Striped, and Spotted hyenas	The long hair coat in brown hyena may lead to overestimation of body weight in this species.
Other			
Chlorambucil	0.16 mg/kg PO EOD [6]	Spotted hyenas	n = 1 case of chronic T-lymphocytic leukemia, given for 5 weeks then stopped for 4 weeks due to thrombocytopenia and epistaxis secondary to presumed bone marrow toxicity. Thrombocytopenia and epistaxis resolved. One dose of L-asparaginase was given then the chlorambucil restarted at 1 mg/kg PO EOD for an additional 67 weeks.
Dexamethasone sodium phosphate	0.5 mg/kg IM, 0.1 mg/kg IM for subsequent doses [1]	Spotted hyenas	n = 1 case of erythema multiforme post vaccination or antibiotic administration.
Diphenhydramine	2 mg/kg IM or PO [1]	Spotted hyenas	n = 1 case of erythema multiforme post vaccination or antibiotic administration.
Famotidine	0.4 mg/kg PO SID [1]	Spotted hyenas	n = 1 case of erythema multiforme post vaccination or antibiotic administration, given for 4 weeks.
L-asparaginase	167 IU/kg IM once [6]	Spotted hyenas	n = 1 case of chronic T-lymphocytic leukemia, one dose given at 9 weeks prior to restarting chlorambucil at a lower dose.

(*Continued*)

Drug name	Drug dose	Species	Comments
Metoclopramide	0.41 mg/kg PO BID [1]	Spotted hyenas	n = 1 case of erythema multiforme post vaccination or antibiotic administration, secondary esophagitis treatment with sucralfate.
Omeprazole	0.82 mg/kg PO SID [1]	Spotted hyenas	n = 1 case of erythema multiforme post vaccination or antibiotic administration.
Prednisone	0.5 mg/kg PO BID × 5d, then tapered to every 48 hr [1]	Spotted hyena	n = 1 case of erythema multiforme post vaccination or antibiotic administration.
	1 mg/kg PO SID [6]	Spotted hyenas	n = 1 case of chronic T-lymphocytic leukemia, given for 9 weeks with oral chlorambucil then an additional 71 weeks with a lower dose of chlorambucil.
Sucralfate	1 g PO TID [1]	Spotted hyenas	n = 1 case of erythema multiforme post vaccination or antibiotic administration.

Species	Weight [1]
Aardwolf *(Proteles cristata)*	7–15 kg
Brown Hyena *(Hyena brunnea)*	37–47.5 kg
Spotted Hyena *(Crocuta crocuta)*	40–86 kg
Striped Hyena *(Hyena hyena)*	25–55 kg

References

1 Hanley, C.S., Simmons, H.A., Wallace, R.S. et al. (2005). Erythema multiforme in a spotted hyena (*Crocuta crocuta*). *Journal of Zoo and Wildlife Medicine* 36 (3): 515–519.

2 Goodnight, A.L., Traslavina, R.P., Emmanuelson, K. et al. (2013). Squamous cell carcinoma of the anal sac in a Spotted hyena (*Crocuta crocuta*). *Journal of Zoo and Wildlife Medicine* 44 (4): 1068–1074.

3 West, G., Heard, D., and Caulkett, N. (2014). Hyenas. In: *Zoo Animal and Wildlife Immobilization and Anesthesia*, 2e (ed. G. West, D. Heard and N. Caulkett), 627–637. Ames, IA: Wiley Blackwell.

4 Miller, R.E. and Fowler, M.E. (2015). Hyenidae. In: *Fowler's Zoo and Wild Animal Medicine*, vol. 8 (ed. R.E. Miller and M. Fowler), 509–514. St. Louis, MO: Elsevier Saunders.

5 Kreeger, T.J., Arnemo, J.M., and Raath, J.P. (2012). *Handbook of Wildlife Chemical Immobilization*, 233–234. Fort Collins, CL, USA: Wildlife Pharmaceuticals Inc.

6 Singleton, C.L., Wack, R.F., Zabka, T.S. et al. (2007). Diagnosis and treatment of chronic T-lymphocytic leukemia in a spotted hyena (*Crocuta crocuta*). *Journal of Zoo and Wildlife Medicine* 38 (3): 488–491.

13

Nondomestic Felids

Drug name	Drug dose	Species	Comments
Antimicrobials and Antifungals			
Amikacin sulfate (Amikin)	10 mg/kg IV q48 hrs × 10d [1]	Florida panthers	n = 1 animal, treatment for dehiscence and postoperative wound management.
Amikacin impregnated (Amiglyde-V) polymethylmethacrylate (Simplex P Bone Cement)	3 rods were formed and placed SQ overlying tibia [1]	Florida panthers	n = 1 animal, treatment for dehiscence and postoperative wound management.
Amoxicillin	11 mg/kg SC SID [2]	African lions	n = 1, 250 kg animal postoperative for surgical repair of hiatal hernia.
	15 mg/kg PO BID [3]	Lions, Tigers	n = 4 animals after surgery for pyometra.
Amoxicillin + Enrofloxacin	A: 17 mg/kg PO BID + E: 8 mg/kg PO BID × 28d [1]	Florida panthers	n = 1 animal, treatment for dehiscence and postoperative wound management.
Amoxicillin/clavulanic acid (Clavamox)	15 mg/kg PO BID × 14d [1]	Florida panthers	n = 1 animal, treatment for dehiscence and postoperative wound management.
	20 mg/kg PO BID [3]	Lions, Tigers	n = 2 animals after surgery for pyometra.
Ampicillin	22 mg/kg IV [3]	Lions, Tigers	n = 4 animals perioperatively receiving ampicillin for pyometra.
Cefazolin	22 mg/kg IV [3]	Lions, Tigers	n = 7 animals perioperatively receiving cefazolin during surgery for pyometra.
	22 mg/kg SC once [4]	Snow leopards	n = 1 animal treated postoperative for stifle surgery, combined with Cefpodoxime proxetil
	22 mg/kg IV [1]	Florida panthers	n = 6 animals, perioperatively for surgery repair of appendicular fractures

(*Continued*)

Zoo and Wild Mammal Formulary, First Edition. Alicia Hahn.

Drug name	Drug dose	Species	Comments
Cefovecin (Convenia)	1 mg/10 kg bodyweight SC [5]	Eurasian lynxes	n = 1 adult female after surgical repair of traumatic patellar luxation
	4 mg/kg SC once every 14d [6]	African lions	n = pharmacokinetic study evaluating 4 and 8 mg/kg. Both doses SC once, resulted in plasma levels above the reported minimum inhibitory concentration for feline common bacterial organisms for 14 days.
	8 mg/kg SC once [7]	African lions	n = 1 female 8 yr old African lion with septic peritonitis, given perioperatively. Postoperative culture of abdominal fluid revealed E. coli responsive to Cefovecin. The cost difference between a 2-week course of oral enrofloxacin and one dose of Cefovecin were similar and thus the high initial cost of Cefovecin was negated.
Cefpodoxime proxetil	7.6 mg/kg PO SID × 14d [4]	Snow leopards	n = 1 animal treated postoperative for stifle surgery, combined with cefazolin
Cephalexin	35 mg/kg PO TID [3]	Large felids	n = 1 animal after surgery for pyometra.
Enrofloxacin associated retinopathy not seen in Tigers and Lions		Tigers, Lions [8]	n = 11 lions and 33 tigers with 81 eyes examined postmortem for potential damage to the outer nuclear retina from enrofloxacin. Cats that had not received enrofloxacin (n = 11) were compared with treated animals (n = 36). The outer nuclear layer thickness or area in treated versus untreated cats was not significantly different. Additionally, no clinical blindness was reported in any of the cats. This study showed no evidence of enrofloxacin-associated thinning of the outer nuclear layer in the lions and tigers evaluated,
Enrofloxacin	1.1 mg/kg SC SID [2]	African lions	n = 1, 250 kg animal postoperative for surgical repair of hiatal hernia
Enrofloxacin	5 mg/kg PO SID [3]	Large felids	n = 2 animals after surgery for pyometra.

Drug name	Drug dose	Species	Comments
Itraconazole (Sporonox 10 mg/ml)	5 mg/kg PO SID [9]	Siberian tigers	n = 1 animal of 6 total felids, diagnosed in Tennessee with Blastomycosis, This animal received Amphotericin B 0.25 mg/kg IV once due to poor appetite, then itraconazole for 30 days with transient improvement but ultimate euthanasia due to suspected hepatotoxicity with histologic blastomycosis lesions in the brain and spinal cord. High CSF concentrations suggest that a lower dose may have provided therapeutic concentrations with less risk of hepatotoxicity.
Marbofloxacin	2 mg/kg PO SID × 7d [5]	Eurasian lynxes	n = 1 adult female postop after surgical repair of traumatic patellar luxation
	2 mg/kg PO SID × 14d [1]	Florida panthers	n = 1 animal, treatment for dehiscence and postoperative wound management
	5 mg/kg PO SID [3]	Large felids	n = 1 animal after surgery for pyometra.
Metronidazole + Omeprazole + Amoxicillin	O: 20 mg SID PO + M: 600 mg PO BID + A: 750 mg PO BID all for 3 weeks [10]	Cheetahs	n = 6, 2.4, captive South African cheetahs with spiral bacterial infection and gastritis. Animals were endoscopically reexamined at 3, 7 and 19 months post treatment and all were improved histologically at 3 mo, many worse at 7 mo but improved at 19 mo. Despite temporary eradication of spiral bacteria, inflammation was not eliminated in any of the animals but the degree was reduced both macroscopically and histologically by 3 months. Some cheetah gained weight and none died of gastritis or developed renal failure (often accompanies) during the study.
Tetracycline + metronidazole + bismuth subsalicylate	T: 500 mg PO QID + M: 250 mg PO QID + B: 300 mg PO QID all concurrently × 7d [11].	Cheetahs	n = 6, 2.4, captive cheetah, 5–10 yrs of age. 3/6 animals had slight improvement in gastritis at 3 weeks post treatment but severity returned at 1 yr post treatment.

(Continued)

Drug name	Drug dose	Species	Comments
Tetracycline + metronidazole + bismuth subsalicylate	T: 500 mg PO BID + M: 500 mg PO BID + B: 600 mg PO BOD × 28d concurrently [12].	Cheetahs	n = 32 cheetah evaluating multiple treatment regimes for treatment of gastritis. Overall, no treatments were successful beyond short-term improvement seen with this protocol and a 45-day protocol with lansoprazole, clarithromycin and amoxicillin. Thus antibiotic treatment for gastritis in cheetah will not cure the issue and should only be prescribed for animals with clinical signs of gastritis such as vomiting and weight loss.
Trimethoprim Sulfamethoxazole	30 mg/kg PO BID × 14d [13]	Leopards	n = 1 postoperative treatment after repair of a hiatal hernia.
	30 mg/kg PO BID [3]	Large felids	n = 1 animal after surgery for pyometra.
Analgesia			
Bupivicaine – 0.125%	6.25 mg given on each side of linea alba between internal oblique and transverse abdominis muscles via ultrasonography [14].	Canadian lynxes	n = 1 Given perioperatively prior to abdominal surgical procedure. Analgesia was from thoracic vertebra 7 – lumbar 1.
Buprenorphine	0.01 mg/kg IV or SC [1]	Florida panthers	n = 1 animal treated post surgical repair of appendicular fractures.
	0.015 mg/kg IM postop, then 0.005 mg/kg IM q8 hrs for 3 doses [14]	Tigers	n = 1 undergoing abdominal surgery.
	0.1–0.2 mg/kg SC BID to QID, IM or PO transmucosal as well [14, 15].	Felids	
	0.02 mg/kg IM [5]	Eurasian lynxes	n = 1, 4 yr old female, 17 kg, diagnosed with hind limb lameness that represented traumatic patellar luxation. Surgical repair performed and during surgery used CRI with ketamine 0.5 mg/kg/hr + fentanyl 0.003 mg/kg/hr IV. Postoperatively gave buprenorphine and meloxicam.
	0.24 mg/kg SC SID × 4d [4]	Snow leopards	n = 1 animal pre and postoperative analgesia for stifle osteochondritis dissecans.
Butorphanol	0.15 mg/kg SC [4]	Florida panthers	Analgesia post surgical repair of fractures

Drug name	Drug dose	Species	Comments
Etodolac	5 mg/kg PO q48 hrs for 5 doses, then q72 hrs [14]	Tigers	n = 1 analgesia.
Gabapentin	3.7 mg/kg PO SID long term [14]	African lions	n = 1 osteoarthritis and presumed intervertebral disc disease.
	4 mg/kg PO SID to BID [4]	Snow leopards	n = 1 animal pre and postoperative analgesia for stifle osteochondritis dissecans. Continued for 15 months post surgery and ultimately combined with Platelet rich plasma intra-articular 2×.
Hydromorphone + ketamine CRI	Continuous IV infusion of H: 0.04 mg/kg/hr + K: 0.6 mg/kg/hr [1]	Florida panthers	n = 1 animal receiving intraoperative analgesia for repair of appendicular fractures.
Lidocaine	20 ml 2% solution given as a brachial plexus block [16]	Cheetahs	n = 1 perioperative brachial plexus block prior to repair of a fractured front limb.
Meloxicam	0.05–0.15 mg/kg PO [4]	Snow leopards	n = 1 animal pre and postoperative analgesia for stifle osteochondritis dissecans.
	0.1 mg/kg IM once [17]	African lions	n = 7 adult captive lions anesthetized for laparoscopic ovariectomy.
	0.1–0.2 mg/kg PO once, then in subsequent days 2–4 give 0.05–0.1 mg/kg SID, from day 5 onward give 0.025 mg/kg q48–72 hrs, PO or SC [14]	Nondomestic felids	Analgesia
	0.1–0.2 mg/kg SC once then 0.1 mg/kg PO SID × 2d [18]	Tigers	n = 7 adult female tigers who underwent laparoscopic ovariectomy, meloxicam was given perioperatively and postoperatively for 2 days for pain control in addition to tramadol 2 mg/kg PO BID.
	0.2 mg/kg PO SID [3]	Lions, Tigers	n = 3 animals after surgery for pyometra.
Meloxicam + tramadol	M: 0.2 mg/kg PO SID + T: 1 mg/kg PO BID [3]	Lions, Tigers	n = 7 animals after surgery for pyometra.
Morphine sulfate	10 ml given as lumbosacral epidural [14]	African lions, Tigers	Lumbosacral epidural analgesia for ovariohysterectomy immediately prior to surgery. One cat that received >11 ml had postoperative dysphoria which responded to an opiod antagonist.
Morphine sulfate + bupivicaine	M: 0.1–0.3 mg/kg + B: 0.3 mg/kg, (not exceeding 6–9 ml total) for epidural analgesia [14]	Nondomestic felids	Epidural analgesia

(*Continued*)

Drug name	Drug dose	Species	Comments
Piroxicam	0.3 mg/kg PO SID × 4d then q48 hrs for subsequent days [14]	Nondomestic felids	Analgesia
Tramadol	2 mg/kg PO BID × 2d [18]	Tigers	n = 7 adult female tigers who underwent laparoscopic ovariectomy, meloxicam was given perioperatively and postoperatively for 2 days for pain control in addition to tramadol 2 mg/kg PO BID.
Tramadol	1–4 mg/kg PO BID short term, 0.8–1.5 mg/kg PO BID long term [14]	Nondomestic felids	Analgesia
Tramadol	4 mg/kg PO TID [1]	Florida panthers	n = 2 animals, analgesia for surgical repair of appendicular fractures.
Anethesia and Sedation			
Butorphanol + medetomidine + midazolam	B: 0.2–0.3 mg/kg + M: 0.05 mg/kg + Mid 0.15–0.2 mg/kg; antagonize with naltrexone 0.7 mg/kg (or 2 × B dose in mg) + atipamezole 0.25 mg/kg (or 5 × M dose in mg) + flumazenil 0.003 mg/kg [19, 20]	African lions	Immobilization may consider adding hyaluronidase 1250 IU to this mixture. Lions can rouse suddenly with medetomidine so be vigilant with monitoring.
Butorphanol + midazolam + dexmedetomidine	B: 0.3 mg/kg + Mid: 0.2 mg/kg + DexM: 0.05 mg/kg IM via dart; antagonize with atipamezole 0.25 mg/kg + flumazenil 0.003 mg/kg IM [17].	African lions	n = 7 adult captive lions anesthetized for laparoscopic ovariectomy. Propofol 4 mg/kg IV titrated to effect allowed intubation.
Detomidine	0.5 mg/kg PO [14]	Tigers	Routinely produces sternal but not lateral recumbency in tigers. Vomiting, salivation, and sinus bradycardia are common adverse effects of oral detomidine.
Dexmedetomidine + butorphanol + midazolam	D: 13.9–17.7 mg/kg + B: 0.19–0.25 mg/kg + Mid: 0.15–0.21 mg/kg IM. Antagonize with atipamezole 0.123–0.127 mg/kg and naltrexone 0.086–0.114 mg/kg IM [21].	Cheetahs	n = 20 cheetah immobilized with combination and resulted in recumbency in 5.5–11.5 min, moderate hypertension initially that resolved overtime and rapid recoveries of 5.4–17 min.

Drug name	Drug dose	Species	Comments
Dexmedetomidine + methadone + midazolam + propofol	Dex: 0.015 mg/kg + Met: 0.3 mg/kg for induction, prior surgery gave Mid: 0.2 mg/kg IV + propofol 1.2 mg/kg IV for surgical plane combined with isoflurane [5]	Eurasian lynxes	n = 1, 4 yr old female, 17 kg, diagnosed with hind limb lameness that represented traumatic patellar luxation. Surgical repair performed and during surgery used CRI with ketamine 0.5 mg/kg/hr + fentanyl 0.003 mg/kg/hr IV. Postoperatively gave buprenorphine 0.02 mg/kg IM. Cefovecin 1 mg/10 kg SC, meloxicam 0.1 mg/kg day of surgery and 0.05 mg/kg for 3 additional days SID. Marbofloxacin 2 mg/kg PO SID × 7d. Immediately postoperative the animal was clinically normal and at recheck exam at 47 days orthopedic exam was normal.
Diazepam	0.15–0.46 mg/kg (20–60 mg/adult tiger or lion) PO 1–3 hrs prior to immobilization [14]	Tigers, Lions	Repeated dosing can cause idiopathic hepatic toxicity
	0.08–0.15 mg/kg IV (10–20 mg/adult lion or tiger) [14]	Tigers, Lions	Sedation
Ketamine	Supplemental 1–3 mg/kg IM or IV [14]	Large Felids	To be used as a supplement during a procedure if the cat begins to move or awaken.
Ketamine + acepromazine	K: 20 mg/kg + A: 0.1 mg/kg [20]	Bobcats	
Ketamine + acepromazine	K: 10 mg/kg + A: 0.2 mg/kg [20]	Servals	
Ketamine + acepromazine	K: 30 mg/kg + A: 0.3 mg/kg IM [20]	Genets	
Ketamine + detomidine	K: 4–5 mg/kg + D: 0.05 mg/kg IM [19]	African lions	Free-ranging, immobilization
	K: 6.7–11.4 mg/kg + D: 0.5 mg/kg sprayed into the mouth [14]	Servals and domestic cats	Sedation or sternal or lateral recumbency. Less reliable in producing recumbency in lions. Vomiting, salivation, and sinus bradycardia are common adverse effects of oral detomidine.
Ketamine + dexmedetomidine	K: 5 mg/kg + Dexmed: 0.02 mg/kg IM, antagonize with atipamezole 0.1 mg/kg IM [20]	Cheetahs	
Ketamine + dexmedetomidine + midazolam	K: 3 mg/kg + Dexmed: 0.0125 mg/kg + Mid: 0.1 mg/kg IM [22]	Tigers	n = 30 tigers given either this 3 drug combo or a combination of K: 3 mg/kg + Dexmed: 0.025 mg/kg. In comparison of both combinations no differences were found in any cardiopulmonary variables or other measurements.

(*Continued*)

Drug name	Drug dose	Species	Comments
Ketamine + medetomidine	K: 5 mg/kg + M: 0.08–0.2 mg/kg IM; antagonize with atipamezole 0.16–0.4 mg/kg IM [14, 20].	Lynxes	Immobilization, supplement with ketamine 2.5 mg/kg. In captive adults may be able to use 50% of the dose for both drugs. In kittens 4–5 weeks of age may consider 5 mg/kg ketamine + 0.08 mg/kg medetomidine.
	K: 3–4 mg/kg + 0.08–0.1 mg/kg IM; antagonize with atipamezole 0.12–0.24 mg/kg IM [14].	Golden cats	Immobilization
	K: 2.2 mg/kg + M: 0.043 mg/kg IM; antagonize with atipamezole 0.25 mg/kg 50% IM 50% SC [14].	Cougars	Immobilization
	K: 2 mg/kg + M: 0.075 mg/kg IM; antagonize with 0.3 mg/kg atipamezole [20].	Cougars	Supplement with ketamine 1 mg/kg as needed.
	K: 2.5 mg/kg + M: 0.03 mg/kg IM [1]	Florida panthers	n = 3 animals sedated for wound care postoperatively.
	K: 3–5 mg/kg + M: 0.05 mg/kg IM; antagonize with atipamezole 0.2 mg/kg IM [10, 16].	Cheetahs	n = 7, 6 animals immobilized at least 4 times each during a study of gastritis treatment. 1 cheetah had a fractured front limb that was repaired.
Ketamine + medetomidine versus ketamine medetomidine midazolam	K: 2 mg/kg + M: 0.05 mg/kg IM (KM). K: 2 mg/kg + M: 0.02 mg/kg + mid: 0.1 mg/kg IM (KMM) [23]	Cheetahs	n = 6 clinically healthy cheetah anesthetized twice, once with KM and a 2nd time with KMM protocol to compare mean arterial resistance index (RI) and pulse pressure index (PPI) to characterize differences in kidney blood flow. In the KM protocol mean arterial pressure was significantly higher but did decrease after atipamezole administration. The PPI was significantly lower throughout the procedure with KM, and with both protocols increased significantly after atipamezole administration. Both the higher blood pressure and the reduced PPI with KM were likely a direct effect of the higher medetomidine dosage, and these findings indicate that lower medetomidine dosages might reduce hypertension and lead to a better PPI in cheetah immobilization.

Drug name	Drug dose	Species	Comments
Ketamine + medetomidine	K: 2.5–3 mg/kg + M: 0.05–0.7 mg/kg IM; antagonize with atipamezole 0.3–0.35 mg/kg (may consider 25% IV and 75% SC) [14, 20]	Panthera spp, cheetahs	Immobilization, supplement with ketamine as needed 1.5 mg/kg. The addition of midazolam at 0.1 mg/kg may reduce convulsions or prevent.
	K: 2.5–4.4 mg/kg + M 0.04–0.08 mg/kg IM; antagonize with atipamezole 0.1–0.24 mg/kg IM) [14]	Jaguars	Immobilization
	K: 2.5–3 mg/kg + M: 0.06–0.08 mg/kg IM; antagonize with atipamezole 0.12–0.35 mg/kg IM [14, 20].	Amur leopards, Cheetahs	Immobilization, supplement with ketamine 2 mg/kg. Consider giving antagonist 1/2 IV and 1/2 IM. If recovered >20 min consider atipamezole up to 0.5 mg/kg.
	K: 2.5–3 mg/kg + M: 0.06–0.08 mg/kg IM; antagonize with atipamezole 0.29–0.4 mg/kg IM [14, 20].	Snow leopards	Immobilization, supplementation with ketamine 2 mg/kg. Consider giving antagonist 1/2 IV and 1/2 IM.
	K: 4 mg/kg + M: 0.1 mg/kg IM; antagonize with atipamezole 0.5 mg/kg (1/2 IV and 1/2 IM) [20]	Asian golden cats	
	K: 2–5.7 mg/kg + M: 0.02–0.08 mg/kg IM; antagonize with atipamezole 0.1–0.35 mg/kg IM [14, 20].	African lions	Immobilization. Supplement with ketamine 1.5 mg/kg. Consider giving antagonist 1/2 IV and 1/2 IM.
	K+ 2.5 mg/kg + M: 0.07 mg/kg IM [19, 20]	Jaguars, African lions	
	K: 200 mg + M: 3 mg total per adult tiger; antagonize with atipamezole 15 mg/adult tiger [14, 24].	Tigers	n = 6 adult tigers, Immobilization
	K: 3 mg/kg + M: 0.018 mg/kg IM, antagonize with atipamezole 0.06 mg/kg 50% IM 50% IV [14, 15].	Sumatran tigers	Immobilization
	K: 2.5 mg/kg + M: 0.03–0.1 mg/kg IM; antagonize with atipamezole 0.12–0.24 mg/kg IM [14].	Amur tigers	Immobilization
	K: 2.5 mg/kg + M: 0.1 mg/kg IM; antagonize with atipamezole 0.5 mg/kg IM [20].	Jungle cats	

(*Continued*)

Drug name	Drug dose	Species	Comments
	K: 5–7 mg/kg + M: 0.03–0.05 mg/kg IM; antagonize with atipamezole at 5 × M dose in mg [19]	African lions	Free-ranging, immobilization
Ketamine + medetomidine + butorphanol	K: 2–2.5 mg/kg + M: 0.04 mg/kg + B: 0.15 mg/kg IM; antagonize with atipamezole 0.2 mg/kg IM [14].	Pallas cats	Immobilization
Ketamine + medetomidine + butorphanol	K: 1–3 mg/kg + M: 0.03–0.047 mg/kg + B: 0.2–0.3 mg/kg IM; antagonize with atipamezole 0.15–0.24 mg/kg 50% IV 50% SC or IM [14, 20].	Servals	Immobilization
	K: 0.8–1.2 mg/kg + M: 0.037–0.058 mg/kg + B: 0.17–0.23 mg/kg IM; antagonized with atipamezole 0.185–0.29 mg/kg 50% IV and 50% SC [25]	Servals	n = 7 (3.4) Servals immobilized with combination and resulted in rapid and smooth induction and recoveries. Minimal cardiopulmonary effects were observed.
Ketamine + medetomidine + midazolam	K: 2.5 mg/kg + 0.046 mg/kg + Mid: 0.1 mg/kg IM. Antagonize with atipamezole 0.23 mg/kg IM [14].	Amur tigers	Immobilization
	M: 0.05 mg/kg + Mid: 1 mg/kg IM in single dart, 10 min later K: 2.5 mg/kg IM in dart or pole syringe as needed. Antagonized with atipamezole 0.25 mg/kg IM [26].	Amur Tigers	n = 4.3 captive Siberia/Amur tigers. This protocol required 1 dart and one pole syringe for a total of 9 ml of total drug. No seizures were seen. Tigers demonstrated initial signs 3.6–3.8 min after medetomidine + midazolam. Sternal recumbency was seen 5.6–6.4 min post ketamine administration. Safe handling was possible at 7–9.3 min post ketamine. Total anesthetic period was for 64–80 min. Heart rate was significantly lower 10–30 min post ketamine, hypertension was also seen 30–60 min post ketamine. 4 animals required oxygen supplementation. During recovery, initial signs were seen at 8–12 min, sternal recumbency at 16–20 min, and standing at 19–23 min.

Drug name	Drug dose	Species	Comments
Ketamine + midazolam + xylazine	X: 0.5 mg/kg + Mid: 1 mg/kg IM, 10 min later K: 10 mg/kg IM. After 60 min antagonized with yohimbine 0.11 mg/kg IM [26].	Amur Tigers	n = 4.3 captive Siberian/Amur tigers. This protocol required 3 darts to deliver the 20 ml for induction. 2 animals experienced seizures. Tigers were sternal 3.3–6.3 min after ketamine and laterally recumbent 8 min after ketamine was administered. Animals were safely handled 10–12 min post ketamine and the procedure lasted from 62–89 min. At 20–30 min post ketamine body temperature was increased and 4 animals received cold water enemas. Blood pressure was increased at 30–60 min post ketamine. Initial signs of recovery post yohimbine were seen 10–22 min and were sternal at 18–30 min and standing at 34–46 min post yohimbine.
Ketamine + midazolam	K: 2–2.5 mg/kg + Mid: 0.1–0.15 mg/kg IM [1]	Florida panthers	n = 2 sedation for postoperative wound management.
	K: 5–10 mg/kg + Mid: 0.1–0.3 mg/kg IM; antagonize with flumazenil [15].	Felids	Use in small felids or debilitated cats. Flumazenil may not be necessary.
Ketamine + midazolam + butorphanol	K: 3–5 mg/kg + Mid: 0.1–0.3 mg/kg + B: 0.1–0.4 mg/kg IM; antagonize with flumazenil and naltrexone [15]	Small felids	Use in small felids or debilitated cats. NOT Recommended for healthy large felids. Flumazenil may not be necessary.
Ketamine + xylazine	K: 2.2–2.6 mg/kg + X: 1.1–1.3 mg/kg IM via dart; antagonize with yohimbine 0.1–0.15 mg/kg IM [27]	Asiatic lions, Tigers, Leopards	n = 52 healthy adult lions, 55 adult leopards and 16 adult male tigers. Immobilization.
	K: 3–10 mg/kg + X: 0.3–1 mg/kg IM; antagonize with yohimbine [15]	Felids	May need to use higher doses in small felids
	K: 3–7 mg/kg + X: 1.1–1.7 mg/kg IM [28]	Leopards	n = 55 (27:28) wild nuisance animals caught via blowdart. No adverse reactions were noted for up to 30 days post immobilization. 50–75 mg ketamine was used for supplementation as needed.
	K: 15 mg/kg + X: 1 mg/kg IM [20].	Margays, Ocelots, Jaguarundis	
	K: 15 mg/kg + X: 0.5 mg/kg IM [20].	Servals	

(*Continued*)

Drug name	Drug dose	Species	Comments
	K: 10 mg/kg + X: 2.2 mg/kg [20]	Snow leopards	
	K: 14.7 mg/kg + X: 1.1 mg/kg IM [14].	Ocelots	Immobilization
	K: 4.6 mg/kg + X: 4 mg/kg IM or K: 6.8 mg/kg + X: 0.4 mg/kg IM; antagonize with yohimbine 0.1 mg/kg SC [14].	Lynxes	Immobilization
	K: 10 mg/kg + X: 1.5 mg/kg IM [20].	Lynxes	
	K: 4 mg/kg + X: 4 mg/kg IM, antagonize with yohimbine 0.125 mg/kg [20]	Iberian lynxes	Supplement with ketamine 2 mg/kg as needed.
	K: 10 mg/kg + X: 2 mg/kg IM [20]	Canadian lynxes	
	K: 27.4 mg/kg + X: 1.9 mg/kg IM [14].	Leopard cats	Immobilization
	K: 24.9 mg/kg + X: 1.7 mg/kg IM [14]	Marbled cats	Immobilization
	K: 29.6 mg/kg + X: 2.1 mg/kg [14]	Golden cats	Immobilization
	K: 19–20 mg/kg + X: 1.6–2 mg/kg IM [14, 20]	Clouded leopards	Immobilization
	K: 25 mg/kg + X: 1 mg/kg IM [20].	Black-footed cats, Wild cats	
	K: 25 mg/kg + X: 2 mg/kg IM [20].	Leopard cats, Marbled cats	Supplement with ketamine 12 mg/kg as needed
	K: 5 mg/kg + X: 1 mg/kg IM [13]	Leopards	n = 1 immobilization for surgical repair of a hiatal hernia.
Ketamine + xylazine	K: 8.4–11 mg/kg + X: 1.8–2 mg/kg IM; antagonize with 0.125 mg/kg yohimbine [14, 20, 29].	Cougars	Immobilization
	K: 13.3 mg/kg + X: 1.2 mg/kg IM [14].	Bobcats	Immobilization, females may require as much as 50% more ketamine than males.
	K: 10 mg/kg + X: 1.5 mg/kg [20]	Bobcats	
	K: 10 mg/kg + X: 1 mg/kg IM [20].	Caracals, Cheetahs	
	K: 6.6–10.8 mg/kg + X: 0.66–0.8 mg/kg IM. Supplement with ketamine 1.1 mg/kg IM; antagonize with yohimbine 0.04–0.13 mg/kg IM [14, 20].	Amur tigers	Immobilization

Drug name	Drug dose	Species	Comments
	K: 4–6 mg/kg + X: less than or equal to 0.2 mg/kg IM [14].	Sumatran tigers	Immobilization, doses of greater than 0.2 mg/kg xylazine result in profound respiratory suppression in this species.
	K: 7.7 mg/kg for males or 11.9 mg/kg for females + M: 0.4 mg/kg IM; antagonize with yohimbine 0.05 mg/kg IM [14].	South Chinese tigers	Immobilization
	K: 7–8 mg/kg + X: 3–4 mg/kg IM; antagonize with yohimbine 0.1–0.125 mg/kg IM [14, 20].	African lions	Immobilization
	K: 10 mg/kg + X: 1 mg/kg IM; antagonize with yohimbine 0.1 mg/kg IM [14].	African lions	Immobilization
	K: 450 mg + X: 110 mg IM [30]	African lions	n = 19 adult female lions. When xylazine was 110 mg or >0.9 mg/kg initially this increased the chances of rapid immobilization and did not require supplemental ketamine after the initial dart.
	K: 6.6 mg/kg + X: 0.066 mg/kg IM. Supplement as needed with ketamine 1.1 mg/kg; antagonize with yohimbine 0.04–0.13 mg/kg IM [14].	Amur leopards	Immobilization
	K: 5–10 mg/kg + X: 1–4 mg/kg IM. Supplement with ketamine 50–70 mg/adult [14, 20].	Leopards	Immobilization
	K: 4–6 mg/kg + X: 0.4 mg/kg IM; antagonize with yohimbine 0.05 mg/kg IM. Supplement with ketamine 1 mg/kg or diazepam 0.01–0.05 mg/kg IV slowly, or midazolam 0.01 mg/kg IV [14].	Tigers	Immobilization
	K: 4 mg/kg + X: 2 mg/kg IM [20]	Jaguars	
Ketamine + xylazine	K: 30 mg/kg + X: 0.5 mg/kg IM [20]	Genets	

(*Continued*)

Drug name	Drug dose	Species	Comments
Ketamine + xylazine + midazolam	K: 9.7 mg/kg + X: 0.49 mg/kg + Mid: 0.1 mg/kg IM; antagonize with yohimbine 0.11 mg/kg IM [14].	Tigers	Immobilization
Medetomidine + butorphanol + midazolam	M: 0.03–0.04 mg/kg + B: 0.04–0.4 mg/kg + Mid: 0.1–0.3 mg/kg IM. (Can substitute medetomidine with dexmedetomidine 0.015–0.02 mg/kg); antagonize with atipamezole 0.18 mg/kg + flumazenil 0.006 mg/kg + naltrexone 0.25 mg/kg IM) [14, 15]	Panthera spp., Cheetah	Immobilization. Fully reversible for <40 min procedures in cheetahs. Sudden early arousals after 40–50 min were observed. As such, avoid or use with extreme caution in larger cats. Supplements may be needed for procedures >30 min. Flumazenil may not be needed.
	M: 0.044–0.058 mg/kg + B: 0.28–0.34 mg/kg + Mid: 0.2–0.3 mg/kg IM; antagonize with naltrexone 0.6–0.7 mg/kg + atipamezole 0.23–0.3 mg/kg + flumazenil 0.0025–0.0039 mg/kg IV or SC [31].	African lions	n = 30, 10.20 free-ranging lions. Lateral recumbency was seen in 5–9.5 min. Mild to moderate hypoxemia seen in 4/30 animals. Recovery was smooth and lions were walking within 1–8.5 min.
Ketamine + medetomidine + butorphanol + midazolam	K: 1–2 mg/kg + M: 0.03–0.04 mg/kg + B: 0.1–0.4 mg/kg + Mid: 0.1–0.3 mg/kg IM. Can substitute medetomidine with dexmedetomidine 0.015–0.02 mg/kg); antagonize with atipamezole + naltrexone ± flumazenil [15]	Felids	Ketamine could instead be given IV shortly after induction. May see spontaneous arousal. Flumazenil may not be necessary.
Midazolam	0.08–0.14 mg/kg (15 mg/adult lion or tiger) PO or IM [14]	Tigers, Lions	Used for premedication or as part of induction protocols
Perphenazine enanthate	3 mg/kg deep IM [14, 32]	Cheetahs	n = 9 captive cheetah, Given perphenazine enanthate or zuclopenthixol acetate or both. The latter two combinations produced ataxia, anorexia, extra pyramidal signs, akathisia, and ptosis. The former alone did not have any appreciable side effects and produced good tranquilization. Perphenazine significantly reduced cats' behavior for 1–6 days. Normal behavior by 14 days post administration. Zuclopenthixol is not recommended for cheetah.

Drug name	Drug dose	Species	Comments
Propofol	1–2 mg/kg IV [14]		For facilitating endotracheal intubation after induction or to provide additional relaxation for a short procedure such as a bandage change. Apnea, cardiovascular effects and risk of rapid, full recovery of a dangerous animal are potential disadvantages.
Saffan (9 mg/ml Alphaxolone + 3 mg/ml alphadolone)	5 ml IV [14]	Panthera spp., Cheetahs	
Telazol	Telazol is NOT approved for use in tigers [14].	Telazol results in prolonged recoveries compared to other drugs in felids.	Tigers: While early literature reporting neurological signs, behavior changes or death in tigers led to the dogma that Telazol was contraindicated, recent reexamination of literature suggests that while adverse effects may occur, scientific literature may not support its contraindication. However the author cannot recommend its use as it is unclear what legal repercussions would be if adverse effects were noted.
Telazol	T: 3 mg/kg + Z: 1.5 mg/kg IM [1]	Florida panthers	n = 1 animal, sedation for postoperative wound management
Telazol	1.6–4.2 or up to 11 mg/kg in small felids IM [15]	Felids	Prolonged recoveries. Use with caution or avoid in tigers.
Telazol	3.8–6.6 mg/kg IM [11]	Cheetahs	n = 6 animals immobilized at least 3 times each during a study of gastritis treatment.
Telazol and flumazenil versus sarmazenil	4 mg/kg IM [20]	Cheetahs	In a few cases cheetah have stopped breathing 60–90 min post Telazol administration and they do not respond to doxapram.
Telazol and flumazenil versus sarmazenil	T: 4.2 mg/kg IM; antagonized with no reversal, flumazenil 0.03 mg/kg IM or sarmazenil 0.1 mg/kg IM 30 min after Telazol administration [33]	Cheetahs	n = 4 cheetah immobilized 3 times 14 days apart. The initial anesthesia was without reversal, the second with flumazenil and the third with sarmazenil. Both reversals significantly shortened the duration of recovery and excitation during recovery. Neither were significantly more efficacious and both can be recommended.

(*Continued*)

Drug name	Drug dose	Species	Comments
Telazol	8.2–15 mg/kg IM [34]	Leopard cats, Clouded leopards, Asiatic golden cats, Marbled cats	n = 28 free-ranging cats immobilized with Telazol and 25 cats immobilized with ketamine 22–31 mg/kg + xylazine 1.46–2.32 mg/kg IM and compared for safety and efficacy. Overall increased dose was correlated with decreased induction time and increased duration of working time but was not correlated with recovery time. Both proved to be efficacious and safe but Telazol is preferred due to decreased volume, faster induction and the lack of muscle rigidity during anesthesia.
	12 mg/kg IM [20]	Marbled cats	Supplement with ketamine 12 mg/kg as needed
	5.5 mg/kg [14]	Ocelots	Immobilization
Telazol	4.4 mg/kg IM [20]	Fishing cats, Asian golden cats	Supplement with ketamine 4.4 mg/kg as needed.
	5 mg/kg IM [14, 20]	Lynxes, Ocelots, Servals, Black-footed cats, Jungle cats, Pampas cats, Wild cats, Genets, Jaguars	Immobilization, supplement as needed with ketamine 2–5 mg/kg.
	4–11.6 mg/kg [14]	Leopard cats	Immobilization
	10 mg/kg [14, 20]	Clouded leopards	Immobilization, supplement with 5 mg/kg ketamine
	1.6–3.6 mg/kg [14]	Panthera spp., Cheetahs, not approved in Tigers	Light anesthesia
	2–7.8 mg/kg [14]	Panthera spp., Cheetahs, not approved in Tigers	Above 3.5 mg/kg deeper anesthesia
	10 mg/kg IM [20]	Bobcats	Supplement with 5 mg/kg ketamine as needed
	4 mg/kg IM [20]	Geoffrey cats, Snow leopards	
	6.6 mg/kg IM [20]	Leopards, Caracals, Jaguarundis	Leopards tend to fight rather than flee so approach cautiously. In Caracal consider supplementing 6.6 mg/kg ketamine as needed. In Jaguarundi 3.3 mg/kg ketamine as needed.

Drug name	Drug dose	Species	Comments
	8 mg/kg IM [20]	Spotted cats	Supplement with ketamine 4 mg/kg as needed.
	8.8 mg/kg [20]	Margays	Supplement as needed with ketamine up to 8.8 mg/kg.
	4–6 mg/kg IM [14, 20]	African lions	Immobilization
Telazol + ketamine	T: 0.6–2.5 mg/kg + K: 4–15.5 mg/kg IM [14].	Cougars	Immobilization
Telazol + ketamine + xylazine	Reconstitute Telazol by adding 400 mg (4 ml) ketamine and 100 mg xylazine (1 ml) for a total of 109 mg/ml of the drug combination with 0.18 mg/ml Telazol + 0.73 mg/ml ketamine + 0.18 mg/ml xylazine. Use 0.023 mg/kg IM in Cheetah; antagonize with 0.1–0.2 mg/kg yohimbine [14].	Panthera spp., Cheetahs, not approved in Tigers	Immobilization
Telazol + ketamine + xylazine	A solution of T: 50 mg/ml + K: 80 mg/ml + X: 20 mg/ml was created and each animal was given 0.03–0.026 ml/kg IM; antagonized with yohimbine [35].	Cheetahs	n = 13 captive cheetah in 32 procedures. Anesthesias were safe with predictable working times, good muscle relaxation and analgesia.
Telazol + medetomidine	T: 0.38–1.32 mg/kg + M: 0.027–0.055 mg/kg IM; antagonize with atipamezole 2.5–5 × the mg of medetomidine used [19, 36].	African lions	n = 17 animals free-ranging subadults, 5.12, 1.5–112 kg, smooth induction and recovery, induced in 3.4–9.5 min, 1 hr working time, no additional drugs needed, walking in 8–26 min when <1 mg/kg Telazol used.
	T: 0.6–1.0 mg/kg + M 0.015–0.025 mg/kg; antagonize with atipamezole [14]	African lions	Immobilization, repeat Telazol dosage at 45 min as needed
	T: 0.08 mg/kg + M: 0.02 mg/kg; antagonize with atipamezole [14].	Amur Tigers	Telazol is NOT approved for use in tigers. While early literature reporting neurological signs, behavior changes or death in tigers led to the dogma that Telazol was contraindicated, recent reexamination of literature suggests that while adverse effects may occur, scientific literature may not support its contraindication. However, the author cannot recommend its use as it is unclear what legal repercussions would be, if adverse effects were noted.

(*Continued*)

Drug name	Drug dose	Species	Comments
	T: 0.5 mg/kg + M: 0.05 mg/kg IM; antagonize with atipamezole [14].	Lynxes	Immobilization
Telazol + medetomidine + propofol or isoflurane	T: 1.2 mg.kg + M: 0.04 mg/kg IM, supplemented with either propofol CRI 0.1 mg/kg/min or isoflurane 1% [37]	Cheetahs	n = 24 adult captive cheetah divided randomly, Both protocols provided acceptable and expected cardiopulmonary values, but propofol resulted in prolonged recovery making it likely unsuitable for long-term anesthesia.
Telazol + medetomidine	T: 1.3–2.3 mg/kg + M: 0.06–0.08 mg/kg IM; antagonize with atipamezole 0.2–0.4 mg/kg IM [19, 20, 38]	African lions	n = 6 free-ranging, Smooth induction in 8–20 min, mild hypoxia, one animal treated for bradypnea, recoveries uneventful, No mortalities during 18 month follow-up.
	T: 2 mg/kg + M: 0.02 mg/kg [20]	Snow leopards	A researcher had good anecdotal success by adding 5 ml of 1 mg/ml medetomidine to a vial of Telazol and administered 0.8 ml to each leopard.
Telazol + romifidine + atropine	T: 2.8–4 mg/kg + R: 0.033–0.047 mg/kg + A: 0.023–0.037 mg/kg IM [39]	Ocelots	n = 8 captive adults, 5.3, protocol produced good immobilization in ocelots with minimal changes over time in cardiovascular parameters.
Telazol + xylazine	T: 5 mg/kg + X: 1 mg/kg IM; antagonize with 0.125 mg/kg yohimbine [20].	Cougars, Little spotted cats	Supplement with ketamine 5 mg/kg as needed in little spotted cats
Xylazine + atropine sulfate	X: 0.5 mg/kg + A: 0.005 mg/kg IM + isoflurane via facemask [40]	Pallas cats	n = 1 captive kitten with neurologic signs, prior to MRI. Propofol 1.5 mg/ml in saline given one drip every 3–5 sec was supportive. The animal had toxoplasmosis and died 2 days later.
Yohimbine	Y: 5–15 mg/adult used to reverse 50–150 mg dose of xylazine [41]	Bengal tigers	n = 6 animals immobilized 5 times each at 2 week intervals with various doses of ketamine + xylazine. Overall yohimbine was effective and resulted in recoveries of 4–6 min versus >60 min when it was not used.

Drug name	Drug dose	Species	Comments
Zuclopenthixol acetate	0.6 mg/kg – not recommended [14, 32]	Cheetahs	n = 9 captive cheetah, Given perphenazine enanthate or zuclopenthixol acetate or both. The latter two combinations produced ataxia, anorexia, extra pyramidal signs, akathisia, and ptosis. The former alone did not have any appreciable side effects and produced good tranquilization. Perphenazine significantly reduced cats' behavior for 1–6 days. Normal behavior by 14 days post administration. Zuclopenthixol is not recommended for cheetah.
	1 mg/kg IM [20]	African lions	
	70 mg adult male, 50 mg adult female [20]	Leopards	
Antiparasitic			
Atropine sulfate + Celostone anti-inflammatory ophthalmic solution	Subconjunctival injection [40]	Pallas cats	n = 1 cat with recurrent anterior uveitis believed secondary to toxoplasma recrudescence that resolved after two injections when clindamycin 25 mg/kg IM BID for 7 days was added during 2nd treatment.
Atropine sulfate + 1% prednisolone acetate ophthalmic suspension + oral clindamycin	Topically given q8 hrs with oral clindamycin 15 mg/kg PO BID × 16d [40]	Pallas cats	n = 1 cat with anterior uveitis during quarantine likely due to toxoplasmosis recrudescence that was successful in stopping clinical signs.
Clindamycin	25 mg/kg IM BID × 7d [40]	Pallas cats	n = 1 cat with recurrent anterior uveitis believed secondary to toxoplasma recrudescence that resolved after two injections when clindamycin was added during 2nd treatment. A second animal with depression and tachypnea was started on clindamycin and died within 24 hrs.
	25 mg/kg PO SID 1 week prior and 1 week after 3 sets of kitten vaccines [40]	Pallas cats	n = 1 kitten, in a collection with many previous juvenile deaths due to toxoplasmosis, given to prevent stress associated with vaccinations leading to clinical signs associated with disease.

(*Continued*)

Drug name	Drug dose	Species	Comments
Fenbendazole	5 mg/kg PO × 5d [42]	Cheetahs	n = 41 captive cheetah, 61 samples 49% positive for Ancylostoma spp., Cystoisospora spp. and Toxascaris leonina. Post treatment all nematodes were cleared, 2 enclosures still had mild cystoisospora present.
Metronidazole + clindamycin	M: 20 mg/kg PO SID × 5d + C: 25 mg/kg IM SID × 14d [40]	Pallas cats	n = 2 kittens with neurologic signs suspected due to toxoplasmosis and also positive for Giardia cysts.
Praziquantel + pyrantel	Use with extreme caution [43]	Cheetahs	n = 16 retrospective case study of animals affected with adverse reactions, and 27 non affected cheetahs who received a combination of praziquantel + pyrantel. 3 reactions were fatal, with the remaining mild to severe. No differences in dose were noted between affected and not affected. No sex predilection occurred but affected cheetah were younger than not for some facilities.
Other			
Alprazolam	0.019 mg/kg PO BID × 42d [4]		n = 1 animal given antianxiety/ sedation trazadone for 6 days after surgery to stifle osteochondritis dissecans, then added alprazolam.
Calcium glubionate	19 mg/kg PO BID [2]	Lynxes	n = 1, 19 kg animal, postoperative treatment after surgical repair of a hiatal hernia.
Cimetidine	1 mg/kg PO TID [2]	Lynxes	n = 1, 19 kg animal, postoperative treatment after surgical repair of a hiatal hernia.
Cinitapride (Cinitiprida)	1 mg PO BID [44]	African lions	n = 1 animal post balloon dilation of esophageal stricture, combined with sucralfate and omeprazole for 30 days
Deslorelin	3–12 mg [45]	Black footed cats, Cheetahs, Leopards	n = 1, 1.0 black footed cat received 3 mg – for 3–4 mo had decreased sperm production, libido and aggression. 4.8 cheetah and 0.1 leopard received 6 mg and males did not have sperm production at 82 days. 0.2 lionesses received 12 mg and returned to estrus 18 months later.

Drug name	Drug dose	Species	Comments
Deslorelin	Cheetah and leopards 6 mg, Lions 12 or 15 mg implants [45]	Cheetahs, African lionesses, and Leopards	n = 31 cheetah (18.13), 10 lion females, and 4 leopards (1 : 3). Deslorelin implants were placed and no adverse side effects were noted. In lions the implant prevented pregnancy for 12–18 months and in the other 2 species for a minimum of 12 months. 21 months after implant, 2 cheetah males still had no live spermatozoa. It is important to remember males are fertile for up to 6 weeks after implant placement and should be kept separate from cycling females during this time.
Doramectin toxicity	Toxicity seen at 0.2–0.5 mg/kg SC once	African lions [46]	n = 10 animals post administration exhibited ataxia, hallucinations, and mydriasis. 2/8 died, the rest responded to supportive therapy and recovered after 4–5 days.
GnRH analogue (Receptal)	0.75 ml IM [47]	Asiatic golden cats	n = 1 animal given drug IM during an artificial insemination procedure to attempt to induce ovulation. 84 days later twin cubs were produced.
Omeprazole	1 mg/kg PO SID × 7d [2]	Cougars	n = 1, 30 kg animal, postoperative treatment after surgical repair of a hiatal hernia.
	40 mg PO SID × 30d [44]	African lions	n = 1 animal post balloon dilation of esophageal stricture, combined with sucralfate and cinitapride for 30 days
Platelet-rich plasma	4–8 ml given intra-articular per affected knee [4]	Snow leopards	n = 2 animals treated after surgery for osteochondritis dissecans.
Porcine Zona Pellucida vaccine	Over 6 wk period: 3 injections of 65μg/pZP with Freunds complete (FCA) or incomplete adjuvant or carbopol [48]	African lions, Asian leopards, Jaguars, Tigers, Snow leopards, Cougars, Siberian lynxes, Canadian lynxes, Servals, Bobcats	n = 27 captive animals, High incidence of injection site reaction with FCA: swelling, lameness or abscessation in five cats; increased irritability and aggression seen in 4 cats; six evaluated for antibodies and all produced antibodies, 2 for greater than 12 mo, All ovariohysterectomized 3–13 mo later and no histopathologic evidence of damage to ovaries, folliculogenesis present in all, and 2/3 females housed with males became pregnant during the study.

(*Continued*)

Drug name	Drug dose	Species	Comments
Probiotic containing Lactobacillus Group 2 and Enterococcus faecium	1 ml PO in food daily of prepared probiotic [49]	Cheetahs	n = 27 juvenile captive cheetahs, with diarrhea, ± mucus and blood, given species specific probiotic for 28 days. Treated cheetahs had significant weight gain and somewhat improved fecal quality with the discontinuation of blood and mucus.
Ranitidine	1.6 mg/kg PO BID [2]	Lynxes	n = 1, 19 kg animal, postoperative treatment after surgical repair of a hiatal hernia.
Sucralfate	1 g PO BID [13]	Leopards	n = 1 postoperative treatment after surgical repair of a hiatal hernia.
	1 g PO BID [44]	African lions	n = 1 animal post balloon dilation of esophageal stricture, combined with cinitapride and omeprazole for 30 days.
	250 mg PO TID [2]	Lynxes	n = 1, 19 kg animal, postoperative treatment after surgical repair of a hiatal hernia.
Tetracosactide (ACTH stimulation test)	500 μg [50]	Cheetahs	n = 8 animals give the medication then tested for ACTH stimulation response. Revealed serum evaluation at 120–180 min is ideal for seeing maximum adrenal stimulation in this species.
Trazodone	7.6 mg/kg PO BID × 6d [4]	Snow leopards	n = 1 animal given anti-anxiety/sedation after surgery for stifle osteochondritis dissecans, Treated for 6 days then increased to 11.4 mg/kg BID × 30d and added alprazolam 0.019 mg/kg PO BID × 42d.
Vincristine	0.2 mg intralesional into a tumor [51]	Pumas	n = 1, 14 year old male puma with right ear pinna tumor. Systemic vincristine 0.5 mg/m^2 iv q7d for 6 treatments and prednisone 2 mg/kg IM q72 hrs for 7 days lead to vomiting, weight loss, and alopecia and did not improve tumor size. So intralesional vincristine 0.2 mg was given q7d for 2 treatments and resulted in complete tumor regression.

Species	Weight
Bobcat *(Felis rufus)*	4–15.3 kg
Black-footed cat *(Felis nigripes)*	1.5–2.75 kg
Cheetah *(Acinonyx jubatus)*	35–72 kg
Fishing cat *(Felis viverina)*	7–14 kg
Flat-headed cat *(Felis planiceps)*	1.6–2.1 kg
Geoffreys cat *(Felis geoffroyi)*	3–9 kg
Genet *(Genetta spp.)*	1–3 kg
Asian Golden cat *(Felis tommincki)*	12–15 kg
Jungle cat *(Felis chaus)*	4–16 kg
Leopard *(Panthera pardus)*	50–80 kg
Leopard cat *(Felis bengalensis)*	2–5 kg
Little spotted cat *(Leopardus tigrinus)*	1.5–3 kg
Marbled cat *(Felis marmorata)*	1.4–5 kg
Pampas cat *(Felis manul)*	3–7 kg
Spotted cat *(Felis tigrina)*	1.75–2.75 kg
Wild cat *(Felis sylvestris)*	3–8 kg
Clouded leopard *(Neofelis nebulosa)*	10–20 kg
Snow leopard *(Panthera uncia)*	25–75 kg
African lion *(Panthera leo)*	100–250 kg
Cougar *(Felis concolor)*	30–75 kg
European lynx *(Felis lynx)*	8–38 kg
Iberian lynx *(Felis pardina)*	10–12 kg
Margay *(Felis tiedii)*	2.6–3.4 kg
Ocelot *(Felis pardalis)*	11–16 kg
Serval *(Felis serval)*	8–18 kg
Tiger *(Panthera tigris)*	Female: 100–160 kg, Male: 140–300 kg
Caracal *(Felis caracal)*	13–19 kg
Jaguar *(Panthera onca)*	64–114 kg
Jaguarundi *(Felis yagouaroundi)*	4.5–9 kg

References

1 Au Yong, J.A., Lewis, D.D., Citino, S.B. et al. (2018). Surgical Management of appendicular long-bone fractures in free-ranging Florida panthers (*Puma concolor coryi*): Six cases (2000–2014). *Journal of Zoo and Wildlife Medicine* 49 (1): 162–171.

2 Hettlich, B.F., Hobson, H.P., Ducote, J. et al. (2010). Esophageal hiatal hernia in three exotic felines (*Lynx lynx, Puma concolore, Panthera leo*). *Journal of Zoo and Wildlife Medicine* 41 (1): 90–94.

3 McCain, S., Ramsay, E., Allender, M.C. et al. (2009). Pyometra in captive large felids: a review of eleven cases. *Journal of Zoo and Wildlife Medicine* 40 (1): 147–151.

4 Huckins, G.L., Chinnadurai, S.K., Ivancic, M. et al. (2018). Osteochondral autograft transfer for treatment of Stifle osteochondritis dissecans in two related snow leopards (*Panthera uncia*). *Journal of Zoo and Wildlife Medicine* 49 (3): 788–793.

5 Devesa-Garcia, V., Baneres-De la Torre, A., Cabezas-Salamanca, M.A. et al. (2016). Surgical correction of traumatic patellar luxation in a Eurasian lynx (*Lynx lynx*). *Journal of Zoo and Wildlife Medicine* 47 (3): 890–894.

6 Flaminio, K., Christensen, J.M., Alshahrani, S.M. et al. (2018). *Proceedings of the Annual American Association of Zoo Veterinarians*. 143.

7 Steel, J., Schumacher, J., Seibert, R. et al. (2012). Cefovecin (Convenia) for the treatment of septic peritonitis in a female lion (*Panthera leo*). *Journal of Zoo and Wildlife Medicine* 43 (3): 678–681.

8 Newkirk, K.M., Beard, L.K., Sun, X. et al. (2017). Investigation of enrofloxacin-associated retinal toxicity in nondomestic felids. *Journal of Zoo and Wildlife Medicine* 48 (2): 518–520.

9 Storms, T.N., Clyde, V.C., Munson, L. et al. (2003). Blastomycosis in nondomestic felids. *Journal of Zoo and Wildlife Medicine* 34 (3): 231–238.

10 Lane, E., Lobetti, R., and Burroughs, R. (2004). Treatment with omeprazole, metronidazole, and amoxicillin in captive South African cheetahs (*Acinonyx jubatus*) with spiral bacteria infection and gastritis. *Journal of Zoo and Wildlife Medicine* 35 (1): 15–19.

11 Wack, R.F., Eaton, K.A., and Kramer, L.W. (1997). Treatment of gastritis in cheetahs (*Acinonyx jubatus*). *Journal of Zoo and Wildlife Medicine* 28 (3): 260–266.

12 Citino, S.B. and Munson, L. (2005). Efficacy and long-term outcome of gastritis therapy in cheetahs (*Acinonyx jubatus*). *Journal of Zoo and Wildlife Medicine* 36 (3): 401–416.

13 Kearns, K.S., Jones, M.P., Bright, R.M. et al. (2000). Hiatal hernia and diaphragmatic eventration in a leopard (*Panthera pardus*). *Journal of Zoo and Wildlife Medicine* 31 (3): 379–382.

14 Ramsay, E.C. (2014). Felids. In: *Zoo Animal and Wildlife Immobilization and Anesthesia*, 2e (ed. G. West, D. Heard and N. Caulkett), 635–646. Ames, IA: Wiley Blackwell.

15 Lamberski, N. (2015). Felidae. In: *Fowler's Zoo and Wild Mammal Medicine* (ed. R.E. Miller and M. Fowler), 467–475. St. Louis, MO: Elsevier.

16 Kimeli, P., Mogoa, E.M., Mwangi, W.E. et al. (2014). Use of brachial plexus blockade and medetomidine-ketamine-isoflurane anaesthesia for repair of radio-ulna fracture in an adult cheetah (*Acinonyx jubatus*). *BMC Veterinary Research* 10: 249.

17 Leclerc, A., Decambron, A., Commere, C. et al. (2018). Laparoscopic ovariectomy with a single-port multiple-access device in seven African lionesses (*Panthera leo*). *Journal of the American Veterinary Medical Association* 252 (12): 1548–1554.

18 Steeil, J.C., Sura, P.A., Ramsay, E.C. et al. (2012). Laparoscopic-assisted ovariectomy of tigers (*Panthera tigris*) with the use of the LigaSure device. *Journal of Zoo and Wildlife Medicine* 43 (3): 566–572.

19 Buss, P. and Miller, M. (2019). Update on Field Anesthesia Protocols for Free-ranging African lions. In: *Fowler's Zoo and Wild Animal Medicine Current Therapy*, vol. 9 (ed. R.E. Miller, N. Lamberski and P.P. Calle), 533–538. St. Louis, MO: Elsevier Saunders.

20 Kreeger, T.J. and Arnemo, J.M. (2012). *Handbook of Wildlife Chemical Immobilization*. China: Kreeger.

21 Woc Colburn, A.M., Murray, S., Hayek, L.C. et al. (2017). Cardiorespiratory effects of dexmedetomidine-butorphanol-midazolam (DBM): A fully reversible anesthetic protocol in captive and semi-free-ranging cheetahs (*Acinonyx jubatus*). *Journal of Zoo and Wildlife Medicine* 48 (1): 40–47.

22 Clark-Prince, S.C., Lascola, K.M., and Shaeffer, D.J. (2015). Physiological and biochemical variables in captive tigers (*Panthera tigris*) immobilised with dexmedetomidine and ketamine or dexmedetomidine, midazolam and ketamine. *Veterinary Record* 177 (22): 570.

23 Stagegaard, J., Horlyck, A., Hydeskoy, H.B. et al. (2017). Ketamine=Medetomidine and Ketamine-Medetomidine-Midazolam anesthesia in captive cheetahs (*Acinonyx jubatus*) comparison of blood pressure and kidney blood flow. *Journal of Zoo and Wildlife Medicine* 48 (2): 363–370.
24 Miller, M., Wever, M., Neiffer, D. et al. (2003). Anesthetic induction of captive tigers (*Panthera tigris*) using a medetomidine-ketamine combination. *Journal of Zoo and Wildlife Medicine* 34 (3): 307–308.
25 Langan, J.N., Schumacher, J., Pollock, C. et al. (2000). Cardiopulmonary and anesthetic effects of medetomidine-ketamine-butorphanol and antagonism with atipamezole in servals (*Felis serval*). *Journal of Zoo and Wildlife Medicine* 31 (3): 329–334.
26 Curro, T.G., Okeson, D., Zimmerman, D. et al. (2004). Xylazine-midazolam-ketamine versus medetomidine-midazolam-ketamine anesthesia in captive Siberian tigers (*Panthera tigris altaica*). *Journal of Zoo and Wildlife Medicine* 35 (3): 320–327.
27 Sontakke, S.D., Umapathy, G., and Shivaji, S. (2009). Yohimbine antagonizes the anesthetic effects of ketamine-xylazine in captive Indian wild felids. *Veterinary anesthesia and analgesia* 36: 34–41.
28 Belsare, A.V. and Athreca, V.R. (2010). Use of xylazine hydrochloride-ketamine hydrochloride for immobilization of wild leopards (*Panthera pardus fusca*) in emergency situations. *Journal of Zoo and Wildlife Medicine* 41 (2): 331–333.
29 Logan, K.A., Thorne, E.T., Irwin, L.L. et al. (1986). Immobilizing wild mountain lions (*Felis concolor*) with ketamine hydrochloride and xylazine hydrochloride. *Journal of Wildlife Diseases* 22 (1): 97–103.
30 Herbst, L.H., Packer, C., and Seal, U.S. (1985). Immobilization of free-ranging African lions (Panthera leo) with a combination of xylazine hydrochloride and ketamine hydrochloride. *Journal of Wildlife Diseases* 21 (4): 401–404.
31 Wenger, S., Buss, P., Joubert, J. et al. (2010). Evaluation of butorphanol, medetomidine, and midazolam as a reversible narcotic combination in free-ranging African lions (*Panthera leo*). *Veterinary Anesthesia and Analgesia* 37 (6): 491–500.
32 Huber, C., Walzer, C., and Slotta-Bachmayr, L. (2001). Evaluation of long-term sedation in cheetah (*Acinonyx jubatus*) with perphenazineenanthate and zuclopenthixol acetate. *Journal of Zoo and Wildlife Medicine* 32 (3): 329–335.
33 Walzer, C. and Huber, C. (2002). Partial antagonism of tiletamine-zolazepam anesthesia in cheetah. *Journal of Wildlife Diseases* 38 (2): 468–472.
34 Grassman, L.I., Austin, S.C., Tewes, M.E. et al. (2014). Comparative immobilization of wild felids in Thailand. *Journal of Wildlife Diseases* 40 (3): 575–578.
35 Lewandowski, A.H., Bonar, C.J., and Evans, S.E. (2002). Tiletamine-zolazepam, ketamine, and xylazine anesthesia of captive cheetah (*Acinonyx jubatus*). *Journal of Zoo and Wildlife Medicine* 33 (4): 332–336.
36 Fahlman, A., Loveridge, A., Wenham, C. et al. (2005). Reversible anaesthesia of free-ranging lions (*Panthera leo*) in Zimbabwe. *Journal of the South African Veterinary Association* 76 (4): 187–192.
37 Buck, R.K., Tordiffe, A.S.W., and Zeiler, G.E. (2017). Cardiopulmonary effects of anaesthesia maintained by propofol infusion versus isoflurane inhalation in cheetahs (*Acinonyx jubatus*). *Veterinary Anesthesia and Analgesia* 44: 1363–1372.
38 Jacquier, M., Aarhaug, P., Arnemo, J.M. et al. (2006). Reversible immobilization of free-ranging African lions (*Panthera leo*) with medetomidine-tiletamine-zolazepam and atipamezole. *Journal of Wildlife Diseases* 42 (2): 432–436.
39 Selmi, A.L., Figueiredo, J.P., Mendes, G.M. et al. (2004). Effects of tiletamine/zolazepam-romifidine-atropine in ocelots (*Leopardus pardalis*). *Veterinary Anesthesia and Analgesia* 31: 222–226.

40 Kenny, D.E., Lappin, M.R., Knightly, F. et al. (2002). Toxoplasmosis in Pallas' cats (*Otocolobus felis manul*) at the Denver Zoological Gardens. *Journal of Zoo and Wildlife Medicine* 33 (2): 131–138.

41 Seal, U.S., Armstrong, D.L., and Simmons, L.G. (1987). Yohimbine hydrochloride reversal of ketamine hydrochloride and xylazine hydrochloride immobilization of Bengal tigers and effects on hematology and serum chemistries. *Journal of Zoo and Wildlife Medicine* 23 (2): 296–300.

42 Meny, M., Schmidt-Kunzel, A., and Marker, L.L. (2012). Diagnosis-based treatment of helminths in captive and wild cheetahs (*Acinonyx jubatus*). *Journal of Zoo and Wildlife Medicine* 43 (4): 934–938.

43 Whitehouse-Tedd, K., Smith, L., Budd, J.A. et al. (2017). Suspected adverse reactions to oral administration of a praziquantle-pyrantel combination in captive cheetahs (*Acinonyx jubatus*). *Journal of the American Veterinary Medical Association* 251 (10): 1188–1195.

44 Ayala, I., Laredo, F., Escobar, M.T. et al. (2018). Benign Idiopathic Esophageal Stricture in a Lion (*Panthera leo*): Dilation by an achalasia balloon. *Journal of Zoo and Wildlife Medicine* 49 (1): 193–195.

45 Bertschinger, H.J., Trigg, T.E., Jochle, W. et al. (2002). Induction of contraception in some African wild carnivores by downregulation of LH and FSH secretion using the GnRH analogue deslorelin. *Reproduction Suppliment* 60: 41–52.

46 Lobetti, R.G. and Caldwell, P. (2012). Doramectin toxicity in a group of lions (*Panthera leo*). *Journal of the South African Veterinary Association* 83 (1): 509.

47 Lueders, I., Ludwig, C., Schroeder, M. et al. (2014). Successful nonsurgical artificial insemination and hormonal monitoring in an asiatic golden cat (*Catopima temminicki*). *Journal of Zoo and Wildlife Medicine* 45 (2): 372–379.

48 Harrenstien, L.A., Munson, L., Chassy, L.M. et al. (2004). Effects of Porcine Zona Pellucida Immunocontraceptives in Zoo Felids. *Journal of Zoo and Wildlife Medicine* 35 (3): 271–279.

49 Koeppel, K.N., Bertschinger, H., van Vuuren, M. et al. (2006). The use of a probiotic in captive cheetahs (*Acinonyx jubatus*). *Journal of the South African Veterinary Association* 77 (3): 127–130.

50 Koster, L.S., Shoeman, J.P., and Meltzer, D.G. (2007). ACTH stimulation test in the captive cheetah (*Acinonyx jubatus*). *Journal of the South African Veterinary Association* 78 (3): 133–136.

51 Sandoval, B.J., Amat, A.C., Sabri, J. et al. (2013). Intralesional vincristine use for treatment of squamous cell carcinoma in a puma (*Puma concolor*). *Journal of Zoo and Wildlife Medicine* 44 (4): 1059–1062.

14

Whales and Dolphins

Drug name	Drug dose	Species	Comments
Antimicrobials and Antifungals			
Amikacin	16.4 mg/kg IM SID, or 7.7 mg/kg IM BID [1]	Belugas	To treat nocardiosis.
	14 mg/kg IM SID or 7 mg/kg IM BID [1]	Small odontocetes, Bottlenose dolphins	
	4.8 mg/kg BID; 7.5–12 mg/kg SID [1, 2]	Killer whales	
	5.8 mg/kg BID [1]	Short-finned pilot whales	
	5000 mg Amikacin mixed with 20 ml sterile saline nebulized SID to BID in 2500 kg animal [2]	Killer whales	
Amoxicillin	2.5–5 mg/kg PO BID [1]	Killer whales, Bottlenose dolphins	
	10 mg/kg PO BID [2]	Killer whales	
	22 mg/kg PO BID [2]	Bottlenose dolphins	
Amoxicillin/clavulanic acid	5–10 mg/kg PO BID [1]	Small odontocetes	
	5–7 mg/kg PO BID [1, 2]	Killer whales	
	10–22 mg/kg PO BID [1, 2]	Beluga whales	
Amphotercin B	1–2 mg/kg PO Sid or liposomal, or microcapsulated, or 2.5 g total dose	Bottlenose dolphins	Liposomal for treatment of zygomycosis; does not have to be liposomal.
Ampicillin	2.25–10 mg/kg PO BID [1]	Killer whales	
Ampicillin/Sulbactam (Unasyn)	10 mg/kg BID [2]	Bottlenose dolphins	
Azithromycin	2.7 mg/kg Loading dose PO once, 1.7 mg/kg maintenance PO BID [1, 2]	Killer whales	

(*Continued*)

Zoo and Wild Mammal Formulary, First Edition. Alicia Hahn.

Drug name	Drug dose	Species	Comments
	6.7 mg/kg loading dose PO, 3.7 mg/kg maintenance PO [1]	Killer whales	Caused anorexia and abdominal discomfort in Beluga calves.
	9.6 mg/kg Loading dose PO once, 5.3 mg/kg PO SID [1]	Small odontocetes	
Carbenicillin	11 mg/kg TID [1]	Killer whales	
	22–44 mg/kg TID [1]	Bottlenose dolphins	
Cefadroxil	11 mg/kg BID [2]	Killer whales	
	22 mg/kg BID [2]	Bottlenose and Commerson's dolphins	
Cefovecin		Bottlenose dolphins	>99% protein-binding levels so likely has an extended duration of action [3].
Cefovecin	8 mg/kg IM [4]	Bottlenose dolphins	Doses evaluated in adult and neonatal dolphins. Plasma concentrations in adults were over MIC 90 for 17 days. For neonatal animals at 8 mg/kg, values stayed over MIC90 for 13 days. However, at 16 mg/kg they were elevated for 17 days.
Cefpodoxime	10 mg/kg PO SID [2]	Bottlenose dolphins	
Ceftazidime	20 mg/kg IM SID [2]	Killer whales, Bottlenose dolphins	
Ceftiofur crystalline-free acid (Excede)	6.6 mg/kg q5–7d [2]	Bottlenose dolphins	
Ceftriaxone	20 mg/kg IM SID [1]	Small odontocetes, Bottlenose dolphins, Beluga whales	
Cefuroxime	20 mg/kg PO BID [1]	Small odontocetes, Bottlenose dolphins, Beluga whales	
	10 mg/kg BID [1]	Killer whales	
	25 mg/kg BID [1]	Commerson's dolphins	
Cephalexin monohydrate	22 mg/kg PO TID [1, 2]	Small odontocetes, Bottlenose and Commerson's dolphins	
	11 mg/kg PO TID [1]	Killer whales	
	15 mg/kg PO TID [1]	Short-finned pilot and Beluga whales	

Drug name	Drug dose	Species	Comments
	33 mg/kg PO TID [1]	Commerson's dolphins	
Cephloridine	6.6 mg/kg IT [1]		
Chloramphenicol	22 mg/kg PO BID [1]		
Ciprofloxacin	8–13 mg/kg PO BID [1]	Killer whales	
	15–29 mg/kg PO BID [1]	Bottlenose dolphins	
	6–9 mg/kg PO BID [1]	Beluga whales	
Clarithromycin	7 mg/kg PO BID [2]	Killer whales	
	8 mg/kg PO TID [2]	Bottlenose dolphins	
Clindamycin	7.7–9.6 mg/kg PO BID [1]	Bottlenose dolphins	
	4.5–5.5 mg/kg PO BID [1]	Killer whales	
	11 mg/kg PO BID [1, 2]	Bottlenose and Commerson's dolphins	
Clindamycin	4.4–7.7 mg/kg PO BID [1]	Short-finned pilot whales	
	7.7 mg/kg PO BID [1]	Beluga whales	
Danofloxacin	8 mg/kg IM SID [2]	Bottlenose dolphins; Beluga whales	
Dihydrostreptomycin	11 mg/kg IM SID [1]		
Doxycycline	1.5 mg/kg PO BID [1]	Small odontocetes, Bottlenose dolphins	
Enrofloxacin	5 mg/kg PO SID [1]	Bottlenose dolphins	
	5 mg/kg BID [1]	Small odontocetes	
	2.5 mg/kg PO BID [1]	Killer and Beluga whales	
	4.5 mg/kg PO BID [1]	Short-finned pilot whale	
Fluconazole	2.8 mg/kg PO SID [1]	Bottlenose dolphins	Histoplasmosis.
	2 mg/kg PO BID [1]	Small odontocetes, Bottlenose dolphins	
	2 mg/kg PO BID [2]	Bottlenose dolphins	
	3.5 mg/kg BID loading dose; then 2.3 mg/kg BID maintenance [2]	Beluga whale calves	
Flucytosine	20 mg/kg PO TID [1]	Bottlenose dolphins	Candidiasis treatment, itraconazole or other azole adjunct, never as a monotherapy.
Gentamicin	4 mg/kg IM SID [1]		Use with caution, nephrotoxicity common.
	1.1 mg/kg IT [1]		
	5 mg/kg IM BID [1]		
	2.5 mg/kg PO TID [1]	Rough-toothed dolphins	Duodenitis treatment.

(*Continued*)

Drug name	Drug dose	Species	Comments
Imipenem	7.7–11.6 mg/kg BID [1]	Beluga whales	
Itraconazole	2.5 mg/kg PO BID [1]	Bottlenose dolphins; Beluga whales; Small odontocetes	Candidiasis treatment, flucytosine adjunct; general antifungal.
	4.6 mg/kg [1]	Bottlenose dolphins	Lobomycosis treatment.
	5 mg/kg PO BID [1]	Bottlenose dolphins	Aspergillosis treatment, associated 2–25 fold increase in liver enzymes.
	5 mg/kg PO BID [1]	Commerson's dolphin	
Itraconazole	1.25 mg/kg PO BID [1]	Killer and Short-finned Pilot whales	
Ketoconazole	1.9 mg/kg PO BID [1]	Beluga whales	Adjunct prednisolone.
	5 mg/kg PO BID [1]	Small odontocetes; Bottlenose dolphins	± adjunct prednisolone.
	4–7 mg/kg PO gradual increase to 10–16 mg/kg PO [1]		
	18 mg/kg PO [1]		Lobomycosis treatment.
	6 mg/kg PO [1]		
Levofloxacin	5 mg/kg PO SID-BID [2]	Killer whales	
	5 mg/kg PO BID; 10 mg/kg PO SID [2]	Bottlenose dolphins	
	8–10 mg/kg PO SID [2]	Short-finned pilot whales	
Linezolid	2.5–5 mg/kg BID [2]	Killer whales	
Meropenem	13 mg/kg IV TID; 20 mg/kg PO TID [2]	Bottlenose dolphins	In conjunction with ciprofloxacin.
Metronidazole	2.5 mg/kg PO BID [2]	Killer whales	
	7 mg/kg PO TID; BID for SW [1]	Small odontocetes, Bottlenose dolphins	
Minocycline	4 mg/kg Loading dose, 2 mg/kg BID maintenance [1]	Small odontocetes, Bottlenose dolphins, Beluga whales	
Nystatin liposomal (Nyotran)	550 ml/160 kg 1 hr IV infusion [2]	Bottlenose dolphins	
Nystatin	7000–14 000 IU/kg PO BID to TID for duration of antibiotic treatment [2, 5]	Cetaceans	Oral candidiasis secondary to antibiotic treatment is common and prophylactic Nystatin treatment during is recommended.
	600 000 IU PO TID [1]		
	600 000 IU PO TID [1]	Rough-toothed dolphins	Duodenitis treatment.
Ofloxacin	5 mg/kg PO BID [1]	Small odontocetes, Bottlenose dolphins	

Drug name	Drug dose	Species	Comments
Posaconazole	2.5–5 mg/kg PO BID [2]	Killer whales, Bottlenose dolphins	
	5 mg/kg PO BID [2]	Pacific white-sided dolphins	
Procaine/benzathine penicillin	10–20 000 IU/kg IM [1]		Occasionally used every other day.
Procaine penicillin G	47 000 IU/kg IM [1]		For diarrhea.
Rifampin	2.5 mg/kg PO BID [1]	Small odontocetes, Bottlenose dolphins, Beluga whales	
	2.2 mg/kg PO BID [1]	Killer whales	
Streptomycin	11 mg/kg IM SID [1]		
Terbinafine	1.25–1.5 mg/kg PO SID [2]	Killer whales	
	2 mg/kg PO SID [2]	Killer whales	
Tetracycline	6.7 mg/kg PO BID [1]		
	22–35 mg/kg PO BID [1]	Killer whales	
	55–65 mg/kg PO BID [1]	Bottlenose dolphins	
	77 mg/kg PO BID [1]	Commerson's dolphins	
	55 mg/kg PO BID [1]	Beluga whales	
Trimethoprim sulfadiazine	30 mg/kg PO SID [1]	Bottlenose dolphins	
	15.7 mg/kg q48 hr [1]	Beluga whale calves	
Trimethoprim sulfadiazine 1:5 and 1:2 (1:2 typically used when Nocardia suspected)	16–22 mg/kg PO SID [1]	Bottlenose dolphins, Small odontocetes	Always give with folic acid, may cause fatal pancytopenia.
	7.7–11 mg/kg PO SID [1]	Killer whales	Always give with folic acid.
	7.7 mg/kg PO SID [1]	Short-finned pilot whales	Always give with folic acid.
	8–16 mg/kg PO SID [1]	Belugas	Always give with folic acid.
	16 mg/kg PO SID [1]	Commerson's dolphins	Always give with folic acid.
Trimethoprim sulfadiazine	22 mg/kg PO SID [1]	Beluga whales	
Trimethoprim sulfamethoxazole	DO NOT use in cetaceans [2]		
Tylosin	32 mg/kg IM SID [1]		Myositis, but efficacious.
	50 mg/kg PO TID [1]		May cause diarrhea.
Vancomycin	1.5–2 mg/kg TID [2]	Killer whales	
	2–3 mg/kg TID [2]	Bottlenose dolphins	
	1–1.5 mg/kg TID PO [1]	Small odontocetes	
	1.1 mg/kg PO BID [1]	Killer whales	

(*Continued*)

Drug name	Drug dose	Species	Comments
Voriconazole	0.27–0.3 mg/kg SID maintained levels of 2–2.7 μg/ml; or 1.5 mg/kg PO BID × 3d then reduce to 0.5 mg/kg SID [2]	Killer whales	Monitor plasma levels closely.
	2.5–3.3 mg/kg PO BID × 3d, then 2.5–3.3 mg/kg q7d [2]	Bottlenose dolphins, Beluga whales	Monitor plasma levels closely.
Analgesia			
Acetominophen	3–5 mg/kg SID PO [6]	Bottlenose dolphins, Orca whales	Monitor transaminases.
Acetylpromazine	100 mg/m body length IV [1]	Cetaceans	Premedication for euthanasia.
Acetylsalicylic acid	5 mg/kg PO as needed, max once daily [2]	Killer whales	For short-term use (5–7 d).
Buscopan	0.3 mg/kg PO BID [2]	Killer whales	
	0.13 mg/kg or 10–20 mg per 70 kg [2]	Bottlenose dolphins	
	0.06 mg/kg BID [2]	Short-finned pilot whales	
Butorphanol	0.05–0.15 mg/kg IM [6, 7]	Bottlenose dolphins, Orca whales	Possible excitatory response seen in one dolphin.
Carprofen	0.5 mg/kg SID PO [6]	Bottlenose dolphins	Gastric ulcerations seen.
Flunixin meglumine	0.25–0.5 mg/kg SID IM [6]	Bottlenose dolphins, Orca whales	Be careful with use in cetaceans as gastric ulcers are common.
Lidocaine 2% + bupivicaine 0.25% local analgesia	L: 1 mg/kg + B: 1 mg/kg [7]	Indo-Pacific dolphins	Infiltrated into the surgical area/tail.
Meloxicam	0.1 mg/kg PO [8]	Bottlenose dolphins	n = 10 adult dolphins given one dose, with a peak plasma concentration at 11 hr and elimination half-life of 70 hr, and detectable drug concentrations up to 7 days. Repeated dosing is cautioned at this time until further multi-dose studies are performed.
Piroxicam	0.08–0.1 mg/kg q6d [2]	Bottlenose dolphins	
Tramadol	0.1–0.4 mg/kg PO, IM or IV BID [6]	Bottlenose, Common, Rough tooth, Spinner, and Spotted dolphins as well as Pygmy and Sperm whales	Titrate up to lowest effective dose, produces good analgesia without change in appetite, drowsiness seen at 0.73 mg/kg.
	0.25–0.5 mg/kg PO SID-BID (<5 d), start low then work up; 0.2 mg/kg SID long-term [2]	Killer whales	

Drug name	Drug dose	Species	Comments
	0.1–0.25 mg/kg PO BID [2]	Bottlenose dolphins	
	0.15–0.25 mg/kg PO SID-BID [2]	Short-finned pilot whales, Beluga whales	
Anesthesia and Sedation			
Atropine	0.02 mg/kg IM [6]	Killer whales, Bottlenose dolphins	Premedication.
Atipamezole	50–200 mg/kg IM IV [6]	Bottlenose dolphins	If medetomidine is 1 mg/ml and atipamezole is 5 mg/ml, can use equal volumes.
Butorphanol	0.05–0.13 mg/kg IM [9]	Bottlenose dolphins	Sedation for tooth extraction, monitor for possible excitation.
	0.1–0.15 mg/kg IM [2]	Killer whales	
	B: 0.2 mg/kg IM. Antagonize with naltrexone 0.3 mg/kg **[6KREEG 187]**	Cetaceans	Captive animals only.
	0.05–0.15 mg/kg IM [5, 6, 10]	Bottlenose dolphins	Sedation adequate for bronchoscopy and minor procedures. Possible reactions when combined with bronchodilators. Onset of action 25 min. Advantage over benzodiazepines is that animals do not seem to override effects if excited prior to administration. Naltrexone given at 0.01 mg/kg IM as antagonist.
Butorphanol; diazepam	0.15 mg/kg IM; 0.1–0.15 mg/kg PO [2]	Killer whales	
	0.06–0.08 mg/kg IM; 0.1 mg/kg PO [2]	Bottlenose dolphins	
Butorphanol; midazolam	0.07 mg/kg IM; 0.06 mg/kg IM [2]	Bottlenose dolphins	
Chlordiazepoxide	0.5 mg/kg IM [1, 6]	Bottlenose dolphins	Reduces anxiety, useful for shipping, no adverse effects.
Diazepam	0.55–0.6 mg/kg PO [6]	Dolphins	Used to help trained dolphins remain still for 35–45 min for imaging. If overdose is seen give flumazenil PO or IV.
	0.1 mg/kg PO [10]	Cetaceans	For anti-anxiety or appetite stimulation.
	0.2 mg/kg IM/PO [10]	Cetaceans	For sedation for transport. Onset of effect is affected by amount of food in stomach and can be 1–4 hrs.

(*Continued*)

Drug name	Drug dose	Species	Comments
	0.05–0.1 mg/kg IV [10]	Cetaceans	Drug can be somewhat irritating and did cause perivascular necrosis of ventral fluke area in one animal.
	0.05–0.15 mg/kg IM [10]	Cetaceans	Sedation. Excited animals are able to override the sedative effects so redosing should be considered carefully as overdosing can occur. Antagonize with flumazenil 0.5 mg/ml at equal volume to benzodiazepine.
	0.1–0.2 mg/kg IM, or 0.25–1 mg/kg PO, or 0.26–0.36 PO [5, 6]	Bottlenose dolphins	Larger doses reserved for research or refractory animals. Keep flumazenil available. IM diazepam is not absorbed as readily as midazolam and as such longer time to drug effect is expected.
	0.1 mg/kg IM or 0.2 mg/kg PO [2]	Killer whales	
	0.15–0.25 mg/kg IM/PO [2]	Bottlenose dolphins	
Diazepam + tramadol	D: 0.13–0.15 mg/kg PO; T: 0.5 mg/kg PO [2]	Killer whales	
Diazepam + meperidine	D: 0.1 mg/kg + Mep: 1 mg/kg + a local anesthetic at surgical site [9]	Cetaceans	Produced almost total immobility for 45 min with maintenance of consciousness and low-normal respiration for laparoscopy procedures.
Etorphine	Euthanasia 0.5 ml/1.5 m in length [11]	Dolphins and Porpoises	For humane euthanasia.
	Euthanasia 4 ml/1.5 m in length [11]	Whales	For humane euthanasia.
Flumazenil	0.005 mg/kg IM PO IV or sublingual [5, 6]	Bottlenose dolphins	When using 5 mg/ml midazolam and 0.5 mg/ml flumazenil, can give equal volumes.
	0.01–0.05 mg/kg IV/IM [2]	Killer whales; Bottlenose dolphins	
Haloperidol	DO NOT USE IN CETACEANS		Severe adverse reactions observed.
Halothane	0.5–3.5% inhalation [6]	Bottlenose dolphins	Higher doses for induction, with lower for maintenance.

Drug name	Drug dose	Species	Comments
Isoflurane	0.5–2% inhalation **[6KREEG 204]**	Bottlenose dolphins	Higher doses for induction, with lower for maintenance.
Ketamine	1.75 mg/kg IM [6]	Bottlenose dolphins	n = 1 case, in combination with medetomidine.
Ketamine + medetomidine	K: 2 mg/kg + M: 0.04 mg/kg. Antagonize with atipamezole 0.2 mg/kg **[6KREEG 187]**.	Cetaceans	
Meperidine	0.1–2 mg/kg IM [5, 6]	Bottlenose dolphins	Given in combination with midazolam, can produce a deep, reversible sedation.
	2 mg/kg IM [1]	Small odontocetes, Bottlenose dolphins, Beluga whales	
	1 mg/kg IM, 0.5–1 mg/kg PO [1]	Killer Whale	
Meperidine + midazolam	Mep: 0.05–2 mg/kg + Mid: 0.1 mg/kg IM **[9, 10,KREEG 204]**	Bottlenose dolphins	Often not reversed unless patient showing signs of extended depression or incoordination.
Medetomidine	10–40 mg/kg IM IV [6]	Bottlenose dolphins	Abolishes sinus arrythmia and causes respiratory suppression and decreased central venous pressure.
Midazolam	0.045–0.1 mg/kg IM [10]	Cetaceans	Sedation. Excited animals are able to override the sedative effects so redosing should be considered carefully as overdosing can occur. Antagonize with flumazenil 0.5 mg/ml at equal volume to benzodiazepine.
	0.05–0.15 mg/kg IM [5, 6]	Bottlenose dolphins	Provides a good plane of sedation for 45–60 min, Use caution with flumazenil for antagonism in non-Tursiops species as may see atrial fibrillation.
	0.045 mg/kg IM [2]	Killer whales	
	0.095 mg/kg IM [2]	Bottlenose dolphins	
Midazolam + butorphanol	M: 0.075 mg/kg IM + B: 0.05 mg/kg IM. Antagonize with flumazenil 0.015 mg/kg IV [7].	Indo-Pacific dolphins	Anesthetic management while surgically debriding a tail abscess.
Midazolam + meperidine	Mid: 0.06 mg/kg + Mep: 1.1 mg/kg IM [9]	Atlantic bottlenose dolphins	n = 1 case with oral mass removal, lidocaine was infiltrated locally around tumor.

(*Continued*)

Drug name	Drug dose	Species	Comments
Naloxone	5–10 mg/kg IM IV [5, 6]	Bottlenose dolphins	For antagonism of butorphanol and meperidine.
Naltrexone	0.005 mg/kg IM IV [5, 6]	Bottlenose dolphins	For opiod antagonism.
	0.1 mg/kg IM [2]	Killer whales, Bottlenose dolphins	
Nitrous oxide	70% Inhalation [6]	Bottlenose dolphins	Light anesthesia.
Pentobarbitol	Euthanasia 60–200 mg/kg [11]	Cetaceans	For humane euthanasia.
Propofol	0.5–3.5 mg/kg IV [6]	Bottlenose dolphins	Onset and duration of effect are injection site dependent.
	3.7 mg/kg IV [12]	Indo-Pacific dolphins	Supplemental to support endotracheal intubation.
	3.5 mg/kg IV, then isoflurane 2% via ET tube [9]	Atlantic bottlenose dolphins	n = 1 case of corneal lesion examination under anesthesia.
	4 mg/kg IV **[6 KREEG 187]**	Cetaceans	
Telazol	T: 2 mg/kg IM or IV **[6 KREEG 187]**	Cetaceans	
Thiopental	10–15 mg/kg IV [6]	Bottlenose dolphins	Requires additional inhalant anesthesia for full induction.
Tramadol + diazepam	T: 0.15–0.2 mg/kg PO + D: 0.15 mg/kg [5]	Cetaceans	Provides sedation adequate for tooth extraction.
Antiparasitic			
Bithionol	4 mg/kg PO q3d × 5 doses [1]		
Dichlorvos	13.2–16.5 mg/kg PO repeat in 7d [1]		
Fenbendazole	11 mg/kg PO [1]	Small odontocetes	
	10 mg/kg PO SID × 3d [2]	Bottlenose dolphins	
Ivermectin	200 µg/kg PO [1]	Small odontocetes	Crassicauda treatment.
Levasimole	DO NOT USE IN CETACEANS [2]		Fatal reactions have been seen in cetaceans. 2 wild caught Beluga whales died shortly after IM injection.
Oxfendazole (Bezelmin)	10 mg/kg [2]	Killer whales	
Praziquantel	10 mg/kg [1]	Small odontocetes	Nasitrema treatment.
	3–10 mg/kg once [2]	Bottlenose dolphins	

Drug name	Drug dose	Species	Comments
Other			
Altrenogest/ Regumate	0.05 mg/kg PO SID [5]	Bottlenose and Pacific white-sided dolphins, Killer and Belugas whales	May prevent ovulation. However, there have been some cases of pregnancy despite treatment and it is unknown if this is due to breakthroughs or drug administration mistakes.
Altrenogest	0.044 mg/kg 20d post partum; 200 mg/kg PO SID for contraception [1, 2]	Killer whales, Bottlenose dolphins	
Ascorbic acid	8 mg/kg PO BID [1]	Killer whales	
Atropine	0.2 mg/kg IM [1, 9]		Often used during anesthesia to decrease reflex bradycardia.
Cimetidine	6 mg/kg PO TID [1]		
	2100 mg PO QID [1]	Killer whales	
	4.5 mg/kg PO BID [1]	Small odontocetes	
	1.5 mg/kg PO SID-BID [2]	Bottlenose dolphins	
Citrate/bicarbonate; use potassium salts for urate stones	1 mEq of each/kg/day (cit. 108 g, bic. 84 mg) [2]	Bottlenose dolphins	
Copper sulfate	4 ppm immersion bath [1]		
Deslorelin/Suprelorin (Implant)	9.4 mg implants [5]	Bottlenose dolphins	Used successfully for 1 yr, anecdotally may have had some failures in other reports.
	9.4 mg implant × 2 per animal once a year [2]	Bottlenose dolphins	Contraception.
	1 × 9.4 mg implant [2]	Commerson's dolphin	Did NOT prevent pregnancy.
Dexamethasone	0.02 mg/kg IM SID [2]	Killer whales	
	0.11 mg/kg PO [1]	Bottlenose dolphins	
	0.025–0.1 mg/kg q48 hrs-BID [2]	Bottlenose dolphins	
	0.02–0.1 mg/kg IM SID [2]	Beluga whales	
	0.025–0.05 mg/kg IM SID [2]	Short-finned pilot whales	
Dimercaptosuccinic acid	11 mg/kg PO BID for 5–7d, for 9 cycles [1]	Bottlenose dolphins	Lead chelation.
Doxapram	1 mg/kg IV [7]	Indo-Pacific dolphins	Given during recovery and allowed animal to regain adequate respiration.
Doxapram	1–2 mg/kg PRN [2]	Killer whales, Bottlenose dolphins	
Epinephrine	0.02 mg/kg IM; 0.02–0.05 mg/kg IM PRN [1, 2]	Small odontocetes; Killer whales, Bottlenose dolphins	

(*Continued*)

Drug name	Drug dose	Species	Comments
Erysipelothrix rhusiopathie vaccine	2 ml IM [5]	Cetaceans	Monitor the animal for 20–60 min post vaccination for reactions. Appropriate vaccination protocol is still under investigation but an initial vaccine, booster 3 weeks later, and then annual vaccination appears prudent, especially in younger cetaceans.
Erythropoietin	63 U/kg twice 48 hrs apart IM [1]	Rough-toothed dolphins	
Esomeprazole	0.05–0.1 mg/kg SID; bid in severe cases [2]	Killer whales	
Exomeprazole	0.1–0.2 mg/kg SID; BID in severe cases [2]	Bottlenose dolphins	
Famotidine	0.3–0.5 mg/kg SID-BID [2]	Killer whales	
	0.5 mg/kg SID-BID [2]	Bottlenose dolphins	
Faropenem	3.5 mg/kg TID [2]	Killer whales	
	4.3–8.6 mg/kg BID-TID [2]	Bottlenose dolphins	
Filgrastim (neupogen)	1–5 µg/kg IM [2]	Killer, Beluga whales, and short-finned pilot whales, Bottlenose dolphins	
Fluoxetine	0.25–0.5 mg/kg PO SID-BID	Bottlenose dolphins	Anti-anxiety.
Folic acid (dose with trimethoprim sulfa)	10 mg BID [1]		
	25–50 mg total dose PO BID [1]	Bottlenose dolphins	
	10–20 mg total dose PO BID [2]	Commerson's dolphins	
	50–100 mg total dose PO BID [2]	Short-finned pilot whales	
	25–100 mg total dose PO BID [2]	Beluga whales	
Folinic acid	0.04–0.06 mg/kg PO BID; 50–150 mg total dose PO BID [2]	Killer whales	
Furosemide	2–4 mg/kg IM [1]	Small odontocetes	
Human chorionic gonadotropin	1000–3000 IU IM SID × 5d [1]	Bottlenose dolphins	To induce ovulation.
Leuprolide acetate	0.075 mg/kg IM q28d [1, 5]	Bottlenose dolphins	Used in males to reduce serum testosterone and produce azospermia. Limited clinical use, use with caution.

Drug name	Drug dose	Species	Comments
Lidocaine 2%	10–20 ml [1]	Bottlenose dolphins	For infra-alveolar nerve block.
Maropitant (Cerenia)	0.3–0.5 mg/kg SID [2]	Killer whales	
Maropitant (Cerenia)	0.5–1.0 mg/kg SID [2]	Bottlenose dolphins	
Megesterol acetete	NOT RELIABLE In male dolphins [5, 12]	Bottlenose dolphins	Not reliable in males as pregnancies occurred, A study of 8 males receiving 0–60 mg PO SID: doses as low as 10 mg strongly suppressed cortisol secretion in nearly all dolphins, caution should be exercised when administering MA to control reproductive behavior in male dolphins.
Pentobarbitol	60–200 mg/kg [11]	Cetaceans	Recommended for euthanasia of stranded marine mammals. Etorphine is another option with less volume. 0.5 ml/1.5 m in dolphins and porpoises and 4 ml/1.5 m in whales.
Pepto-Bismol			Scale to humans, PO [1].
PgF2 alpha (dinoprost tromethamine, Lutalyse)	25 mg BID × 3d to lyse retained CL (Corpus luteum) [2]	Killer whales	
	15 mg BID × 3d to lyse retained CL [2]	Bottlenose dolphins	
	5 mg BID × 3d to lyse CL [2]	Pacific white-sided dolphin	
Prednisone	0.03–0.1 mg/kg SID-BID [2]	Killer and Beluga whales, Bottlenose dolphins,	
Prednisolone	0.01 mg/kg PO SID [1]		Adjunct to ketoconazole.
Prednisolone sodium succinate	1–10 mg/kg IM IV [1]	Small odontocetes	For treatment of shock.
Pregnant mare serum gonadotropin (PMSG)	1200 IU on day 1 IM, Day 3: 400 IU PMSG, day 7: 1000 IU hCG, OR 1500 IU PGMS on day 1 IM and repeat in 48 hrs [1]	Bottlenose dolphins	
Ranitidine	2 mg/kg PO BID [1]	Small odontocetes	
	1–1.5 mg/kg SID-BID [2]	Bottlenose dolphins	
S-adenosyl-methionine (SAM-e)	1600–2000 mg total PO SID [2]	Bottlenose dolphins	
Simethicone	5000 mg total PO BID [2]	Killer whales	
	160–400 mg total PO BID [2]	Bottlenose dolphins	

(*Continued*)

Drug name	Drug dose	Species	Comments
Sucralfate	1 g PO QID [1]	Rough-toothed dolphins	Duodenitis treatment.
	20–15G PO BID-TID [2]	Killer whales	
	4–5G PO BID-TID [2]	Beluga whales	
	2–2.5G PO BID-TID [2]	Bottlenose dolphins	
Thiamine	1 mg/kg IM SID followed by oral [1]		
	2–4 mg/Kcal feed PO SID [1]		2 hr before feeding.
	25–35 mg/kg fish PO SID [1]		
Vitamin E/Selenium	0.06 mg/kg (based on selenium) IM once [2]	Bottlenose dolphins	
Vitamin E	100 IU/kg fish PO SID [1]	Killer whales	
Yunnan Baiyao	250 mg/100 lbs body weight PO SID [2]	Bottlenose dolphins	

Species	Weight [5, 6]
Bottlenose dolphin *(Tursiops truncatus)*	90–315 kg
Pacific white-sided dolphin *(Lagenohynchus obliquidens)*	60–160 kg
Orca whale *(Orcinus orca)*	500–5600 kg
Beluga whale *(Delphinapterus leucas)*	300–1600 kg
False killer whale *(Pdeudorca crassidens)*	430–800 kg
Rough-toothed dolphins *(Steno bredanensis)*	90–150 kg

Acknowledgments

The author would like to thank SeaWorld Parks and Entertainment for contributing to this chapter.

References

1 Dierauf, L.A. and Gulland, F.D. (2001). *CRC Handbook of Marine Mammal Medicine*, 709–714. Florida: CRC Press.
2 SeaWorld Parks and Entertainment (2018). Personal communication.
3 Valitutto, M. (2001). Protein-binding of Cefovecin (Convenia) in 25 zoological species: a predictor for extended duration of action. *Annual Proceedings of the American Association of Zoo Veterinarians*. 48.
4 Garcia-Parraga, D., Gilabert, J.A., Valls, M. et al. (2012). Updates on the pharmacokinetics of Cefovecin (Convenia®) in marine mammals. *Annual Proceedings of the International Association of Aquatic Animal Medicine*.

5 Dold, C. (2015). Cetaceans. In: *Fowler's Zoo and Wild Animal Medicine*, vol. 8 (ed. R.E. Miller and M. Fowler), 423–434. St. Louis, MO: Elsevier Saunders.

6 Dold, C. and Ridgeway, S. (2014). Cetaceans. In: *Zoo Animal and Wild Immobilization and Anesthesia*, vol. 2 (ed. G. West, D. Heard and N. Caulkett), 679–692. Ames, IA: Wiley Blackwell.

7 Tamura, J., Yanagizawa, M., Endo, Y. et al. (2017). Anesthetic management of an Indo-Pacific Bottlenose dolphin (*Tursiops aduncus*) requiring surgical debridement of a tail abscess. *Journal of Zoo and Wildlife Medicine* 48 (1): 200–203.

8 Simeone, C.A., Nollens, H.H., Meegan, J.M. et al. (2014). Pharmacokinetics of single dose oral meloxicam in bottlenose dolphins (*Tursiops truncatus*). *Journal of Zoo and Wildlife Medicine* 45 (3): 594–599.

9 Higgins, J.L. and Hendrickson, D.A. (2013). Surgical procedures in pinniped and cetacean species. *Journal of Zoo and Wildlife Medicine* 44 (4): 817–836.

10 Walsh, M.T., Reidarson, T., McBain, J. et al. (2006). Sedation and anesthesia techniques in cetaceans. *Annual Proceedings of the American Association of Zoo Veterinarians*. 237–239.

11 Greer, L. and Rowles, T. (2000). Humane euthanasia of Stranded Marine Mammals. *Annual Proceedings of the American Association of Zoo Veterinarians*. 374–375.

12 Houser, D.S., Champagne, C.D., Jensen, E.D. et al. (2017). Effects of oral megestrol acetate administration on the hypothalamic-pituitary-adrenal axis of male bottlenose dolphins (*Tursiops truncatus*). *Journal of the American Veterinary Medical Association* 251 (2): 217–223.

15

Seals, Sea Lions, and Walruses

Drug name	Drug dose	Species	Comments
Antimicrobials and Antifungals			
Amikacin	7 mg/kg IM BID [1]	California sea lions	
	10–15 mg/kg IM SID [2]	California sea lions	
	7.7 mg/kg IM BID [1, 3]	Walruses	
Amoxicillin	20 mg/kg IV once in intravertebral extradural vein [1, 4]	Harbor and Northern elephant seal pups	n = 8 Northern Elephant seal pups and 10 Harbor seal pups ranging from 1–6 mo of age and 39–61 kg and 9–18.5 kg respectively. Drug half-lives were 1.15–3.61 hrs and 0.45–2.63 hours respectively.
	22 mg/kg PO BID [1]	California sea lions, Harbor seals, Elephant seals	
Amoxicillin/ clavulanic acid (Clavamox)	12.5–20 mg/kg PO BID in combination with ketoconazole 3–10 mg/kg PO SID for 7–21d [5]	Southern elephant seals	Treatment of captive Southern elephant seals at Taronga Zoo for oral candidiasis. Topical Mycostatin applied with paintbrush SID resulted in more rapid and longer regression of lesions.
	15–20 mg/kg PO BID [3]	California sea lions, Harbor seals	
	22 mg/kg PO BID [1]	California sea lions, Harbor seals, Elephant seals	
Amoxicillin	22 mg/kg PO BID [3]	Walruses	
Amoxicillin trihydrate	20 mg/kg PO BID × 21d [6]	Harbor seals	n = 1, 29 yr old female undergoing gastrotomy for foreign bodies. Postoperatively on injectables for 7 days until eating then started on amoxicillin × 21d in addition to ciprofloxacin for 7 days.

(Continued)

Drug name	Drug dose	Species	Comments
Ampicillin	22 mg/kg IM, IV, PO TID [1]	Pinnipeds	
Azithromycin	10 mg/kg PO SID [2]	California sea lions	
Cefovecin (Convenia)	4 mg/kg IM [7]	Patagonian and California sea lions	n = 10 Patagonian Sea lions and one California Sea lion – plasma levels above MIC90 for approximately 57 days.
	4 mg/kg IM [7]	Walruses	n = 1 animal, plasma levels stayed above MIC90 for >50 days.
	8 mg/kg IM once [3]	California sea lions, Harbor seals	
Ceftazidime	20 mg/kg IM BID [3]	California sea lions, Harbor seals	
Ceftiofur crystalline free acid (Excede)	6.6 mg/kg IM q5d [2]	Phocid seals and California sea lions	
Ceftiofur crystalline free acid (Excede)	6.6 mg/kg SC q5d, or 5 mg/kg SC SID [3]	California sea lions	
Ceftiofur sodium	2 mg/kg IM SID [2]	California sea lions	
	2.45 mg/kg IM SID [8]	California sea lions	n = 1 animal with sarcocystis-related rhabdomyolysis, acute renal failure, and leukocytosis.
Ceftriaxone	20 mg/kg IM SID [3]	California sea lions	
Ceftriaxone sodium	23 mg/kg IM SID [6]	Harbor seals	n = 1, 29 yr old female undergoing gastrotomy for foreign bodies. Pre and postoperatively on enrofloxacin as well as ceftriaxone sodium for 7 days until eating then switched to oral antibiotics.
Cefuroxime	10–15 mg/kg PO BID [1, 3]	Walruses	
	20–22-mg/kg PO BID to TID [3]	California sea lions	
Cephalexin	20 mg/kg PO TID [3]	California sea lions	
	22 mg/kg PO TID [1]	California sea lions	
Cephaloridine	8.8 mg/kg IT BID [1]	California sea lions	IT = Intratracheal administration.
Chloramphenicol	4.2 mg/kg IV, PO, TID [1]	Harbor seals	
	20–30 mg/kg PO BID to TID [1]	California sea lions	

Drug name	Drug dose	Species	Comments
Ciprofloxacin	6.25 mg/kg PO BID × 7d [6]	Harbor seals	n = 1, 29 yr old female undergoing gastrotomy for foreign bodies. Postoperatively on injectables for 7 days until eating then started on amoxicillin for 21 days in addition to ciprofloxacin for 7 days.
	9.8 mg/kg PO SID × 5d [9]	Northern elephant seals	n = 1 animal postoperative repair of a hiatal hernia.
	7.5 mg/kg PO BID [1, 3]	Walruses	
	20 mg/kg PO BID [3]	California sea lions, Harbor seals	
	Ophthalmic TID to QID [1]	Harbor seals	Treatment of keratitis, subpalpebral lavage in addition to fluconazole and atropine.
Clindamycin	7.3 mg/kg PO BID [1, 3]	Walruses	
	8–11 mg/kg PO BID [1]	California sea lions	
	10 mg/kg PO BID [2]	Northern fur seals	
	12 mg/kg PO BID [3]	California sea lions, Harbor seals	
Danofloxacin	7 mg/kg SC q72 hr [8]	California sea lions	n = 1 animal with sarcocystis-related rhabdomyolysis and acute renal failure and leukocytosis.
	10 mg/kg SC SID [3]	California sea lions, Harbor seals	
Doxycycline	2–5 mg/kg PO BID [2]	California sea lions, Phocid seals, Northern Fur seals	
	8–11 mg/kg PO BID [3]	California sea lions, Harbor seals	
	10–20 mg/kg SID PO [10]	Northern elephant seals	n = 18 juvenile seals without ocular disease. Within 1 hr of administration doxycycline was measurable within the tear film and remained in tears for at least 6 days after the end of dosing. Plasma levels reached levels that should be appropriate for systemic infections but were not studied further in this study.
Enrofloxacin	2.2 mg/kg PO BID [3]	Walruses	
	5 mg/kg PO BID [3]	California sea lions, Harbor seals	

(*Continued*)

Drug name	Drug dose	Species	Comments
	2.5–5 mg/kg PO BID [1]	California sea lions	
	3.3 mg/kg PO BID [1]	Walruses	
	3.75 mg/kg PO BID [2]	Pinnipeds	
	5 mg/kg IM SID [6]	Harbor seals	n = 1, 29 yr old female undergoing gastrotomy for foreign bodies. Pre and postoperatively on enrofloxacin as well as ceftriaxone sodium for 7 days until eating then switched to oral antibiotics.
	10 mg/kg IM SID [2]	California sea lions	
Erythromycin	5.5 mg/kg PO BID [1]	Pinnipeds	
Fluconazole	0.5 mg/kg PO BID [1]	Pinnipeds	
	Ophthalmic TID - QID [1]	Harbor seals	Treatment for keratitis with subpalpebral lavage in addition to ciprofloxacin and atropine.
Gentamicin	0.75 mg IT BID × 2d, then SID [1]	Pinnipeds	IT = intratracheal administration.
Griseofulvin	15 mg/kg PO SID × 45d [1]	Pinnipeds	
	5000 mg/day PO 4 wks [1]	Australian sea lions	
Imipenem	2.5–5 mg/kg BID [3]	California sea lions	
Isoniazid	2 mg/kg PO SID [1]	Gray seals	
Itraconazole	1.5–2 mg/kg PO SID [1, 3]	Walruses	
	0.5–1 mg/kg PO BID [1]	Other pinnipeds	
Itraconazole	3–5 mg/kg PO SID to BID [3]	Harbor seals	
Ketoconazole	10 mg/kg IM, PO SID [1]	Pinnipeds	Monitor liver enzymes.
	4.4 mg/kg PO BID [1, 3]	Walruses	
	1 mg/kg PO BID [1]	Other pinnipeds	
Levofloxacin	5 mg/kg PO SID [2]	Pinnipeds	
	5 mg/kg PO SID [3]	Walruses	
Marbofloxacin	5 mg/kg PO SID [11]	Harbor seals	n = 55 animals 33.22, juvenile seals, 5 mg/kg SID would be expected to be efficacious in treating susceptible bacteria except Pseudomonas.
	5 mg/kg SID IM or PO [2]	Steller sea lions	
Metronidazole	10 mg/kg PO TID [1]	California sea lions	

Drug name	Drug dose	Species	Comments
	10–15 mg/kg PO BID [3]	Walruses	
	10–20 mg/kg PO BID [3]	California sea lions	
	15 mg/kg PO BID [2]	California sea lions	To decrease dose frequency.
Mycostatin	Applied topically SID with paintbrush for 30 days [5]	Southern elephant seals	Treatment of captive Southern elephant seals at Taronga Zoo for oral candidiasis – resulted in more rapid and longer regression of lesions than the combination of oral Clavamox and ketoconazole.
Neomycin	20 mg/kg PO TID [1, 3]	California sea lions	
Nystatin	7–14 000 U PO BID to TID [3]	Walruses, California sea lions	
	600 000 U PO TID [1]	Pinnipeds	
Penicillin G	9090 IU/kg PO BID [1]	California sea lions	
Penicillin benzathine/ procaine	4545–9090 IU/kg IM SID [1]	Pinnipeds	
Procaine/benzathine penicillin	10–20 000 IU/kg IM SID [1]	California sea lions	Occasionally used EOD.
Penicillin benzathine	30 000 IU/kg IM SID [1]	California sea lions	
Rifampin	5 mg/kg PO SID [1]	Pinnipeds	
Tetracycline	4.5 mg/kg PO TID [1]	California sea lions	
	12.5 mg/kg PO SID [1]	Pinnipeds	
	22 mg/kg PO SID [1, 3]	California sea lions	
	44 mg/kg PO BID [1, 3]	Walruses	
Trimethoprim sulfadiazine	3.6 mg/kg PO BID [1]	California sea lions	
	4.5 mg/kg PO BID [1]	Harbor seals	
Trimethoprim sulfadiazine 1:5 or 1:2 solution	10–12 mg/kg PO SID [3]	Walruses	1:2 typically used when Nocardia is suspected.
Trimethoprim sulfadiazine	10–13 mg/kg PO SID [1]	Walruses	
Trimethoprim sulfadiazine 1 : 5 or 1 : 2 solution	10–20 mg/kg PO SID [3]	California sea lions	1 : 2 typically used when Nocardia is suspected.
Trimethoprim sulfadiazine	22–30 mg/kg PO SID [1]	California sea lions	

(*Continued*)

Drug name	Drug dose	Species	Comments
Voriconazole	1.8 mg/kg PO SID [12]	Pacific walruses	n = 1 animal with coccidioidomycosis, treated initially with Clavamox but minimal improvement combined with fungal assay results lead to a change to voriconazole and improvement over 3 months to stable condition.
Analgesia			Caution with NSAIDS use >72 hrs in Pinnipeds as may result in gastric ulceration in some species.
Buprenorphine	0.12–2 mg/kg SC once or q3–6d PRN [3]	California sea lions	
Buprenorphine sustained release	0.12 mg/kg SC [13]	Northern elephant seals	n = 26 juveniles, max concentration of 1.21 ng/ml detectable 12 hr post administration. Cellulitis or abscesses at the injection site were present in 6/23 seals between 24 and 168 hr post administration and thus should be used with caution in this species.
Butorphanol	0.055 mg/kg IM [14]	Northern elephant seals	Provided sedation for 3 hrs and detectable plasma concentrations for up to 5 hrs post injection.
	0.05–0.2 mg/kg IM [14]	Otariid seals	Used for mild sedation and analgesia.
Carprofen (Rimadyl)	1–1.25 mg/kg PO SID [3]	California sea lions	
Carprofen	3–4 mg/kg PO SID × 5d [15]	California sea lions	n = 10 animals with traumatic injuries, osteoarthritis, pneumonia, or keratitis with blepharospasm. There were no deleterious clinical side effects in this study. All animals continued to eat and interact with others. Animals with trauma or osteoarthritis-associated lameness showed improvement and there was documented reduction in blepharospasm.
	2 mg/kg IM [16]	Walruses	n = 2 cases for post anesthetic procedure analgesia for 3–5 days.
Flunixin meglumine	0.25–0.5 mg/kg IM SID [3]	Walruses, California sea lions	Use lowest effective dose.
	Caution [14]	Southern elephant, Harbor and Gray seals	To treat ocular inflammation and musculoskeletal disorders. Anorexia was reported if used for >72 hrs presumably due to gastric inflammation/ulceration.
Gabapentin	1–4 mg/kg PO SID [2]	Pinnipeds	Suggest to use with tramadol and an NSAID – all at very low doses-very effective analgesia.
Indomethacin	0.1–0.3 mg/kg PO initial, then 0.1–0.2 mg/kg PO q12–24 hrs, or 0.45 mg/kg q48 hrs [1]	California sea lions, Northern elephant seals	

Drug name	Drug dose	Species	Comments
Lidocaine hydrochloride 2%	4 mg/kg given in 2 points ventrolateral and ventromedial with a 20ga 1 1/2″ needle [17]	California sea lions	Technique was created with 10 CSL cadavers, then attempted on 26 anesthetized animals prior to euthanasia and one case of clinical ocular disease. The retrobulbar block was 76.9% successful, meaning a blepharospasmic globe returned to at least halfway to central orientation. No systemic adverse effects. Lidocaine 2–3 ml was injected by SC infiltration lateral to the orbital rim – used in 5 blepharospasmic animals and successful in 60% – meaning reduction of blepharospasm for up to 3 hrs. Success was dependent more on location rather than dose.
Meloxicam	0.05–0.1 mg/kg [2]	Pinnipeds	
	0.1 mg/kg PO SID [2]	Seals, California sea lions, Steller sea lions	
	0.1–0.2 mg/kg PO SC SID [3]	California sea lions, Harbor seals	
	0.1 mg/kg PO SID [16]	Walruses	n = 3 animals for 3–5 days post anesthetic procedures.
Profenal (NSAID)	Ophthalmic BID [1]	Hawaiian monk seals	
Tramadol	0.1–0.25 mg/kg PO SID to BID [3]	Walruses	Up to 0.8 mg/kg utilized BID without adverse effects.
	1 mg/kg PO BID to TID [3]	California sea lions	Up to 4 mg/kg, single dose, used with no adverse effects.
	2 mg/kg PO q6–8 hrs [18]	California sea lion	n = 15 wild sea lions given a single dose of tramadol (pharmacokinetic not dynamic study). Overall based on dosing simulations 4 mg/kg q8–12 hrs may also be adequate but requires further study.
	2–4 mg/kg PO BID [2]	Pinnipeds	
Anethesia and Sedation			
Azaperone + xylazine	A: 0.57–2 mg/kg + X: 0.57–2 mg/kg IM dart [14]	South African fur seals	n = 15 animals, 7% mortality, sufficient for branding, short immobilization time.
Atipamezole	0.04 mg/kg IV [14]	Southern elephant seals	Failed to arouse from ketamine + medetomidine anesthesia.
	0.2–0.3 mg/kg IM [3]	California sea lions	Typically 5–7.5 × medetomidine dose in mg.
Butorphanol	B: 0.05–0.2 mg/kg IM [3]	California sea lions, Harbor seals	

(*Continued*)

Drug name	Drug dose	Species	Comments
	B: 0.05–0.2 mg/kg IM [14]	Otariid seals	Used for mild sedation and analgesia.
	B: 0.2 mg/kg IV, followed by isoflurane 1.5–2% inhaled [14].	Harbor seals	Atropine is routinely given 0.02 mg/kg IV at induction.
Butorphanol	B: 0.055 mg/kg IM [14]	Northern elephant seals	Provided sedation for 3 hrs and detectable plasma concentrations for up to 5 hrs post injection.
	B: 0.4 mg/kg IM [14, 19]	Harbor seals	Given as deep IM injection into gluteal region 5–20 min prior to procedure and animals are sufficiently relaxed in approx 10 min, for radiographs or skin scrapings. The addition of mild manual restraint and 1–2% lidocaine for regional analgesia for blubber biopsies is well tolerated. The addition of diazepam 0.2 mg/kg facilitates deep muscle biopsies, endoscopic exams and evaluations of the head and eyes. Some lethargy is seen for 1–4 hrs post procedure but animals are responsive to commands and will eat and swim within 1 hr.
Butorphanol + diazepam	B: 0.4 mg/kg IM, followed by D: 0.2 mg/kg IV [14]	Harbor seals	Sufficient for deep muscle biopsy or endoscopy.
Butorphanol + medetomidine	B: 0.2 mg/kg + M: 0.05 mg/kg IM [3]	California sea lions	
Butorphanol + medetomidine + midazolam	B: 0.1–0.2 mg/kg + M: 0.04–0.05 mg/kg + Mid: 0.1–0.15 mg/kg IM [3]	California sea lions	
Butorphanol + midazolam	B: 0.05–0.1 mg/kg + Mid: 0.1–0.2 mg/kg IM [3]	Walruses	
	B: 0.2 mg/kg + Mid: 0.15 mg/kg IM [3]	Harbor seals	
Carfentanil	C: 2.4–2.7 mg given IM via dart. Antagonized with naltrexone 175–350 mg IM in lip when approachable, and additional 175–350 mg given at conclusion of procedure [20].	Pacific walruses	n = 17 adult wild bulls, carfentanil provided reliable immobilization within 7–21 min. Then when first approached given naltrexone and all but one had smooth reversal of effects in 10–20 min (5 min in one, likely given IV injection). Additional naltrexone given at conclusion of procedure to ensure complete reversal. All but one animal remained hauled out for several hours in sternal or lateral recumbency after antagonism. No adverse effects. Some larger males had less complete immobilization due to weight. 4 animals were intubated and maintained on isoflurane for diagnostic sampling and transmitter attachment.

Drug name	Drug dose	Species	Comments
Diazepam	D: 0.1–0.2 mg/kg IV [21]	Phocids <30 kg	
	D: 0.15 mg/kg IM [14]	Hawaiian monk seals	Given prior to mask induction with isoflurane.
	D: 0.1–0.2 mg/kg PO for Transport sedation. 0.15–0.2 mg/kg IM for sedation [14].	California sea lions	Used prior to transport to aid in physical restraint.
	D: 0.1–0.22 mg/kg PO [2]	California sea lions	
Diazepam	D: 0.15 mg/kg IM or 0.2 mg/kg PO; antagonize with flumazenil 0.01–0.04 mg/kg IV or IM [3]	California sea lions	
	D: 0.25–0.35 mg/kg IM [14]	Fur seals	Sedation
Diazepam + isoflurane	D: 0.15–2 mg/kg IV, followed by isoflurane 0.5–2% inhaled [14].	Harbor seals	Atropine is routinely given 0.02 mg/kg IV at induction.
Etorphine	7.8 mg total regardless of body size; antagonize with naltrexone 250 mg IM after tag attachment [22].	Atlantic Walrus	n = 40 adult male walruses, for attaching system loggers on tusks and collection of biologic samples. 27 animals were intubated and ventilated during recovery. Induction was on average 4–7 min, and recovery within 4–8 min. Some animals had severe acidosis and hypercarbia. Darting to recovery was 12–19 min.
Flumazenil	D: 0.01–0.04 mg/kg IM or IV [3]	Harbor seals	
	D: 0.01–0.1 mg/kg IM [3]	Walruses	
	0.1–0.5 mg/kg IM [14]	Crabeater seals	To reduce recovery time after midazolam + meperidine anesthesia. However, not full reversal so higher doses may be needed. 1 mg per 20–25 mg benzodiazepine was used to reverse zolazepam in a Southern elephant seal.
Haloperidol	0.11 mg/kg PO BID [1]	California sea lions	
Halothane	0.75–5% inhaled [14]	California sea lions	n = 30 animals, 3% mortality.
Isoflurane	0.75–3% inhaled [14, 23]	California sea lions	n = 115 animals, 0% mortality.
	0.8–4% inhaled [14]	Hooker's sea lions	n = 29 animals, 0% mortality.
	1.2–4% Inhalation [14]	New Zealand fur seals	

(Continued)

Drug name	Drug dose	Species	Comments
	N/A [14]	South American sea lions	n = 7 animals, 0% mortality.
Ketamine	0.15–0.25 mg/kg IM, then halothane 1–4% inhaled [14]	Weddell seals	For physiologic studies, anesthesia not described.
	K: 1.9–2.8 mg/kg IM [14]	South African fur seals	n = 58 animals, 0% mortality. Sufficient for tooth extraction, some tremors noted.
	K: 2 mg/kg IM; supplement with K: 1 mg/kg IM as needed [23]	Subantarctic fur seals	May consider atropine 0.02 mg/kg IM to decrease secretions. For long procedures you may wish to intubate and use gas anesthesia.
	K: 2.1 mg/kg IM; supplement with K: 1 mg/kg IM [23]	Northern sea lions	May consider atropine 0.02 mg/kg IM to decrease secretions. For long procedures you may wish to intubate and use gas anesthesia.
	K: 4.3–7.8 mg/kg IM dart [14],	South African fur seals	n = 27 animals, 19% mortality, variable anesthesia.
Ketamine	K: 5 mg/kg IM [23]	Northern elephant seals	May consider atropine 0.02 mg/kg IM to decrease secretions. For long procedures you may wish to intubate and use gas anesthesia.
	K: 5 mg/kg IM; supplement with K: 2.5 mg/kg as needed [23]	Ringed seals	If seal becomes anoxic due to prolonged apnea, intubate with cuffed endotracheal tube and ventilate. Doxopram IV may also be given.
	K: 6.8–7 mg/kg IM dart [14]	Antarctic fur seals	n = 30 animals, No mortalities, but muscle tremors seen.
Ketamine + detomidine	K: 2–4.3 mg/kg + D: 0.04–0.055 mg/kg, Followed by isoflurane 1–5% inhaled [14].	California sea lions	n = 4 animals, 0% mortalities.
Ketamine + diazepam. Give diazepam with a separate syringe to prevent precipitation.	K: 1.5 mg/kg + D: 0.05 mg/kg [23]	Harbor seals	May consider atropine 0.02 mg/kg IM to decrease secretions. For long procedures you may wish to intubate and use gas anesthesia.
	K: 2.16–6.67 mg/kg + D: 0.04–0.28 mg/kg IM or IV [14]	Juan Fernandez fur seals	n = 12 IM, 10 IV, 17% mortalities with IM, 0% with IV. Decreased induction and recovery times with IM than when used IV, variable plane of anesthesia with IV induction there was deeper immobilization.
	K: 3.6 mg/kg + D: 0.12 mg/kg; supplement with 1.8 mg/kg ketamine [23]	Guadalupe fur seals	The drug combo may be given IV but should be reduced by 50% and heart rate and core body temp monitored carefully.

Drug name	Drug dose	Species	Comments
	K: 4.5 mg/kg + D: 0.14 mg/kg IM [23]	Galapagos Fur seals	May consider atropine 0.02 mg/kg IM to decrease secretions. For long procedures or if animal is anoxic you may wish to intubate and use gas anesthesia.
	K: 6 mg/kg + D: 0.2 mg/kg; supplement with K: 3 mg/kg as needed [23]	Crabeater seals Gray seals, Harp seals, Hooded seals	If seal becomes anoxic due to prolonged intubate with cuffed endotracheal tube and ventilate. Doxopram IV may also be given. Use needles over 60 mm long to penetrate blubber layer. Opioids are not recommended as they can cause prolonged apnea which must be antagonized to avoid death.
	K: 7 mg/kg IM, D: 0.22 mg/kg IM [23].	Northern fur seals	May consider atropine 0.02 mg/kg IM to decrease secretions. For long procedures you may wish to intubate and use gas anesthesia.
Ketamine + medetomidine	K: 1.5–2 mg/kg + M: 0.035–0.04 mg/kg IM [3]	California sea lions	
	K: 2 mg/kg + M: 0.1 mg/kg IM; antagonize with atipamezole 0.5 mg/kg IM [23]	New Zealand fur seals, Southern fur seals	
	K: 2.5 mg/kg + M: 0.07–0.14 mg/kg IM [14]	Northern elephant seals	Bradycardia, prolonged recovery, poor reversibility, variable plane of anesthesia.
Ketamine + medetomidine	K: 2.5 mg/kg + M: 0.14 mg/kg IM; supplemental K: 1.25 mg/kg as needed; antagonize with atipamezole 0.7 mg/kg IM [14, 23]	California sea lions	n = 35 animals, 0% mortalities, Variable anesthesia,. Another 16 animals were immobilized with the same doses plus 1–5% isoflurane with no additional mortalities.
Ketamine + midazolam or diazepam	K: 8 mg/kg + Mid or D: 0.22 mg/kg IM [23]	Leopard seals	If using diazepam, give in a separate syringe. May consider atropine 0.02 mg/kg IM to decrease secretions. For long procedures you may wish to intubate and use gas anesthesia.
	K: 10 mg/kg + M or D: 0.22 mg/kg IM [23]	California sea lions, Northern elephant seals, Southern fur seals	If using diazepam, give in a separate syringe. May consider atropine 0.02 mg/kg IM to decrease secretions. For long procedures you may wish to intubate and use gas anesthesia.
Ketamine + midazolam	K: 2.7 mg/kg + Mid: 0.02 mg/kg IM [14]	Southern elephant seals	
	K: 1 mg/kg + Mid: 0.1 mg/kg IM dart [14, 23]	South American fur seals	n = 1 no mortality,.

(*Continued*)

Drug name	Drug dose	Species	Comments
	K: 2 mg/kg + Mid: 0.1 mg/kg IM [23]	Weddell Seals	Maintain anesthetized animals in lateral not sternal recumbency to assist respiration. If seal becomes anoxic due to prolonged apnea, intubate with a cuffed endotracheal tube and manually ventilate. Doxopram IV may be given.
Ketamine + xylazine	K: 3 mg/kg + X: 0.5 mg/kg IM [14, 23]	Southern elephant seals	Some apnea treated with 2 mg/kg doxapram.
	K: 3 mg/kg + X : 1 mg/kg IM; supplement with K: 1 mg/kg and X: 0.2 mg/kg IM; antagonize with yohimbine 0.2 mg/kg [23]	Weddell seals	Maintain anesthetized animals in lateral not sternal recumbency to assist respiration. If seal becomes anoxic due to prolonged apnea, intubate with a cuffed endotracheal tube and manually ventilate. Doxopram IV may be given.
	K: 3.1–11.4 mg/kg + X: 0.3–1.7 mg/kg IM dart [14],	Subantarctic fur seals	n = 32 animals, 13% mortality, variable anesthesia.
	K: 4 mg/kg + X: 0.75 mg/kg IM [23]	Gray seals	May consider atropine 0.02 mg/kg IM to decrease secretions. For long procedures you may wish to intubate and use gas anesthesia. For prolonged apnea manually ventilate. Also could consider Doxopram IV.
	K: 4.2–5.2 mg/kg + X: 0.6–0.9 mg/kg IM dart [14]	South African fur seals	n = 7 animals, 29% mortality, xylazine doses estimated.
	K: 7–7.6 mg/kg + X: 0.58–0.62 mg/kg IM [14]	Antarctic fur seals	n = 45, 7% mortalities,.
	K: 3.8–10.8 mg/kg + X: 0.7–2 mg/kg IM [14]	Antarctic fur seals	n = 14 animals, 14% mortalities. Poor sedation with ketamine < or equal to 5.6 mg/kg.
	K: 7 mg/kg + X: 0.6 mg/kg IM; supplement with K:3.5 mg/kg [23]	Antarctic fur seals	May consider atropine 0.02 mg/kg IM to decrease secretions. For long procedures you may wish to intubate and use gas anesthesia.
Ketamine + xylazine	K: 4 mg/kg + X: 0.5 mg/kg; supplement with K: 2 mg/kg as needed [23].	California sea lions, Galapagos Fur seal	May consider atropine 0.02 mg/kg IM to decrease secretions. For long procedures you may wish to intubate and use gas anesthesia.
	K: 5.6–7.8 mg/kg + X: 0.5–1.3 mg/kg IM [14]	Antarctic fur seals	n = 7 animals, 0% mortality.
Medetomidine	0.07 mg/kg IM [14]	Sea lions	Sedation for electroencephalography due to lack of interference with brain wave patterns.

Drug name	Drug dose	Species	Comments
Medetomidine + ketamine	M: 0.06 mg/kg IM, followed 15 min later by K: 2 mg/kg IM [14]	Gray seals, Harbor seals	Apnea and bradycardia were common. Antagonize with atipamezole, 30 min after last ketamine dose. In Harbor seals, ventilation and careful cardiac monitoring required.
	M: 0.14 mg/kg + K: 2.5 mg/kg IM; antagonize with atipamezole 0.2 mg/kg IM. Premedicate with Atropine 0.02 mg/kg IM [14].	California sea lions	Provided effective and safe immobilization. Disadvantages include moderately variable anesthetic depth, large injection volume with commercial products and cost.
Medetomidine + Telazol	M: 0.07 mg/kg + T: 1 mg/kg IM; antagonize with atipamezole 0.2 mg/kg IM [14].	California sea lions	Provided reversible, reliable anesthesia with lower injection volume and cost than ketamine + medetomidine.
Midazolam	Mid: 0.3–0.5 mg/kg IM, supplemented by isoflurane inhaled [14]	Weddell seals	Dose rates from study on estimated body weights.
	Mid: 0.26–0.85 mg/kg IM, with supplemental isoflurane 1–5% inhaled for induction [14].	Crabeater seals	
	0.15–2 mg/kg IM for moderate sedation. 0.4–0.5 mg/kg IM for heavy sedation [14].	Phocids	Higher doses are useful for larger species when physical restraint is dangerous and stressful.
	0.2 mg/kg IM [24]	Juvenile Harp seals	n = 11 seals, aged 3.5–11 wks of age and 22–41.5 kg. Midazolam at 0.2 mg/kg versus 0.1 mg/kg followed by 4% mask induction with isoflurane provided a greater level of sedation, and better tolerance of endotracheal placement and maintenance with spontaneous breathing during recovery.
Midazolam + butorphanol	Mid: 0.1 mg/kg + B: 0.1 mg/ks combined and given IV [21]	Phocids <30 kg	
	Mid: 0.1–0.25 mg/kg + B: 0.1–0.25 mg/kg IM, followed by net and mask induction with isoflurane [25]	Otarids >30 kg	
Midazolam + butorphanol + medetomidine	Mid: 0.1 mg/kg + B: 0.15 mg/kg + M: 0.035 mg/kg IM [25]	Otarids >80 kg	Supplement with isoflurane in oxygen by mask or ET tube,.
	Mid: 0.2–0.26 mg/kg + B: 0.2–0.4 mg/kg + M: 0.01–0.013 mg/kg IM + isoflurane 0.5–2% inhaled [14].	California sea lions	n = 2 animals anesthetized 13 times. Reversal with atipamezole, flumazenil, and naltrexone.

(*Continued*)

Drug name	Drug dose	Species	Comments
Midazolam + meperidine	Mid: 0.15–0.4 + Mep: 1–3 mg/kg IM [14]	Crabeater seals	Degree of sedation was unpredictable. Additional ketamine 1.3–2 mg/kg IM or 1 mg/kg IV was used in 2 animals.
Midazolam + meperidine	Mid: 0.04 mg/kg + Mep: 2.25–3.55 mg/kg IM [14]	Southern elephant Seals	Rapid recovery after naloxone or naltrexone administration.
Midazolam + meperidine (± atropine)	Mid: 0.1 mg/kg + Mep:2.2 mg/kg IM [23]	Walruses	Atropine 0.04 mg/kg IM, SC, or IV is recommended to prevent bradycardia. Use 8–10 cm needles to deliver drugs into epaxial muscles caudal to the last rib and cranial to pelvis or muscles of the forelimb.
Midazolam + meperidine	Mid: 0.1–0.2 mg/kg + Mep: 2–3 mg/kg IM (given as separate injection into gastrocnemius muscle with 9 cm 18ga needles); antagonize with flumazenil 0.002 mg/kg IM and naltrexone 1 mg/kg IM [16].	Walruses	n = 3 captive animals anesthetized for 6 procedures, fasted for 24 hr. After sedation with M/M combo an IV catheter was placed in the extradural intravertebral vein and propofol given to effect. Orotracheal intubation was performed and anesthesia maintained with isoflurane and IPPV.
Midazolam + meperidine + ketamine	Mid: 0.04 mg/kg + Mep: 4 mg/kg IM followed by K: 1.5–2.3 mg/kg IV [14]	Southern elephant seals	Initial ketamine dose 2.3 mg/kg followed by incremental doses of 1.5 mg/kg IV to maintain anesthesia for 1 hour.
Midazolam + meperidine + thiopentone	Mid: 0.04 mg/kg + Mep: 2.25–3.55 mg/kg IM + T: 3.4 mg/kg IV [14]	Southern elephant seals	Good induction of 5 minutes duration after thiopentone, allowing intubation. Antagonize with naltrexone or naloxone.
Naltrexone	0.1 mg/kg IM [3]	Walrus	
	0.1–0.4 mg/kg IM [3]	California sea lions, Harbor seals	
Propofol	2–6 mg/kg IV [14, 26]	Harbor Seals	n = 30 Harbor seal pups and 2 adults and two Northern elephant seal pups at 5 mg/kg. Optimal short-acting anesthetic, some apnea seen. Supplemental isoflurane at 2–5% allows intubation. Primary disadvantage is large volumes required for animals >40 kg.
Proprioprornazine	1–2 mg/kg IM [1]	Pinnipeds	
Telazol	0.8–1 mg/kg IM or IV [25]	Phocids	Supplement with isoflurane in oxygen by mask or ET tube.
	T: 0.8 mg/kg IV [14]	Northern elephant seals	Atropine added routinely 0.02 mg/kg IV at induction. IV Telazol provides 15 min anesthesia for intubation, then can supplement with isoflurane as needed.
	T: 1 mg/kg IM or IV [27]	Northern elephant seals	n = 46 animals in 66 procedures, resulted in heavy sedation.

Drug name	Drug dose	Species	Comments
	T: 1 mg/kg IM or 0.6 mg/kg IV [23]	Weddell seals	If physically possible IV Telazol results in shorter induction time, faster recovery, and decreased mortality versus IM administration.
Telazol	T: 0.83 mg/kg IV after receiving atropine 0.02 mg/kg IM. Intubated and maintained on isoflurane [6].	Harbor seals	n = 1 animal undergoing gastrotomy to remove foreign bodies. Procedure lasted 2.5 hr total and used ventilation at 6 breaths per minute with 7–1200 ml of oxygen per breath with <25 mmHg inspiratory pressure. Initial evaluation and suture removal conducted with butorphanol 0.05–0.066 mg/kg IM.
	0.3–1.1 mg/kg [14]	Weddell seals	n = 30 seals, Depth of anesthesia variable, 6 had prolonged apnea, and 3 mortalities reported, a lack of antagonist was considered a disadvantage.
	T: 0.5–1 mg/kg IM [14]	Gray seals	Considered reliable and safe, some require ventilation. Lower dose range used for electroejaculation procedures. However, some required additional IM doses.
	T: 1 mg/kg IM [23]	Crabeater seals	If seal becomes anoxic due to prolonged apnea, intubate with cuffed endotracheal tube and ventilate. Doxopram IV may also be given.
	0.46 mg/kg IV [14]	Southern elephant seals	Satisfactory immobilization for gastric lavage and sampling.
	T: 0.7–1 mg/kg IM [14]	Southern elephant seals	Dose rate >1 mg/kg result in multiple studies in apnea, tremors, hallucinations, and mortalities.
	T: 0.77–1.25 mg/kg given IM. Then IV catheter placed in extradural intravertebral vein and supplements given as needed [5].	Southern elephant seals	n = 5 captive animals, fasted for 24 hrs, 20 l/min oxygen nasal insufflation, and avoiding hyperthermia with morning procedures, hosing animal with cold water and packing ice around flippers.
	T: 0.7–1.9 mg/kg IM [14, 23]	Subantarctic fur seals	n = 49 animals, 4% mortality, Prolonged recoveries, apnea requiring artificial respiration. May consider atropine 0.02 mg/kg IM to decrease secretions. For long procedures you may wish to intubate and use gas anesthesia.
	T: 0.9–1.3 mg/kg IM [14]	Subantarctic fur seals	Top-up doses of Telazol have been associated with increased mortality. However, supplemental doses of ketamine have not.

(Continued)

Drug name	Drug dose	Species	Comments
	T: 1 mg/kg IM; supplement with ketamine 1 mg/kg as needed [23].	Southern elephant seals	Could instead give 0.5 mg/kg Telazol IV, but animals may show apnea for 2–15 min. Can give Doxopram IV if animal becomes anoxic.
	T: 1.2 mg/kg IM; supplement with ketamine 1 mg/kg as needed [23]	Northern fur seals	May consider atropine 0.02 mg/kg IM to decrease secretions. For long procedures you may wish to intubate and use gas anesthesia.
	T: 1.2–1.7 mg/kg IM dart [14]	Subantarctic fur seals	n = 172 animals, respiratory depression, 3% mortalities.
Telazol	T: 1.4 mg/kg; supplement with T: 0.7 mg/kg as needed. Consider antagonizing with flumazenil 0.006 mg/kg IM [23].	Leopard seals	May consider atropine 0.02 mg/kg IM to decrease secretions. For long procedures you may wish to intubate and use gas anesthesia.
	T: 1.43 mg/kg IM dart [14]	South American fur seals	n = 32 animals, 0% mortality, partial reversal with flumazenil. An additional 4 animals given 0.81 mg/kg ketamine as supplement due to insufficient sedation.
	T: 1.5 mg/kg IM; supplement with ketamine 1 mg/kg as needed [23].	Harbor seals, South American fur seals	May consider atropine 0.02 mg/kg IM to decrease secretions. For long procedures you may wish to intubate and use gas anesthesia.
	T: 1.7 mg/kg IM [14]	California sea lions	n = 60 animals, 0% mortalities but apnea seen. Given 10 min after atropine 0.02 mg/kg IM. Top-up doses of Telazol have been associated with increased mortality. However, supplemental doses of ketamine have not.
	T: 1.7 mg/kg IM; supplement ketamine 1 mg/kg IM as needed [23]	Galapagos fur seals, Southern fur seals	Do not give additional Telazol for supplementation. May consider atropine 0.02 mg/kg IM to decrease secretions. For long procedures you may wish to intubate and use gas anesthesia. Doxopram IV may also be given.
	T: 1.6–3.3 mg/kg + isoflurane inhaled [14].	Steller's sea lions	n = 51 animals, 10% mortality.
	T: 1.8–8.1 mg/kg IM [14]	Steller's sea lions	n = 29 animals, 21% mortality, best results 1.8–2.5 mg/kg.
	T: 2 mg/kg IM or (1.2–1.4 mg/kg IM) [14]	Leopard seals	Apnea, bradycardia, and mortalities seen. Seals were not intubated or ventilated during study. Parenthetical doses in another study were most reliable.
	T: 2 mg/kg IM [23]	Subantarctic fur seals	Higher doses may be required for seals in poor body condition.

Drug name	Drug dose	Species	Comments
	T: 2.2 mg/kg IM [23]	Northern elephant seals	May consider atropine 0.02 mg/kg IM to decrease secretions. For long procedures you may wish to intubate and use gas anesthesia.
	T: 2.75 mg/kg IM; antagonize with flumazenil 1 mg for every 20–25 mg Telazol [14].	South American sea lions	n = 13 animals, 0% mortality.
	T: 2 mg/kg IM [23]	Walruses	n = 3 animals. Smooth induction 14–29 min, and recovery, but can be prolonged at 75–220 min. 1/3 animals died during recovery.
	T: 2 mg/kg IM [23]	Northern sea lions, New Zealand fur seals	Do not supplement additional Telazol. If induction is rapid, be prepared to stimulate respiration chemically or manually. May consider atropine 0.02 mg/kg IM to decrease secretions. For long procedures you may wish to intubate and use gas anesthesia.
Telazol	T: 2 mg/kg IM; supplement as needed with ketamine 1 mg/kg IM [23]	Southern sea lions	Monitor closely for hyperthermia, particularly when ambient temperature is >20 °C or 68 °F. If becomes anoxic due to prolonged apnea, intubate with cuffed endotracheal tube and manually ventilate. Can also use Doxopram IV.
Telazol + butorphanol	T: 0.9 mg/kg IV + B: 0.1 mg/kg IV [9].	Northern elephant seals	n = 1 animal immobilized 2 × with Telazol 0.8 mg/kg IV and once with the addition of butorphanol for surgery to repair a hiatal hernia.
Telazol + ketamine	T: 1.15 mg/kg + K: 0.27 mg/kg IM dart [14]	South American fur seals	n = 8, 0% mortality, partial reversal with flumazenil.
Telazol + medetomidine	T: 1 mg/kg + M: 0.04 mg/kg IM; antagonize with atipamezole 0.2 mg/kg IM [23]	California sea lions	May consider atropine 0.02 mg/kg IM to decrease secretions. For long procedures you may wish to intubate and use gas anesthesia.
	T: 1 mg/kg + M: 0.07 mg/kg IM [14]	California sea lions	n = 17 animals, additional 22% with supplemental 1–5% isoflurane, 0% mortalities. Reliable anesthesia, antagonize with atipamezole. Ataxia and disorientation during recovery seen in some animals.

(*Continued*)

Drug name	Drug dose	Species	Comments
	T: 1 mg/kg + M: 0.07 mg/kg IM [28]	California sea lions	n = 23 animals 8.15, Time to max effect was 3–7 min, only one animal was not sufficiently anesthetized, 16/23 were intubated without additional medication, 7 required isoflurane via mask for full induction to allow intubation. Total immobilization time was 25–62 min, Recovery time post atipamezole (0.2 mg/kg IM) was 2–14 min. Prolonged recoveries with muscle fasciculations and shaking noted in 6/23 animals. One animal died during procedure and no gross or histologic causes of death were identified.
Xylazine	0.8–2.8 mg/kg IM [14]	Leopard seals	Variable plane of anesthesia with lower dose, mortalities with higher doses.
Yohimbine	0.06 mg/kg IV [14]	Southern elephant seals	To hasten recovery from a ketamine + xylazine sedation.
	0.5 mg/kg IM [14]	Weddell seals	Hastened recovery from a ketamine + xylazine + diazepam procedure.
Antiparasitic			
Dichlorvos	9.7–11.5 mg/kg, PO (Tablet), or 29.3–32.8 mg/kg PO (Capsule) [1]	Northern fur seals	Caution for organophosphate toxicity.
Fenbendazole	11 mg/kg PO SID × 2 doses [1]	Northern elephant seals, California sea lions	
	15–20 mg/kg PO SID × 3d [3]	California sea lions	
Ivermectin	100–200 μg/kg SC [1]	Northern fur seals	
Ivermectin	200 μg/kg SC [1]	California sea lions, Northern elephant seals, Harbor seals	Tremors observed in Guadalupe fur seal after administration.
Ivermectin (Equavalan)	0.2 mg/kg IM once or 0.1 ml/100 lb bwt in adults once a week [3]	California sea lions	
Levamisole	15 mg/kg SC [1]	California sea lions, Northern elephant seals	
	8 mg/kg PO [1]	California sea lions	
Ponazuril	11 mg/kg PO SID [8]	California sea lions	n = 1 animal with sarcocystis-related rhabdomyolysis and acute renal failure.
Praziquantel	5–7 mg/kg PO q10d for 2 doses [3]	California sea lions	

Drug name	Drug dose	Species	Comments
Other			
Acetylcysteine	20% solution nebulized BID to QID [1]	Pinnipeds	
Acetylcysteine + Isoproterenol	400 mg IT BID-QID [1]	Pinnipeds	Nebulized in 12–15 ml saline with 1 : 50000 isoproterenol.
Adrenaline	1 ml of 1 : 1000 given intracamerally in the eye [29]	New Zealand fur seals	n = 1 animal with bilateral phacofragmentation, where intracameral adrenaline was the only drug successful at producing pupillary dilation (prednisone PO, pancuronium atropine topically were not successful) atropine sulfate was injected episclerally as well to maintain dilation. Eyes remained partially dilated for approximately 7 days post surgery.
Aluminum hydroxide	30–90 mg/kg PO [1]	California sea lions	For treatment of leptospirosis and associated renal changes.
Aminophylline	5.5 mg/kg IV, IM, PO Bid to TID [1]	California sea lions, Harbor seals, Northern elephant seals	
Atropine	0.02 mg/kg PRN [3]	California sea lions, Harbor seals	
	0.2 mg/kg IM [1, 14]		Often used 10 min prior to anesthesia to decrease reflex bradycardia.
Calcitonin nasal spray	5 IU/kg q72 hrs [8]	California sea lions	n = 1 animal with sarcocystis related rhabdomyolysis and acute renal failure and later hypercalcemia that responded to calcitonin.
Castor oil + Dry mustard	1.2 ml/kg of 4 : 1 ratio PO [1]	Pinnipeds	
Cimetidine	6.7 mg/kg PO × 7d [6]	Harbor seals	n = 1, 29 yr old female undergoing gastrotomy for foreign bodies. 7 days postop started feeding and treating with cimetidine for 7 days.
Cimetidine	5–15 mg/kg PO TID [1]	California sea lions	For treatment of animals with leptospirosis.
Cisatracurium	0.2 mg/kg IV intermittently to maintain eye position. Antagonized with Edrophonium 0.1 mg/kg IV slowly over 5 min [16]	Walruses	n = 1 animal undergoing ophthalmic surgery. Was successful at keeping eye in central position.
Depo-Provera (Depo medroxyprogesterone acetate)	400 mg Injection [30]	Gray seals	Depo-Provera DID NOT prevent ovulation in 3/7 animals when given 1 wk postpartum or prior to expected ovulation. Drug serum levels peaked at 2 weeks and were undetectable at 6 weeks.

(*Continued*)

Drug name	Drug dose	Species	Comments
Deslorelin acetate implant	0.5 mg/kg SQ annually [2]	Pinnipeds	For contraception: Caution: may not be immediately reversible.
Dexamethasone	0.1 mg/kg SID [3]	California sea lions, Harbor seals	
	0.2–1 mg/kg IM, PO SID [1]	California sea lion, Elephant seals	
	2.2 mg/kg IV [1]	California sea lions	For treatment of shock.
Dextrose	100 ml/kg/d SQ or RO [1]	California sea lions	For treatment of animals with leptospirosis.
	500 mg/kg IP [31]	Hypoglycemic yearling California sea lions	For treatment of hypoglycemia, increased glucose serum levels by 50 mg/dl for up to 2 hrs.
Dobutamine	0.2–2 μg/kg/min IV [32]	Pinnipeds	Lower dose than terrestrial mammals.
Doxapram	1–2 mg/kg PRN [3]	California sea lions	
	>5 mg/kg not recommended [14]	Southern elephant seals	Resulted in shaking and hyperresponsive animals when used as an antagonist for a ketamine diazepam anesthetic procedure.
Ephedrine	0.05–0.1 mg/kg IV [32]	Pinnipeds	Positive inotrope.
Epinephrine	0.02–0.05 mg/kg PRN [3]	California sea lions, Harbor seals	
Famotidine	0.5 mg/kg PO or IM SID [3]	California sea lions, Harbor seals	
	0.5 mg/kg SC or IM [2, 8]	California sea lions	n = 1 animal with sarcocystis related rhabdomyolysis and acute renal failure.
	0.9 mg/kg IM SID [9]	Northern elephant seals	n = 1 animal prior to surgical repair of hiatal hernia.
Ferrocon (Iron) supplement	1.5 mg/kg PO SID [3]	California sea lions	
	1.5 mg/kg PO SID [2]	Steller sea lions	For iron deficiency anemia.
Fluoxetine HCl (5HT reuptake inhibitor – antianxiety)	0.2–1.2 mg/kg PO SID [1]	California sea lions, Steller sea lions	Treatment for regurgitation and flank sucking.
Furosemide	2.5–5 mg/kg IM, IV, PO BID [1]	Harbor seals, California sea lions	
Gastrograffin (diatrizoate meglumine + diatrizoate sodium solution)	2 ml/kg delivered via endoscopy biopsy port [9]	Northern elephant seals	n = 1 animal for imaging due to suspicion of hiatal hernia.

Drug name	Drug dose	Species	Comments
Hydrogen peroxide	5 ml/kg PO PRN [1]	Pinnipeds	
Insulin	Hagedorn neutral protamine insulin: 0.35 U/kg IM SID [33]	California sea lions	n = 1 captive adult male with chronic pancreatitis which led to hyperglycemia, glucosuria and increased fructosamine levels treated initially with Hagedorn insulin with 1″ 25ga needle in caudal gluteal muscles for 6 days, then BID for a few weeks. Glycemic control was fair to good based on fructosamine levels.
Insulin	Glargine insulin: 0.5–0.75 U/kg IM SID [33]	California sea lions	n = 1 captive adult male, initially treated with Hagedorn, but switched to Glargine insulin. Provided glucose concentrations within reference range within 6 hrs of administration, Fair to good regulation reported via fructosamine levels.
Isoetharine	90 mg nebulized in 1% solution PRN [1]	Pinnipeds	For treatment of bronchospasm.
Isoproterenol	1:50000 IT [1]	Pinnipeds	
Isuprel	0.4 mg/kg PO BID to TID, or 0.5 ml nebulized BID to QID [1]	California sea lions	Bronchodilator.
Leuprolide acetate	0.075 mg/kg IM monthly [2]	Males: California sea lions, Steller sea lions, Northern fur seals	For males for contraception and to decrease male to male aggression during breeding season.
	0.09–0.12 mg/kg IM q28d [1]	California sea lions	May cause injection site pain.
	18.75 mg (5 doses of 3.75 mg reconstituted with 3 ml diluent) [34]	Northern fur seals	n = 2 females in a captive colony, injections given monthly for 6 months during breeding season and prevented pregnancy for 2 years.
	22.5 mg (0.09–0.12 mg/kg) IM depot via hand injection in pelvic limb or dart monthly from April to Sept. Reconstituted with 1.5–9 ml diluent [35].	California sea lions	n = 3 males from 10 to 23 yrs. old, 1 animal had injection site pain, lameness, and swelling as well as moderate to marked anorexia and depression. Treating with flunixin meglumine for 3–7 days post injection improved symptoms.
Maropitant (Cerenia)	0.5–1 mg/kg SID PO or SC [3]	California sea lions, Harbor seals	
Maropitant	1 mg/kg SC or 2 mg/kg PO [8]	California sea lions	n = 1 animal with sarcocystis related rhabdomyolysis and acute renal failure.
Maropitant (Cerenia)	1 mg/kg PO or SC SID [2]	Pinnipeds	

(Continued)

Drug name	Drug dose	Species	Comments
Megestrol acetate	0.3–0.5 mg/kg PO BID [1]	Pinnipeds	
Metoclopramide	0.5–1 mg/kg PO BID to TID [3]	California sea lions, Harbor seals	
	0.2 mg/kg IM TID [9]	Northern elephant seal	n = 1 animal prior to surgical repair of hiatal hernia.
	0.2 mg/kg PO BID [2]	Pinnipeds	
	0.5 mg/kg SC [8]	California sea lions	n = 1 animal with sarcocystis related rhabdomyolysis and acute renal failure.
Mirtazapine	15 mg for smaller seal/sea lion, or 30 mg for adult sea lion; given PO SID in AM [2]	Pinnipeds	Appetite stimulant. Can also crush tablet and give rectally.
Norepinephrine	0.1–0.5 μg/kg/min [32]	Pinnipeds	Vasopressor.
Omeprazole	1 mg/kg PO SID [2]	Pinnipeds	
Ondansetron	0.3 mg/kg SC SID [2]	Pinnipeds	
Oxytocin	20–40 USP units IM [1]	Pinnipeds	
Phenobarbitol	1–1.5 mg/kg PO SID-BID [1]	California sea lions	Treatment of idiopathic seizures.
Phenylephrine	1–3 μg/kg/min IV [32]	Pinnipeds	Vasopressor.
Prednisone	Up to 0.5 mg/kg PO SID [2]	Pinnipeds	Dose dependent on reason for treatment.
	1 mg/kg PO SID to BID [3]	California sea lions, Harbor seals	
Primidone	2.5 mg/kg PO TID loading or initial control; 1–2.5 mg/kg PO SID maintenance [1]	Pinnipeds	
Pyridoxine (Vit. B6)	0.25 mg/kg PO SID [1]	Pinnipeds	
Ranitidine	1 mg/kg PO BID [3]	California sea lions, Harbor seals	
	1 mg/kg PO BID [33]	California sea lions	n = 1 captive adult male with chronic pancreatitis, managed with daily ranitidine combined with metronidazole 10 mg/kg PO BID and an all-capelin diet to reduce fat content.
Simethicone	40 mg PO BID [3]	Harbor seals	
	80–250 mg/kg PO BID to TID [3]	California sea lions	
	1000–2000 mg PO BID to TID [3]	Walruses	

Drug name	Drug dose	Species	Comments
Sodium chloride	3 g/kg fish SID; 100–200 mg/kg PO, IP [1]	Pinnipeds	For maintenance.
Temeril-P (5 mg Trimeprazine + 2 mg prednisolone)	3 tablets PO BID [2]	California sea lions, adult male	
Theophylline	8.9 mg/kg loading; 6.1 mg/kg maintenance [1]	Pinnipeds	
Thiacetarsamide	0.44 mg/kg IV slow drip twice [1]	Pinnipeds	Arsenical for heartworm treatment and trematodes in canids.
Thiamine	1 mg/kg IM SID; 2–4 mg/kcal feed PO SID 2 hr prior to feeding; 25–35 mg/kg fish PO SID at feeding [1]	Pinnipeds	
Ursodeoxycholic acid	10 mg/kg PO SID [33]	California sea lions	n = 1 captive adult male with chronic pancreatitis and subsequent diabetes mellitus. When cholestatic disease was apparent started on ursodeoxycholic acid. A few months later the animal died with chronic pancreatic fibrosis and bile duct fibrosis and abscessation of the gall bladder.
Vitamin A	300–600 IU/d PO [1]	Northern fur seals	
Vitamin B Complex (based on Thiamine)	2 mg/100 lbs (150 mg/ml) [2]	Pinnipeds	
Vitamin E	100 IU/kg PO in fish [1]		High levels (50 000 IU/D) may increase Vitamin E req.
	100 mg/day PO in fish [1]	Harbor seals	Adult males.
Vitamin E and Selenium	S: 2.5 mg/kg, Vit E: 50 mg/ml: 1 ml per 100 lbs [2]	Pinnipeds	
Whole Blood transfusion	300 ml of whole blood given IO into trochanteric fossa of femur [36]	Guadalupe fur sea given blood from a healthy California sea lion	n = 1 animal, undergoing rehabilitation with a PCV of 6% prior to transfusion, 12% after and 38% prior to release 10 weeks later. This animal was also given vitamins, antibiotics, steroids and iron in addition to whole blood.
Yunnan Baiyo herbal supplement	250 mg capsules: 3 capsules PO BID for adult female Steller sea lion, 2 capsules PO BID for Male adult California sea lion [2]	Steller sea lions, California sea lions	

Species	Weight
California sea lion *(Zalophus californianus)*	Female: 50–100 kg Male: 200–400 kg
Northern Steller sea lion *(Eumetopias jubatus)*	Female 270 kg, Male 1000 kg
Southern sea lion *(Otaria flavescens)*	Female: 140 kg, Male: 200–350 kg
Antarctic fur seal *(Arctocephalus gazella)*	Female: 30–51 kg, Male: 126–160 kg
Crabeater seal *(Lobodon carcinophaga)*	200–300 kg
Galapagos fur seal *(Arctocephalus galapagoensis)*	Female: 27 kg, Male: 64 kg
Gray seal *(Halichoerus grypus)*	Female: 105–186 kg, Male: 170–310 kg
Guadalupe fur seal *(Artocephalus townsendi)*	Female: 50 kg, Male: 140 kg
Harbor seal *(Phoca vitulina)*	Female: 50–150 kg, Male: 70–170 kg
Harp seal *(Phoca greonlandica)*	120–135 kg
Hooded seal *(Cystophora cristata)*	Female: 145–300 kg, Male: 200–400 kg
Leopard seal *(Hydrurga leptonyx)*	Female: 225–290 kg, Male: 200–455 kg
New Zealand fur seal *(Arctocephalus forsteri)*	Female: 40–70 kg, Male: 120–185 kg
Northern elephant seal *(Mirounga angustirostris)*	Female: 900 kg, Male: 2000–2700 kg
Northern fur seal *(Callorhinus ursinus)*	Female 43–50 kg, Male: 181–272 kg
Ringed seal *(Pusa hispida)*	61–142 kg
South American fur seal *(Arctocephalus australis)*	Female: 30–60 kg, Male: 150–200 kg
Southern elephant seal *(Mirounga leonine)*	Female: 359–900 kg, Male: 2000–3700 kg
Southern fur seal	Female: 36–122 kg, Male: 134–363 kg
Southern (Subantarctic) fur seal *(Arctocephalus tropicalis)*	21–68 kg
Weddell seal *(Leptonychotes weddellii)*	350–475 kg
Atlantic walrus *(Odobenus romarus rosmarus)*	Female: 400–560 kg, Male: 900 kg
Pacific walrus *(Odobenus rosmarus divergens)*	Female: 800 kg, Male: 2000 kg

References

1 Dierauf, L. and Gulland, F.M.D. (2001). *CRC Handbook of Marine Mammal Medicine.* CRC Press.

2 Mystic Aquarium (2018). Personal communication.

3 SeaWorld Parks and Entertainment (2018). Personal communication.

4 Gulland, F.M., Stoskopf, M.K., Johnson, S.P. et al. (2000). Amoxicillin pharmacokinetics in harbor seals (*Phoca vitulina*) and northern elephant seals (*Mirounga angustirostris*) following single dose intravenous administration: implications for interspecific dose scaling. *Journal of Veterinary Pharmacology* 23 (4): 223–228.

5 Vogelnest L. and Hulst, F. (1996). The Veterinary management of Southern Elephant seals (*Mirounga leonine*) at Taronga Zoo. *Proceedings of the American Association of Zoo Veterinarians.*

6 Dunker, F., Haulena, M., Crawford, G. et al. (2001). Anesthesia and Postoperative Care for Gastrotomy in a Harbor Seal (*Phoca vitulina*). *Proceedings of the American Association of Zoo Veterinarians.*

7 Garcia Parraga, D., Gilabert, J.A., Valls, M. et al. (2012). Updates on the pharmacokinetics of Cefovecin (Convenia) in Marine mammals. *Proceedings of the International Association for Aquatic Animal Medicine.*
8 Alexander, A.B., Hanley, C.S., Duncan, M.C. et al. (2015). Management of Acute renal failure with delayed hypercalcemia secondary to Sarcocystis neurona-induced myositis and Rhabdomyolysis in a California Sea lion (*Zalophus californianus*). *Journal of Zoo and Wildlife Medicine* 46 (3): 652–656.
9 Greene, R., Van Bonn, W.G., Dennison, S.E. et al. (2015). Laparoscopic gastropexy for correction of a hiatal hernia in a northern elephant seal (*Mirounga angustirostris*). *Journal of Zoo and Wildlife Medicine* 46 (2): 414–416.
10 Freeman, K.S., Thomasy, S.M., Stanley, D. et al. (2013). Population pharmacokinetics of doxycycline in the tears and plasma of northern elephant seals (*Mirounga angustirostris*) following oral drug administration. *Journal of the American Veterinary Medical Association* 243 (8): 1170–1178.
11 Kukanich, B., Huff, D., Riviere, J. et al. (2007). Naïve averaged, Naïve pooled, and population pharmacokinetics of orally administered Marbofloxacin in juvenile harbor seals. *Journal of the American Veterinary Medical Association* 230 (3): 390–395.
12 Schmitt, T.L. and Proctor, D.G. (2014). Coccidioidomycosis in a Pacific walrus (*Odobenus rosmarus divergens*). *Journal of Zoo and Wildlife Medicine* 45 (10): 173–175.
13 Molter, C.M., Barbosa, L., Johnson, S. et al. (2015). Pharmacokinetics of a single subcutaneous dose of sustained release buprenorphine in northern elephant seals (*Mirounga angustirostris*). *Journal of Zoo and Wildlife Medicine* 46 (1): 52–61.
14 Lynch, M. and Bodley, K. (2014). Phocid seals. In: *Zoo Animal and Wild Immobilization and Anesthesia* (ed. G. West, D. Heard and N. Caulkett), 647–660. Ames, IA: Wiley Blackwell.
15 Dold, C., Haulena, M., and Gulland, F.M.D. (2004). Pharmacokinetics of oral Carprofen in the California Sea lion (*Zalophus californianus*). *Proceedings of the American Association of Zoo Veterinarians.*
16 Kaartinen, J., Lair, S., Walsh, M.T. et al. (2018). Anesthesia of aquarium-housed walrus (*Odobenus rosmarus*): a case series. *Journal of Zoo and Wildlife Medicine* 49 (2): 435–443.
17 Gutierrez, J., Simeone, C., Gulland, F. et al. (2016). Development of retrobulbar and auriculopalpebral nerve blocks in California Sea lions (*Zalophus californianus*). *Journal of Zoo and Wildlife Medicine* 47 (1): 236–243.
18 Boonstra, J.L., Barbosa, L., Van Bonn, W.G. et al. (2015). Pharmacokinetics of tramadol hydrochloride and its metabolite O-desmethyltramadol following a single, orally administered dose in California Sea lions (*Zalophus californianus*). *Journal of Zoo and Wildlife Medicine* 46 (3): 476–481.
19 Tuomi, P.A. (2000). Butorphanol and butorphanol/diazepam administration for analgesia and sedation of harbor seals (*Phoca vitulina*). *Proceedings of the International Association for Aquatic Animal Medicine.*
20 Tuomi, P.A., Mulcahy, D.M., and Garner, G.W. (1996). Immobilization of Pacific Walrus (*Odobenus rosmarus divergens*) with carfentanil, naltrexone reversal, and Isoflurane anesthesia. *Proceedings of the International Association for Aquatic Animal Medicine.*
21 Van Bonn, W.G. (2015). Pinnipeds. In: *Fowler's Zoo and Wild Animal Medicine*, vol. 8 (ed. R.E. Miller and M. Fowler), 436–449. St. Louis, MO: Elsevier Saunders.
22 Olberg, R., Kovacs, K.M., Bertelsen, M.F. et al. (2017). Short duration immobilization of Atlantic walrus (*Odobenus romarus rosmarus*) with etorphine, and reversal with naltrexone. *Journal of Zoo and Wildlife Medicine* 48 (4): 972–978.
23 Kreeger, T.J. and Arnemo, J.M. (2012). *Handbook of Wildlife Chemical Immobilization*. China: Kreeger.

24 Lair, S., Pang, D., Rondenay, Y. et al. (2005). Anesthesia of juvenile harp seals (*Phoca greonlandica*) with midazolam and Isoflurane. *Proceedings of the International Association for Aquatic Animal Medicine.*

25 Haulena, M. (2014). Otariid seals. In: *Zoo Animal and Wild Immobilization and Anesthesia* (ed. G. West, D. Heard and N. Caulkett), 661–672. Ames, IA: Wiley Blackwell.

26 Gulland, F.M.D. and Gage, L.J. (1997). Preliminary trials of the use of propofol for general anesthesia of Phocid seals. *Proceedings of the International Association for Aquatic Animal Medicine.*

27 Champagne, C.D., Houser, D.S., Costa, D.P. et al. (2012). The effects of handling and anesthetic agents on the stress response and carbohydrate metabolism in northern elephant seals. *PLoS One* 7 (5): 1–13.

28 Haulena, M., Gulland, F.M.D., and Spraker, T.R. (1999). A comparison of the use of Medetomidine plus Ketamine and Medetomidine plus Telazol (tiletamine and zolazepam) to immobilize California Sea lions (*Zalophus californianus*). *Proceedings of the International Association for Aquatic Animal Medicine.*

29 Barnes, J. and Smith, J.F. (2002). Bilateral Phacofragmentation in a New Zealand Fur seal (*Arctocephalus forsteri*). *Proceedings of the American Association of Zoo Veterinarians.*

30 Seely, A. and Ronald, K. (1991). The effect of Depo-Provera on reproduction in the Grey seal (*Halichoerus grypus*). *Proceedings of the American Association of Zoo Veterinarians.*

31 Fravel, V.A., Van Bonn, W., Gulland, F. et al. (2016). Intraperitoneal dextrose administration as an alternative emergency treatment for hypoglycemic yearling California Sea lions (*Zalophus californianus*). *Journal of Zoo and Wildlife Medicine* 47 (1): 76–82.

32 Colitz, C.M.H. and Bailey, J.E. (2019). Lens diseases and anesthetic considerations for ophthalmologic procedures in Pinnipeds. In: *Fowler's Zoo and Wild Animal Medicine Current Therapy*, vol. 9 (ed. R.E. Miller, N. Lamberski and P.P. Calle), 610–617. St. Louis, MO: Elsevier Saunders.

33 Meegan, J.M., Sidor, I.F., Steiner, J.M. et al. (2008). Chronic pancreatitis with secondary diabetes mellitus treated by use of insulin in an adult California Sea lion. *Journal of the American Veterinary Medical Association* 232 (11): 1707–1712.

34 Calle, P.P., Smith, J., and McClave, J. (2005). The use of Leuprolide acetate for male contraception in a Northern Fur Seal (*Callorhinus ursinus*) colony. *Proceedings of the American Association of Zoo Veterinarians.*

35 Calle P.P., Stetter, M.D., Raphael, B.L. et al. (1997). Use of depo leuprolide acetate to control undesirable male associated behaviors in the California Sea lion (*Zalophus californianus*) and California Sea otter (*Enhydra lutris*). *Proceedings of the International Association for Aquatic Animal Medicine.*

36 Gage, L.J., Beckman, K., Wickham, D. et al. (1996). Transfusion of a Guadalupe Fur Seal (*Arctocephalus townsendi*) with California Sea lion (*Zalophus californianus*) blood. *Proceedings of the International Association for Aquatic Animal Medicine.*

16

Manatees and Dugongs

Drug name	Drug dose	Species	Comments
Antimicrobials and Antifungals			Oral or stomach tube delivered antibiotics may result in loss of normal intestinal flora and associated diarrhea and hypermotility [1].
Amikacin	7 mg/kg IM or PO BID [1, 2]	Manatees	
Amoxicillin	10–11 mg/kg SID or 7 mg/kg BID PO [3]	Florida manatees	
Ampicillin	5.5 mg/kg PO SID [2]	Sirenians	
Ceftiofur	2 mg/kg IM SID [4]	Dugongs	n = 1 animal in rehabilitation, given for 12 days then released.
Ceftiofur crystalline-free acid (Excede)	4–10 mg/kg SC [2, 5]	Florida manatees	n = 2 animals treated for pneumothorax and pneumoperitoneum.
	6.6 mg/kg SC q5d [3]	Florida manatees	
Ceftriaxone	22 mg/kg IM SID [1, 2]	Manatees	
Cephalexin	40 mg/kg PO SID [2]	Sirenians	
Ciprofloxacin	10 mg/kg PO SID [3]	Florida manatees	
Danofloxacin	6–8 mg/kg IM q48 hr [2, 3]	Sirenians	
Enrofloxacin	5 mg/kg PO BID [3]	Florida manatees	
Gentamicin	2.5 mg/kg PO TID or 4.4 mg/kg IM SID [2]	Manatees	
Itraconazole	2.5 mg/kg PO BID [2, 3]	Manatees	
Metronidazole	7 mg/kg PO BID [2, 3]	Sirenians	For treatment of hemorrhagic coliis, adjunct to gentamicin.
Oxytetracycline	3–9 mg/lb/day IM SC [1]	Manatees	Animals have been treated with standard cattle doses: for bacterial pneumonia 5–9 mg/kg is used and for foot rot or other less severe infections 3–5 mg/kg is used.

(Continued)

Zoo and Wild Mammal Formulary, First Edition. Alicia Hahn.

Drug name	Drug dose	Species	Comments
	4.5 mg/kg IM BID [2]	Dugongs	
	15 mg/kg IM BID [2]	Sirenians	
Penicillin G (benzathine procaine)	22 000 IU/kg IM SID [1, 2]	Manatees	
	25 000 IU/kg IM or SC SID [2]	Dugongs	
Tetracycline	55 mg/kg IM BID [2]	Manatees	
Trimethoprim sulfadiazine 1:5 or 1:2	20 mg/kg PO SID × 28d [3]	Florida manatees	1:2 ratio of drugs used for Nocardia suspicion.
Trimethoprim sulfamethoxazole	18–22 mg/kg PO BID [3]	Florida manatees	
	21.5 mg/kg PO SID × 8d [2]	Sirenians	
Tulathromycin	2.5 mg/kg SQ q7d [2, 3]	Sirenians	
Sulfasalazine	10 mg/kg IM BID [2]	Manatees	
Analgesia			
Flunixin meglumine	0.3 mg/kg IV once or 0.07 mg/kg IM once [2]	Sirenians	
Flunixin meglumine	0.5–1.1 mg/kg IM [3]	Florida manatees	
Ketoprofen	1–2 mg/kg IM [2, 6, 7]	Sirenians	For severe abdominal pain, use caution in dehydrated animals to prevent adverse effects on kidneys.
	2 mg/kg SID [3]	Florida manatees	
	2 mg/kg IM caudal epaxial at the level of peduncle [2, 5]	Florida manatees	n = 2 manatees treated for pneumothorax and pneumoperitoneum.
Lidocaine 2%	local infusion to effect [7]	Florida manatees	Local analgesia.
Tramadol	1 mg/kg PO SID [2, 3]	Sirenians	
Anethesia and Sedation			IM effect onset time is generally 15–20 min but can be up to 25 min. IM injections are given with 90 mm 18ga spinal needles into gluteal muscles. IV and IM injections: the skin is cleaned with iodine surgical solution for 3 min prior to injection to minimize iatrogenic contamination. IM injections in calves with 21 ga 3.75–5 cm needles Ideally fasted for 24 hrs prior to anesthesia.
Atipamezole	1 mg/20 mg xylazine IV, or 1 mg/2 mg detomidine IV, or 5 mg/1 mg detomidine IM [6, 7]	Florida manatees	To antagonize xylazine or detomidine.

Drug name	Drug dose	Species	Comments
Butorphanol + diazepam	B: 0.01–0.025 mg/kg IV + Dia: 0.01–0.025 mg/kg IV [6, 7]	Florida manatees	For mild to moderately painful procedures, give butorphanol 10 min prior to diazepam.
Butorphanol + detomidine	B: 0.015 mg/kg + D: 0.015 mg/kg IM [3]	Florida manatees	
Butorphanol + midazolam	B: 0.04–0.06 mg/kg + Mid: 0.1 mg/kg IM [6] [7],	Florida manatees	For anesthesia induction or short procedures in fractious individuals.
	B: 0.03–0.07 + Mid: 0.06–0.1 mg/kg IM [3]	Florida manatees	
	B: 0.1 mg/kg + Mid: 0.1 mg/kg [6, 7]	Florida manatees	For anesthesia induction in severely fractious individuals, results in very deep sedation, use with caution.
Detomidine	0.005–0.01 mg/kg [6, 7]	Florida manatees	Moderate sedation, beware of narrow therapeutic index.
Detomidine + butorphanol	D: 0.025–0.005 mg/kg + B: 0.005–0.01 mg/kg [6, 7]	Florida manatees	In combo with detomidine for minor surgical procedures or anesthetic induction.
	D: 0.0086 mg/kg + B: 0.0086 mg/kg [6, 7]	Florida manatees	For heavier sedation, ± intubation, excellent analgesia and muscle relaxation, beware of narrow therapeutic index.
Detomidine + midazolam + butorphanol	D: 0.017 mg/kg + Mid: 0.07 mg/kg + B: 0.017 mg/kg IM [5]	Florida manatees	n = 1 animal, sedated then transported for radiographs and computed tomography.
Diazepam	D: 0.05–0.1 mg/kg PO; antagonize with flumazenil 0.008–0.05 mg/kg IV or IM [3]	Florida manatees	
Diazepam	0.08 mg/kg [8]	West Indian manatees	To assist with intubation prior to isoflurane anesthesia.
	15–20 mg/450 kg animal PO BID [6, 7]	Sirenians	To alleviate anxiety and enhance appetite in rehabilitation animals.
	0.02–0.035 mg/kg IV [6, 7]	Florida manatees	For nonpainful diagnostics.
	0.066 mg/kg IM [6, 7, 9]	Florida manatees	For tranquilization for 60–90 min.
	0.02–0.035 mg/kg IM [1]	Dugongs	For mild and pre-operative sedation.
Flumazenil	1 mg/20 mg midazolam or diazepam IV or in equal volume as midazolam/diazepam given IM [6, 7]	Florida manatees	For reversal of midazolam or diazepam.
	F: 0.008–0.05 mg/kg IV or IM [3]	Florida manatees	
Isoflurane	Supplement via intubation or mask induction via facemask [6]	Florida manatees	
Meperidine	0.5–1 mg/kg IM [6, 7, 9]	Florida manatees	By itself or in combo with midazolam (0.045 mg/kg IM) for more painful procedures or anesthetic induction.

(*Continued*)

Drug name	Drug dose	Species	Comments
Meperidine + midazolam	Mep: 0.5–1 mg/kg + Mid: 0.045 mg/kg IM [6, 7, 9]		For more painful procedures.
	Mep: up to 1 mg/kg + Mid: 0.066 mg/kg IM; antagonize with flumazenil and naloxone [10]	Florida manatees	For light general anesthesia and restraint.
Midazolam	M: 0.02–0.05 mg/kg IM [5, 6, 7]	Manatees and Florida manatees	Mild to moderate sedation, upper end of dose has 60–90 min sedation, 0.07 mg/kg used for sedation prior to radiographs and computed tomography.
	M: 0.05–0.072 mg/kg [6, 7]	Florida manatees	Sedation for 20–30 min at peak effect for endoscopy, freeze branding or noninvasive procedures.
	M: 0.045–0.08 mg/kg [9, 10]	Florida manatees	The lower end of range lasted 60–90 min.
	M: 0.05–0.15 mg/kg IM [3]	Florida manatees	
	0.08 mg/kg [6, 7]	Florida manatees	Anesthetic induction and intubation.
	0.02–0.05 mg/kg IM [1]	Dugongs	For mild or pre-operative sedation.
Naltrexone	N: 0.1–0.4 mg/kg IM [3]	Florida manatees	
	1–2 mg/1 mg butorphanol IV or IM to reverse butorphanol, or an equal volume dose IM to reverse meperidine [6, 7]	Florida manatees	For reversal.
Pethidine	up to 1 mg/kg IM [1]	Manatees	In conjunction with benzodiazepines for fractious individuals for procedures that require analgesia.
Xylazine	0.05–0.1 mg/kg IM [6, 7]	Florida manatees	Moderate sedation, beware of narrow therapeutic range.
Yohimbine	Reversal: 1 mg/5–10 mg xylazine IV or IM, or 2–3 mg/1 mg detomidine IV or IM [6, 7]	Florida manatees	Reversal of xylazine or detomidine.
Antiparasitic			
Fenbendazole	10 mg/kg PO once [9]	Manatees	
	10–15 mg/kg PO once [2, 7]	Manatees	For treatment of nematode infestation.
	10 mg/kg PO SID × 3d [3]	Florida manatees	
Ivermectin	200 µg/kg PO once [2]	Manatees	

Drug name	Drug dose	Species	Comments
Ivermectin + praziquantel (Eqvalan gold)	200 mg/kg PO SID, repeated in 21d [11]	Antillean manatees	n = 1 case of an adult female manatee, 274 kg, exhibiting signs and nasal parasite *Pulmonicola cochleotrema*. Four days post treatment clinical signs decreased and were absent by 7 days.
Praziquantel	10–20 mg/kg PO once [2, 7]	Manatees	For treatment of trematode infestations.
	8–16 mg/kg PO [2]	Manatees	For treatment of trematodes.
	8–16 mg/kg PO once or repeat in 14d [3]	Florida manatees	
Other			
Atropine	0.02 mg/kg Total dose, 1/4 IV and 3/4 SC once [2, 3]	Sirenians	For treatment of brevitoxicosis.
Bismuth subsalicylate (Pepto Bismol)	12 mg/kg PO once, then 6 mg/kg PO SID × 5d [2]	Sirenians	
Dexamethasone	0.25–0.5 mg/kg IM SID [1]	Manatees	Used to stimulate the appetite and decrease inflammation.
	0.05–0.1 mg/kg SID [3]	Florida manatees	
	2 mg/kg IM [2]	Sirenians	
Epinephrine	0.02–0.05 mg/kg as needed [3]	Florida manatees	
Mineral oil	2 ml/kg (up to 1 l total) [3]	Florida manatees	
	2–3 ml/kg (up to 1.5 l total) [9]	Manatees	For constipation, given via stomach tube. GI transit time is 7–10 days so 3–4 doses of oil may be necessary. Warm freshwater enemas as well may remove compacted fecal material distally.
Simethicone	80 mg total dose, PO BID-TID [2, 3]	Manatees	For gas relief in calves.
Sodium chloride tablets	10–15 g PO SID in adults, 1 g PO BID in calves [3]	Florida manatees	
Vitamin B1 (thiamine)	1 mg/kg IM SID, follow with oral dosing [2].	Sirenians	For treatment of thiamine deficiency.
	2–4 mg/kcal feed PO SID, give 2 hrs prior to feeding [2]	Sirenians	For supplementation when supplements are administered prior to feeding.
Vitamin B1 (Thiamine)	25–35 mg/kg of fish PO SID at main feeding [2]	Sirenians	For supplementation when supplements are administered at time of feeding.
Vitamin C (Ascorbic acid)	1 mg/kg PO SID [2]	Sirenians	
Vitamin E	100 IU/kg of fish PO SID [2]	Sirenians	

Species	Weight [8, 6]
Dugong *(Dugong dugong)*	Adult 250–300 kg, calves 20–35 kg
West African manatee *(Trichechus senegoiensis)*	<500 kg
Amazonian manatee *(Trichechus inunguis)*	450–480 kg
Antillean manatee *(Trichechus manatus monotus)*	up to 1000 kg
West Indian manatee *(Trichechus monatus latirostris)*	400–1775 kg, males 400–600, females up to 1600, calves 18–45 kg

Acknowledgments

The author would like to thank SeaWorld Parks and Entertainment for contributing to this chapter.

References

1 Vogelnest, L. and Woods, R. (2008). Dugong. In: *Medicine of Australian Mammals* (ed. L. Vogelnest and R. Woods). Victoria, Australia: Csiro Publishing.

2 Dierauf, L.A. and Gulland, F.D. (2018). *CRC Handbook of Marine Mammal Medicine*, 607–674. Florida: Taylor & Francis Group, LLC.

3 SeaWorld Parks and Entertainment (2018). Personal communication.

4 Blyde, D.J. and Mackie, J. (2017). Relocation of a wayward Dugong (*Dugong dugon*). *An. Proc. Int. Assoc. Aq. An. Med.*

5 Gerlach, T.J., Sadler, V.M., and Ball, R.L. Conservative management of pneumothorax and pneumoperitoneum in two Florida manatees (*Trichechus manatus latirostris*). *Journal of Zoo and Wildlife Medicine* 44 (4): 996–1001.

6 Nolan, E.C. and Walsh, M.T. (2014). Sirenians (*Manatees* and *Dugongs*). In: *Zoo Animal and Wild Immobilization and Anesthesia* (ed. G. West, D. Heard and N. Caulkett), 693–702. Ames, IA: Wiley Blackwell.

7 Walsh, M.T. and deWit, M. (2015). Sirenia. In: *Fowler's Zoo and Wild Animal Medicine*, vol. 8 (ed. R.E. Miller and M. Fowler), 450–456. St. Louis, MO: Elsevier Saunders.

8 Kreeger, T.J., Arnemo, J.M., and Raath, J.P. (2002). *Handbook of Wildlife Chemical Immobilization*, vol. 205, 250. Fort Collins, Colorado: Wildlife Pharmaceuticals Inc.

9 Dierauf, L.A. and Gulland, F.D. (2001). *CRC Handbook of Marine Mammal Medicine*, 939–960. Florida: CRC Press.

10 Brunson, D.B. (2015). Comparative Anesthesia and analgesia of aquatic mammals. In: *Veterinary Anesthesia and Analgesia: The fifth edition of Lumb and Jones* (ed. K.A. Grimm, L.A. Lamont, W.J. Tranquilli, et al.), 777–783. Wiley.

11 Borges, J.C., Jung, L.M., Santos, S.S. et al. (2017). Treatment of Pulmonicola cochleotrema infection with Ivermectin-Praziquantel combination in an Antillean manatee (*Trichechus manatus manatus*). *Journal of Zoo and Wildlife Medicine* 48 (1): 217–219.

17

Elephants

Drug name	Drug dose	Species	Comments
Antimicrobials and Antifungals			
Amikacin	6–8 mg/kg IM SID [1, 2, 3]	African elephants	n = 3. Anecdotally one elephant at 7 mg/kg IM SID × 21d developed elevated creatinine and casts in the urine that resolved after stopping the medication.
Amoxicillin	11 mg/kg IM SID [3, 4]	Asian elephants	n = 5
Amoxicillin trihydrate	5.5–11 mg/kg [2, 5]	Asian elephants	n = 10 all male. No side effects reported.
Ampicillin	8 mg/kg PO BID to TID [3, 6]	Asian elephants	n = 3 above MIC for 8 hrs. Weights estimated.
Ceftiofur short-acting (Naxcel)	1.1 mg/kg IM BID to TID, or 1.1 mg/kg IV SID [3, 7]	Asian elephants	n = 4, 3 adult females. It is suggested when using the higher dose to reconstitute powder with less volume than the label indicates.
Ceftiofur long-acting (Excede)	6.6 mg/kg SC q7–10 d	Asian elephants	n = 11, 4.7, healthy, 11–45 yrs of age. 3/11 had reactions with 2/3 showing a 13 × 18 cm or smaller swelling that resolved on own, and 1/3 with a 5 cm sterile abscess that healed after lancing. Same researchers looked at the same dose in 2 adult African elephants SC in flank area and found earlier Tmax and lower AUC but similar median terminal half-lives [3, 8].
Ceftiofur (Excenel)	2 g (0.55 mg/kg) via intravenous regional perfusion diluted with heparinized saline, then followed with 60 ml heparinized saline IV [9]	Asian elephants	n = 1 tourniquet placed, then intravenous regional perfusion EOD for total of 70 treatments for the treatment of digital osteitis.

(Continued)

Zoo and Wild Mammal Formulary, First Edition. Alicia Hahn.

Drug name	Drug dose	Species	Comments
Cefoxitin + gentamicin IV, trimethoprim sulfamethoxazole and phenylbutazone PO	Perfusate: 1 ml Heparin added to 5 ml Saline and 10 mg lidocaine, combined with 2 g cefoxitin reconstituted with saline to 20 ml and gentamicin 2 g reconstituted to 50 ml with saline. This was given IV after tourniquet applied proximally. T: 48 g PO BID for 4 wks, P: 5 g PO BID × 7d [10]	Asian elephants	n = 1, 19 yr old female. Right carpal sole abscess. Received intravenous regional perfusion with cefoxitin and gentamicin for 2 treatments separated by 15d and in between supplemented with trimethoprim sulfamethoxazole.
Enrofloxacin	2.5 mg/kg PO SID [3, 11, 12]	Asian elephants	n = 6 rectal administration of this dose does not achieve therapeutic levels in African elephants (seen in a separate study of 0.3 African elephants).
	1.07–1.25 mg/kg PO BID [13]	Not specified	n = 1 no adverse effects noted after 2 wks.
	1.5–2.8 mg/kg PO SID [13]	Asian elephants	n = 1
Gentamicin sulfate	4.4 mg/kg IV or IM SID [13]	Not specified	IV injection can be diluted with 10% saline. Appears to maintain blood levels consistent with human treatment recommendations for 24 hrs.
Metronidazole	15 mg/kg rectally SID [3]	Asian elephants	n = 1 sick animal.
Metronidazole	15 mg/kg rectally q8–24 hrs [14, 15]	Asian elephants	n = 5 adult females. Absorbed well rectally. One elephant defecated 8 min post administration and had poor absorption; however, a second elephant defecated at 87 min post administration and had similar absorption to other elephants in study.
Oxytetracycline long-acting (LA 200)	18–20 mg/kg IM q48 hrs [3, 16, 17]	African elephants	n = 18 healthy calves (600–980 kg).
Penicillin G (benzathine) and Procaine penicillin	2273 IU/kg IM q48 hrs or 4545 IU/kg IM 96 hrs [3, 18]	African elephants	n = 5 healthy adult females. Dosing dependent on organisms targeted. Use higher dose every 36 hrs for Clostridia, and q24 hrs for *Pasteurella multocida*.
Sulfadimethoxine ormetoprim	16.2–18.5 mg/kg PO BID on day 1, then 9.25 mg/kg PO BID thereafter [13]	Not specified	Regimen used × 30d with positive results and no adverse effects. For more serious infections, could consider 23–26.4 mg/kg on day 1 and 13 mg/kg thereafter. Diarrhea may result with higher dose but will resolve with the discontinuation of treatment.
Trimethoprim sulfamethoxazole	22 mg/kg PO 2–6× daily [2, 3, 19]	Asian and African elephants	n = 3. In horses BID dosing is appropriate. African elephants require 4–6×/day dosing to maintain trough concentrations above MIC. Anecdotal favorable responses have been reported with BID dosing, however.

Drug name	Drug dose	Species	Comments
Tylosin	12 mg/kg SID × 5d [20]	Not specified	To treat acute Mycoplasma infections.
Antimicrobials used for treatment of Mycobacterial infections	See this website for most current recommendations on treating Mycobacterium infections in elephants: http://www.nasphv.org/Documents/ElephantTB NASPHV.pdf [21]		
Antiviral			
Famciclovir	8–15 mg/kg PO or rectal q8 hrs [22]	Asian elephants	n = 6, 1.5, 4.5–9 yrs of age. Range of both routes of administration resulted in concentrations considered therapeutic in humans taking this medication.
	6.7 mg/kg PO or rectally after initial 8 g bolus on day 1, and continued for 14–30d [23]	Asian elephants	n = 2 calves. First known calves successfully treated after developing clinical signs and viremia.
	12 mg/kg PO TID × 10d, then BID × 6d and SID for final 10d based on PCR and clinical response [24]	African elephants	n = 1, 5 yr old male. Clinical hemorrhagic EEHV case, treated successfully.
Local Anesthetic			
Procaine HCl 1–2%		Not specified	Infiltration. Duration 45–60 min [2, 25].
Lidocaine HCl 2%		Not specified	Infiltration. Epidural, spinal, topical. Duration 60–120 min [2, 25].
Mepivicaine HCl		Not specified	Infiltration. Duration 90–180 min [2, 25].
Bupivacaine HCl		Not specified	Infiltration. Epidural, topical. Duration 240–480 min [2, 25].
Analgesia			
Butorphanol tartrate	0.015 mg/kg IV or IM [26]	Asian elephants	Analgesia without sedation.
Butorphanol tartrate	0.007–0.13 mg/kg [2, 27]	African elephants	Adult, captive.
Flunixin meglumine	1 mg/kg SID (route not specified) [28–29]	Not specified	Anecdotal doses have been reported in a survey of zoo veterinarians. No studies available at this time.
Ibuprofen	6 mg/kg PO BID [3, 30]	Asian elephants	n = 10
	7 mg/kg PO BID [3, 30]	African elephants	n = 10
Ketoprofen	1–2 mg/kg PO or IV q24–48 hrs [3, 31]	Asian elephants	n = 5, 2.3, healthy adults. Food and water not withheld. Long-term safety not determined.
Morphine sulfate	3–6 mg/100 kg QID [20]	Not specified	3–6 mg/100 kg for sedation and analgesia. Doses of 6–20 mg/100 kg have also been reported but likely provide greater sedation.

(*Continued*)

Drug name	Drug dose	Species	Comments
Phenylbutazone	3 mg/kg PO q48 hrs [3, 32, 33]	Asian elephants	n = 8. Eliminated slower in Asian elephants thus given every 48 hrs. 2 reported cases of segmental gangrene and ear sloughing post IV use.
	2 mg/kg PO SID [3, 32]	African elephants	n = 10
	1–2 mg/kg PO SID or 2–4 mg/kg rectally EOD [3, 32]	Asian elephants	n = 1, 32 yr old with left hind limb lameness was given 1–2 mg/kg SID PO or rectally EOD. Had noticeable improvement and no negative side effects long term (10 mo).
	1.7 mg/kg PO BID [32]	Asian elephants	n = 1, 19 yr old. Severe sole abscess surgically treated. Had "good" results.
Anesthetic			
Acepromazine	0.004–0.06 mg/kg IM or IV with 100 mg Xylazine/metric ton bw IM [2, 34]	Asian and African elephants	Do not expose animal to sunlight for long periods as photosensitization has been reported as a triangle on the dorsal aspect of the neck when >0.06 mg/kg was combined with xylazine.
	0.1 mg/kg IM [35]	Asian elephants	If combined with other drugs, dose can be reduced by up to 50%.
	0.004–0.005 mg/kg (total 10–30 mg) IM, IV [27]	African or Asian elephants	Sedation
Acepromazine and xylazine	A: 150 mg + X: 350 mg [35]	Asian elephants	n = 2 adult females at 2500–3000 kg., recumbent immobilization in 12–15 min. Duration 60 min. Good for minor surgeries.
Atipamezole HCl	1 mg atipamezole for every 12 mg xylazine IM or IV slowly [2, 34]	Asian elephants	
	5–10 mg will reverse 100 mg xylazine [36]	Not specified	IM or slowly given IV.
Atipamezole HCl	8–14 μg/kg [37]	Asian elephants	n = 1, 5000 kg male. Standing sedation performed 3 times with IV xylazine (X: 33–72 μg/kg) for treatment of foot abscesses. Partial reversal with atipamezole as listed here made the animal more responsive to voice commands while heavily sedated.
Azaperone	0.08–0.09 mg/kg IM [38]	African elephants	Standing sedation.
	0.017–0.046 mg/kg IM [38]	Asian elephants	Standing sedation.
	0.06–0.15 mg/kg IM [38]	African elephants	Standing sedation.
	0.067 mg/kg IM [38]	African elephants	Standing sedation.

Drug name	Drug dose	Species	Comments
	0.024–0.038 mg/kg IM [2]	Asian elephants	Short-acting tranquilizer.
	0.056–0.107 mg/kg IM or IV [2]	African elephants	Short-acting tranquilizer.
Butorphanol + azaperone for standing sedation	B: 0.003 mg/kg IV mixed with A: 0.12 mg/kg; or B: 0.006–0.014 mg/kg IV 24–73 min after A: 0.068–0.12 mg/kg [39].	African elephants	n = 2+, adult aggressive females. For moderate surgical procedures. Reversal with naloxone 0.004 mg/kg IV in higher butorphanol range only.
Butorphanol + azaperone	B: 10 mg total dose + A: 0.12 mg/kg IM [2]	African elephants	n = 1
Butorphanol + xylazine for aggressive adult elephants	IM xylazine at total doses of 700–1000 mg/adult elephant (approximate dosages of 0.2–0.3 mg/kg) followed by intravenous butorphanol at doses of 50–180 mg/adult elephant (approximate dosages of 0.01–0.03 mg/kg) [39]	African elephants	Depending on size and temperament.
Butorphanol tartrate + xylazine for standing sedation	Adult male: X: 0.16 mg/kg IM + B: 0.036 mg/kg IV given 26 min later [39].	African elephants	n = 1 for two procedures. 2nd procedure 2 yrs later required additional 0.004 mg/kg butorphanol at 77 min. Rated as fair.
	Adult female: X: 0.035 mg/kg IV + B: 0.005 mg/kg IV. 14 min later, additional X: 0.014 mg/kg and B: 0.003 mg/kg given IV [39].	African elephants	n = 1 for two procedures., In 2nd procedure, gave 0.14 mg/kg xylazine IM followed by 0.014 mg/kg butorphanol 44 min later. Rated as fair.
	B: 0.004 mg/kg IV + X: 0.1 mg/kg IM [40]	African elephants	n = 1, 8 yr, 1500 kg. For radiography of a broken tusk.
Carfentanil (naltrexone reversal)	0.0021 mg/kg, supplement with 0.0005 mg/kg if needed; antagonize with naltrexone 0.08 mg/kg [41].	African elephants	Agitated or aggressive animals may require higher doses.
	Calves: 1 mg. Adults: 3 mg + 1500 IU hyaluronidase; antagonize with naltrexone 100 mg per mg carfentanil used [42].	African elephants	n = 37 wild (n = 4 calves 4–6 yrs, n = 29 adults). Recumbency in 10–14 min. Recovery in 2–9 min.
Carfentanil	0.002–0.004 mg/kg (total 5–12 mg) [2, 27]	Asian elephants	
	0.0013–0.0024 mg/kg (total 3–12 mg) [2, 27]	African elephants	
	0.002–0.0026 mg/kg IM [43]	African elephants	n = 16
Carfentanil (nalmefene hydrochloride reversal)	0.0018–0.0022 mg/kg IM; antagonize with 0.045–0.079 mg/kg nalmefene [44]	African elephants	n = 8. Recumbent in 6–14 min. Recovered in 1–4.2 min. Resulted in high blood pressure and not recommended as only agent in immobilizing African elephants.
Detomidine	0.0055 IM [2]	Asian elephants	

(*Continued*)

Drug name	Drug dose	Species	Comments
Detomidine + butorphanol for standing sedation (yohimbine and naltrexone for reversal)	D and B: 14.7–16.2 μg/kg in a 1 : 1 ratio; antagonize with Y: 73–98 μg/kg and N: 49–98 μg/kg IV and 74–98 μg/kg IM (1/3–1/2 naltrexone to be given IV) [45]	African elephants	n = 3, 1.2, captive. 14 procedures over 5 yrs. Evening before only half ration of hay and water ad libitum offered. 6 procedures that were more involved required additional 4–7.3 μg/kg supplements of each drug 1–2× depending on procedure. 5 procedures had mild adverse effects post with abdominal distention ± transient anorexia that resolved with exercise and flunixin meglumine.
Detomidine + butorphanol	D: 0.04–0.06 mg/kg + B: 0.03–0.06 mg/kg IM [46]	Asian elephants	Bulls. Standing sedation for minor procedures.
	D: 0.02–0.03 mg/kg IM + B: 0.02–0.03 mg/kg IM [3]	Asian elephants	Young calf. Standing sedation, but may cause very young elephants to lie down.
	D: 0.013–0.02 mg/kg + B: 0.013–0.02 mg/kg IM [3]	African elephants	Standing sedation.
Etorphine	0.0015–0.003 mg/kg IM (total dose 6–20 mg) [2]	African elephants	Opioid narcotics elevate blood pressure and may cause a fatal pink foam syndrome in wild African elephants. Combining with azaperone may counteract.
	0.015–0.003 mg/kg IM [3]	African elephants	Immobilization.
Etorphine (nalmefene reversal)	0.0027–0.0036 mg/kg IM; antagonize with nalmefene hydrochloride 0.027–0.049 mg/kg given IV and SC [43]	African elephants	n = 6. Recumbency in 22–40 min. Standing post reversal in 0.7–2.1 min.
Etorphine	Mixed with 1 l of Saline and given as CRI at 2.5 mg/hr IV [47]	African elephants	n = 45 free-ranging bulls.
Etorphine + hyaluronidase (diprenorphine reversal)	E: 9.5 ± 0.5 mg + H: 2000 IU; antagonize with diprenorphine 23.3 ± 1.5 mg IV and 11.7 ± 0.5 mg IM or 24 mg IV total [48].	African elephants	n = 20 (2.18), free-ranging. All induced. Recumbent within 15 min. Standing post reversal within 10 min.
Etorphine + azaperone + halothane (diprenorphine reversal)	Premed A: 120 mg and E: 1 mg IM, then induction with E: 2 mg IM. Halothane intranasal as supplement; antagonize with 5 mg diprenorphine [49].	African elephants	n = 2, 5 yr old males for dental procedures.
Etorphine + azaperone + CRI etorphine (naltrexone and diprenorphine reversal)	E: 11–15 mg IM + A: 30–60 mg IM. CRI: E: 0.0104 mg/ml in saline given at 2.5 mg/hr; antagonize with N: 50 mg IV and D: 36–42 mg IV [50].	African elephants	n = 14 free-ranging bulls. All induced completely. Laparoscopic vasectomies performed with 57–125 min surgeries. All standing post reversal in 3–5 min.
Haloperidol	40–100 mg/animal IM or PO BID [51]	Asian elephants	Captive
Hyaluronidase	See carfentanil + hyaluronidase protocol [42]		

Drug name	Drug dose	Species	Comments
	1000–3000 IU/dart [52]	African elephants	To improve absorption of induction drugs.
Hyaluronidase + etorphine hydrochloride	H: 2000 IU + E: 9–10 mg IM via dart [48]	African elephants	n = 20 wild adults immobilized for translocation.
	H: 4500 IU + E: 11.3–11.9 mg/animal via dart, 2nd immobilization increased etorphine to 15 mg/animal and had more rapid inductions [53].	African elephants	n = 16 free-ranging adult females.
Medetomidine	0.003–0.005 mg/kg IM [2, 41]	Asian elephants	Sedative
Nalmefene	26 × the amount of carfentanil used [54, 55]	African elephants	A dose each of IV and SC or IV and IM.
Naloxone HCl	10 mg total dose in small elephants; up to 30–50 mg in adults [20, 51, 56]	African and Asian elephants	IV or divided into IV and IM.
Naltrexone HCl	50–100 mg per 1 mg narcotic [38, 42, 52, 54, 57]	Not specified	IV or divided into IV and IM.
Tolazoline HCl	0.5 mg/kg IV, or 2 mg tolazoline per mg xylazine [52, 54, 58]	Not specified	
Perphenazine enanthate	100–300 mg total dose IM [2]	African elephants	
	200–250 mg total dose IM [2]	Asian elephants	n = 4 adult, 1800–3800 kg.
Telazol	3 mg/kg [2, 41]	African elephants	n = 1. Recumbent in 2 min and recovered in 6 hrs.
Xylazine	Adult: 0.08–0.1 mg/kg IM [2]	African elephants	Sedation. Best in combination with other drugs for juveniles.
	Adult: 0.15–0.2 mg/kg IM [2]	African elephants	Immobilization, best in combination with other drugs for juveniles.
Xylazine + acepromazine	X: 0.12 mg/kg IM + A: 0.05 mg/kg IM [2]	Asian elephants	Immobilization.
Xylazine + butorphanol	X: 0.035–0.16 mg/kg IM + B: 0.005–0.036 mg/kg IM [3]	African elephants	Sedation. IM or IV. Can give separately with xylazine IM first, then butorphanol IV 20 min later or together IV.
Xylazine + ketamine	X: 0.1 mg/kg IM + K: 0.3–0.7 mg/kg IM [2]	Asian elephants	Adult, sedation.
	X: 0.12 mg/kg + K: 0.12 mg/kg IM [2]	Asian elephants	Adult, immobilization.
	X: 0.12 mg/kg + K: 0.33 mg/kg IM [2]	Asian elephants	Juvenile, immobilization.
Xylazine + ketamine	X: 0.06–1.4 mg/kg + K: 0.47–0.73 mg/kg IM [2]	African elephants	Sedation
	X: 0.14 mg/kg + K: 1.14 mg/kg IM [2]	African elephants	Juvenile, sedation.

(Continued)

Drug name	Drug dose	Species	Comments
Xylazine + ketamine (tolazoline reversal)	X: 0.2 mg/kg IM + K: 1–1.5 mg/kg IM; antagonize with T: 0.5 mg/kg IV [58]	African elephants	n = 15 Immobilization. Recumbent within 10–19 min. Standing post reversal within 3 min. No relapses post reversal.
Xylazine + ketamine + diazepam + isoflurane (yohimbine reversal)	X: 0.1 mg/kg IM. 20 min later K: 0.4 mg/kg + D: 0.013 mg/kg IV. Isoflurane via ET for supplement; antagonize with Y: 2.5 mg IM and IV [59]	Asian elephants	n = 1, <1 yr of age, 198 kg. Surgical repair of umbilical hernia.
Zuclophenthixol acetate	480 mg followed by 500 mg at 5 hr [2]	Asian elephants	n = 1
Antiparasitic			
Albendazole	2.5 mg/kg orally once [51, 60, 61]	Asian elephants	
Fenbendazole	5 mg/kg PO, q3 wks [62, 63]	Asian elephants	n = 7 (two case reports), captive. Treatment led to declining egg counts of strongyles and paramphistomes in 2 days. When repeated in 3 wks led to clearance of infestation.
	2–2.5 mg/kg PO as a single dose [51, 60, 61]	Asian elephants	
	5 mg/kg PO once [64, 65]	Asian elephants	n = 4 (two case studies). Infected with *Murshida murshida* and cleared fecal samples of eggs within 10 days in all elephants.
Ivermectin	0.2–.0.4 mg/kg PO [3]	African elephants	n = 6
	5 ml 1% ivermectin syrup, instilled in each ear canal q2 wks for six treatments [66]	African elephants	n = 2 wild born elephants in captivity for 25 yrs. Mucoid discharge from external ear. Microscopically revealed mite *Loxoaneotus bassoni*.
	0.059–0.087 mg/kg orally using the injectable preparation, may retreat at 5–6 wks [67].	African and Asian elephants	n = 4 African, n = 5 Asian. Treatment for elephant lice. Within 48–72 hrs lice were easier to remove manually. 7 days post treatment no lice.
Levamisole	2.5–3 mg/kg PO single dose [51, 60, 61, 68]	Asian elephants	For treatment of strongyles.
Mebendazole	2.5–7 mg/kg PO [51, 68, 69]	Asian elephants	For treatment of strongyles. In one study of 3 elephants, within 4 days post treatment fecal exams were negative for nematodes in all 3 and flukes in 2/3 animals, and within 3 days post administration adult parasites were recovered in feces. Generally given once only.
Oxibendazole	2.5 mg/kg PO once [51, 60, 61]	Asian elephants	For helminthiasis.

Drug name	Drug dose	Species	Comments
Praziquantel	2.5–4.0 mg/kg PO [51, 61]	Asian elephants	For cestodiasis.
Thiabendazole	20–32 mg/kg PO once [51, 60, 61, 68]	Asian elephants	For helminthiasis. The anthelmintic efficacy of six drugs was compared under field conditions against strongylosis in elephants. Mebendazole at 3 and 4 mg/kg, levamisole 3 mg/kg and Morantel tartrate 5 mg/kg were proven to be 100% effective. Mebendazole at 2 mg/kg and 2.5 mg/kg, thiabendazole at 32 mg/kg, Bephenium hydroxynaphthoate at 25 mg/kg, and disophenol at 3 mg/kg were found to be effective only in 79.1–92.2, 88.1–100, 84.6–95.3, 85.9–100 and 68.3–84% of cases respectively.
Emergency Drugs			
Atropine sulfate	0.02–0.04 mg/kg IV, IM, SC [70]	Asian elephants	n = 1. Anesthetized for cesarean section to remove dead calf. Premedication with azaperone. 90 min later administered IV atropine as well as IM etorphine and excitement and agitation resulted.
Calcium gluconate or borogluconate	0.7 mEq/kg slowly IV [71]	Not specified	For hypocalcemia.
Diazepam	0.1–0.2 mg/kg IV or 400–800 mg total IM [2]	Not specified	To control seizures.
Dobutamine	250 mg/l of saline, given at 5 μg/kg/min [72]		Used for elephants with low mean blood pressure <54 mmHg.
Doxapram	0.5 mg/kg IV or under the tongue (calf) at 5 min intervals or 0.22 mg/kg in adults [2]	Elephant calves or African elephant adults	Based on equine dosing.
Epinephrine HCl	0.1 mg/kg IV, IM [2]	Not specified	1 mg/ml concentration. Based on equine dosing.
	0.1 ml/kg [70]	Elephant calves	1 : 1000 solution.
Lidocaine	0.25–0.5 mg/kg IV, q15 min as needed [2]	Not specified	For ventricular arrhythmia.
Prednisolone	1 mg/3 kg bw [20]	Not specified	For the treatment of heatstroke.
Sodium bicarbonate	0.5–1 mEq/Kg slowly IV [2]	Not specified	For metabolic acidosis.
Other			
Cabergoline	1 mg PO 2×/wk [73]	Asian and African elephants	In one Asian elephant, successfully decreased prolactin levels associated with hyperprolactinemia and the elephant resumed normal estrus cycling. In 6 African elephants treated, levels decreased in most but no return to cycling was reported.

(Continued)

Drug name	Drug dose	Species	Comments
Calcium	95 mg/kg of bw SID [74]	Asian elephants	n = 10. Dose higher than previous recommendation of 45 mg/kg SID, for daily supplementation.
Calcium magnesium borogluconate	750 ml IV infusion with 12 g calcium borogluconate [71]	Asian elephants	n = 1 in dystocia.
Chlorphenirimine maleate	1700–2300 mg/animal [51]	Asian elephants	
Chlorpromazine	2000 mg PO BID [75]	Asian elephants	n = 1 adult male. Sedation/calming effect for an elephant used in ceremonies in India that was agitated around crowds of people. The medication worked well and the animal was treated for 6 mo. Agitation returned when medication was discontinued.
Dexamethasone	1 mg/5 kg bw [20]	Not specified	For the treatment of heatstroke.
Domperidone	2 g/day PO SID × 14d, then 3.5 g/day PO SID × 8 wks [76]	African elephants	n = 1. Authors experience in giving orally to female adult elephant that had given birth 9 yr previously but offspring was still nursing. Gave domperidone to collect milk for bottle feeding for an orphaned elephant. Using in conjunction with oxytocin for milk let down may have been more successful as well as collecting milk >4×/day. At peak production were obtaining 0.5–1 l/day but collecting only 2×/day.
Estradiol cypionate	10 mg IM + 200 IU oxytocin IV [77]	Asian elephants	n = 1. Given on day 15 postpartum. An additional 10 IU oxytocin the next day facilitated the removal of a retained placenta.
Leuprolide acetate to control musth	37.5–45 mg SC given premusth [78]	Asian elephants	n = 1, 52 yr old male. Over an 81 mo period, 12 injections total were given every 2–34 mo. A pattern of 2 short intervals and a 3rd progressively longer interval were noted over time. The 1st and 3rd injections did not have desired effect but the other 10 suppressed musth behavior. If injection was not given very early or premusth, testosterone levels dropped but behavior did not. Long-term effects and potential reversibility of testosterone suppression are unknown.
Oxytocin	20–30 IU IM or IV initially, increase in increments of 20–30 IU every 20–30 min as needed [70].	Not specified	For labor induction in dystocia case.

Drug name	Drug dose	Species	Comments
	0.013 mg/kg IV, or 50–100 IU IM or SC, or IV if needed [71, 79]	Asian elephants	n = 1. Still required vestibulotomy, but author felt this dose was safe to prevent uterine rupture or placental displacement.
	40–60 IU IV [70]	Not specified	For milk let down. Give one injection when needing to nurse or collect milk for bottle feeding.
Rabies (killed monovalent vaccine)	4 ml IM given as 2 doses 9 days apart then boostered annually [80]	Asian elephants	n = 16
	2 ml given once, then boostered every 1–2 yrs based on titers [81]	African elephants	n = 14, 4.10, healthy, captive, 0.9–38 yr of age. No adverse effects.
Tetanus toxoid vaccine	1 ml IM/SC [82]	Asian elephants	n = 22, age 24–56 yrs. All previously vaccinated with same tetanus toxoid equine vaccine 4 yrs prior and all but 2 still maintained some titer prior to study. All animals increased in titer indicating a response to vaccine. Older animals mounted a larger response.
Vitamin E/ Selenium	To achieve the mean value for circulating alpha-tocopherol in captive elephants (0.5 μg/ml), feed must provide at least 1.0, and more like 2.0–2.5 IU vitamin E/kg body mass (approximately 130–167 IU/kg diet) [83, 84, 85, 86, 87]	Free ranging African elephant levels revealed 0.34–0.88 μg/ml and did not vary significantly across sex or age class [86]. 26 captive female Asian elephants at a work camp in Nepal had a range of 0–23–1.57 μg/ml alpha-tocopherol levels [87].	Both elephants and rhinoceros appear to have limited absorption of dietary vitamin E, perhaps due to minimal dietary lipid levels in zoo feeds. Elephants with deficiency have heart lesions similar to those of swine with microangiopathy. Analysis of serum or plasma from 35 elephants confirmed common occurrence and persistence of low circulating alpha-tocopherol levels. Concentrations averaged <0.3 μg/ml despite prolonged supplementation with D,L-alpha-tocopherol acetate, the most common vitamin E supplement for animal diets. Further experimental work demonstrated that supplementing the diet with D,L- or D-alpha-tocopherol acetate or D-alpha tocopherol to provide up to 62 IU/kg body weight (BW) increased circulating blood alpha-tocopherol by <0.2 μg/ml.
Zinc carbonate	2 g/day PO [18]	Asian elephants	n = 1. One elephant with skin lesions responded well.

Species	Weight [30, 34]
African Elephant *(Loxodonta africana)*	Female: 2000–4000 kg; Male 4000–6000 kg
Asian Elephant *(Elephas maximas)*	Female: 2300–3700 kg; Male: 3700–4500 kg

References

1 Lodwick, L.J., Dubach, J.M., Phillips, L.G. et al. (1994). Pharmacokinetics of Amikacin in African elephants (*Loxodonta africana*). *Journal of Zoo and Wildlife Medicine* 25 (3): 367–374.

2 Mikota, S.K. (2006). Therapeutics. In: *Biology, Medicine, and Surgery of Elephants* (ed. M.E. Fowler and S.K. Mikota), 211–231. Ames, IA: Wiley Blackwell.

3 Wiedner, E. (2015). Proboscidae. In: *Zoo and Wild Animal Medicine, Current Therapy*, vol. 8 (ed. R.E. Miller and M. Fowler), 517–532. St. Louis, MO: Elsevier Saunders.

4 Schmidt, M.J. (1978). Penicillin G and amoxicillin in elephants: a study comparing dose regimens administered with serum levels achieved in healthy elephants. *Journal of Zoo and Wildlife Medicine* 9 (4): 127–136.

5 Sinphithakkul, P., Klangkaew, N., Sanyathitiseree, P. et al. (2016). Pharmacokinetics of amoxicillin trihydrate in male Asian elephants (*Elephas maximus*) following intramuscular administration. *Journal of Veterinary Pharmacology and Therapeutics* 39 (3): 287–291.

6 Rosin, E., Schultz-Darken, N., Perry, B. et al. (1993). Pharmacokinetics of ampicillin administered orally in Asian elephants (*Elephus maximus*). *Journal of Zoo and Wildlife Medicine* 24 (4): 515–518.

7 Dumonceaux, G., Isaza, R., Kock, E.D. et al. (2005). Pharmacokinetics and i.m. bioavailability of ceftiofur in Asian elephants (*Elephas maximus*). *Pharmacology & Therapeutics* 28 (5): 441–446.

8 Adkesson, M.J., Junge, R.E., Allender, M.E. et al. (2012). Pharmacokinetics of a long-acting ceftiofur crystalline-free acid formulation in Asian elephants (*Elephas maximus*). *American Journal of Veterinary Research* 73 (10): 1512–1518.

9 Dutton, C.J., Delnatte, P.G., Hollamby, S.R. et al. (2017). Successful treatment of digital osteitis by intravenous regional perfusion of ceftiofur in an African elephant (*Loxodonta africana*). *Journal of Zoo and Wildlife Medicine* 48 (2): 554–558.

10 Ollivet-Courtois, F., Lecu, A., Yates, R.A. et al. (2003). Treatment of a sole abscess in an Asian elephant (*Elephas maximus*) using regional digital intravenous perfusion. *Journal of Zoo and Wildlife Medicine* 34 (3): 292–295.

11 Miller, J. and McClean, M. (2008). Pharmacokinetics of Enrofloxacin in African elephants (*Loxodonta africana*) after a single rectal dose. *Proceedings of the AAZV ARAV Joint Conference*. 224–225.

12 Sanchez, C.R., Murray, S.Z., Isaza, R. et al. (2005). Pharmacokinetics of a single dose of enrofloxacin administered orally to captive Asian elephants (*Elephas maximus*). *American Journal of Veterinary Research* 66 (11): 1948–1953.

13 Olsen, J.H. (1999). Antibiotic therapy in elephants. In: *Zoo and Wild Animal Medicine, Current Therapy*, vol. 4 (ed. M.E. Fowler and R.E. Miller), 533–541. St. Louis, MO: Saunders/Elsevier.

14 Gulland, F.M. and Carwardine, P.C. (1987). Plasma metronidazole levels in an Indian elephant (*Elephas maximus*) after rectal administration. *Veterinary Record* 120 (18): 440.

15 Sander, S.J., Siegal-Willot, J.L., Ziegler, J. et al. (2016). Pharmacokinetics of a single dose of metronidazole after rectal administration in captive Asian elephants (*Elephas maximus*). *Journal of Zoo and Wildlife Medicine* 47 (1): 1–5.

16 Bush, M., Stoskopf, M.K., Raath, J.P. et al. (2000). Serum oxytetracycline concentrations in African elephant (*Loxodonta africana*) calves after long-acting formulation injection. *Journal of Zoo and Wildlife Medicine* 31 (1): 41–46.

17 Limpoka, P., Chai Anan, S., Sirivejpandu, R. et al. (1987). Plasma concentrations of oxytetracycline in elephants following intravenous and intramuscular administration of Terramycin/LA injectable solution. *Acta Veterinaria Brno* 56: 173–179.

18 Schmidt, M.J. (1989). Zinc deficiency, presumptive secondary immune deficiency and hyperkeratosis in an Asian elephant: A case report. *Proceedings of the American Association of Zoo Veterinarians*. 23–31

19 Page, C.D., Mautino, M., Derendorf, H.D. et al. (1991). Comparative pharmacokinetics of trimethoprim-sulfame-thoxazole administered intravenously and orally to captive elephants. *Journal of Zoo and Wildlife Medicine* 22 (4): 409–416.
20 Schmidt, M. (1986). Elephants (Proboscidea). In: *Zoo and Wild Animal Medicine* (ed. M.E. Fowler), 911–912. Philadelphia, PA: Saunders.
21 Recommendations for the diagnosis, treatment, and management of tuberculosis (*Mycobacterium tuberculosis*) in elephants in human care (2017). http://www.nasphv.org/Documents/ElephantTB_NASPHV.pdf (accessed 30 November 2018).
22 Brock, P., Isaza, R., Hunter, R.P. et al. (2012). Estimates of the pharmacokinetics of famciclovir and its active metabolite penciclovir in young Asian elephants (*Elephas maximus*). *American Journal of Veterinary Research* 73 (12): 1996–2000.
23 Schmitt, D.L., Hardy, D.A., Montali, R.J. et al. (2000). Use of Famciclovir for the treatment of endotheliotrophic herpesvirus infections in Asian elephants (*Elephas maximus*). *Journal of Zoo and Wildlife Medicine* 31 (4): 518–522.
24 Bronson, E., McClure, M., Sohl, J. et al. (2017). Epidemiologic evaluation of elephant endotheliotropic herpesvirus 3B infection in an African elephant (*Loxodonta africana*). *Journal of Zoo and Wildlife Medicine* 48 (2): 335–343.
25 Fowler, M.E. and Mikota, S.K. (2006). Chemical restraint and general anesthesia, section I: chemical restraint. In: *Biology, Medicine, and Surgery of Elephants* (ed. M.E. Fowler and S.K. Mikota), 91–110. Ames, IA: Wiley Blackwell.
26 Ingram, L.M., Isaza, R., Koch, D.E. et al. (2005). Pharmacokinetics of intravenous and intramuscular butorphanol in Asian elephants (*Elephas maximus*). *Annual Proceedings of the American Association of Zoo Veterinarians*. 70–71.
27 Fowler, M.E. (1995). Elephants. In: *Restraint and Handling of Wild and Domestic Animals*, 265–269. Ames, IA: Iowa State University Press.
28 Mortenson, J. (1998). Determining dosages for anti-inflammatory agents in elephants. *Annual Proceedings of the American Association of Zoo Veterinarians*. 477–479.
29 Mortenson, J. and Sierra, S. (1998). Determining dosages for antibiotic and anti-inflammatory agents in elephants. *Proceedings of the First North American Conference on Elephant Foot Care and Pathology*. 50–55.
30 Bechert, U. and Christensen, J.M. (2007). Pharmacokinetics of orally administered ibuprofen in African and Asian elephants (*Loxodonta africana* and *Elephas maximus*). *Journal of Zoo and Wildlife Medicine* 38 (2): 258–268.
31 Hunter, R.P., Isaza, R., and Koch, D.E. (2003). Oral bioavailability and pharmacokinetic characteristics of ketoprofen enantiomers after oral and intravenous administration in Asian elephants (*Elephas maximus*). *American Journal of Veterinary Research* 64 (1): 109–114.
32 Bechert, U., Christensen, M., Nguyen, C. et al. (2008). Pharmacokinetics of orally administered phenylbutazone in African and Asian elephants (*Loxodonta africana* and *Elephas maximus*). *Journal of Zoo and Wildlife Medicine* 39 (2): 188–200.
33 Miller, R.M. (1977). Segmental gangrene and sloughing of elephants' ears after intravenous injection of phenylbutazone. *Veterinary Medicine, Small Animal Clinician* 72 (4): 633–637.
34 Cheeran, J.V., Chandrasekharan, K., and Radhakrishnan, K. (2002). Tranquilization and translocation of elephants. *Journal of Indian Veterinary Association Kerala* 7 (3): 42–46.
35 Nayar, K.N.M., Chandrasekharan, K., and Radhakrishnan, K. (2002). Management of surgical affections in captive elephants. *Journal of Indian Veterinary Association Kerala* 7 (3): 55–59.
36 Rietschel, W., Hildebrandt, T., Goritz, F. et al. (2001). Sedation of thai working elephants with xylazine and atipamezole as a reversal. a research update on elephants and rhinos. *Proceedings of the International Elephant and Rhino Research Symposium*. 121–123.

37 Honeyman, V.L., Cooper, R.M., and Black, S.R. (1998). A protected contact approach to anesthesia and medical management of an Asian elephant (*Elephas maximus*). *Annual Proceedings of the American Association of Zoo Veterinarians*. 338–341.
38 Horne, W.A. and Loomis, M.R. (2014). Elephants. In: *Zoo Animal and Wildlife Immobilization and Anesthesia*, 2e (ed. G. West, D. Heard and N. Caulkett), 703–717. Ames, IA: Wiley Blackwell.
39 Ramsay, E. (2000). Standing sedation and tranquilization in captive African elephants (*Loxodonta africana*). *Annual Proceedings of the American Association of Zoo Veterinarians*. 111–114.
40 Heard, D.J., Jacobson, E.R., and Brock, K.A. (1986). Effects of oxygen supplementation on blood gas values in chemically restrained juvenile African elephants. *Journal of American Veterinary Medical Association* 189 (9): 1071–1074.
41 Kreeger, T.J., Arnemo, J.M., and Raath, J.P. (2002). *Handbook of Wildlife Chemical Immobilization*, 183–184. Fort Collins, Colorado: Wildlife Pharmaceuticals Inc.
42 Karesh, W.B., Smith, K.H., Smith, F. et al. (1997). Elephants, buffalo, kob, and rhinoceros: immobilization, telemetry, and health evaluations. *Annual Proceedings of the American Association of Zoo Veterinarians*. 296–230.
43 Jacobson, E.R., Heard, D.J., Caligiuri, R. et al. (1987). Physiologic effects of etorphine and carfentanil in African elephants. *Proceedings of the 1st International Conference of Zoological and Avian Medicine*. Oahu, Hawaii (6–11 September 1987) Madison, Wisconsin: Omnipress. 525–527.
44 Jacobson, E.R., Kollias, G.V., Heard, D.J. et al. (1988). Immobilization of African elephants with carfentanil and antagonism with nalmefene and diprenorphine. *Journal of Zoo Animal Medicine* 19 (1–2): 1–7.
45 Neiffer, D., Miller, M., Weber, M. et al. (2005). Standing sedation in African elephants (*Loxodonta africana*) using detomidine-butorphanol combinations. *Journal of Zoo and Wildlife Medicine* 36 (2): 250–256.
46 Bouts, T., Dodds, J., Berry, K. et al. (2017). Detomidine and butorphanol for standing sedation in a range of zoo-kept ungulate species. *Journal of Zoo and Wildlife Medicine* 48 (3): 616–626.
47 Marais, H.J., Hendrickson, D.A., Stetter, M. et al. (2013). Laparoscopic vasectomy in African savannah elephant (*Loxodonta africana*); surgical technique and results. *Journal of Zoo and Wildlife Medicine* 44 (4s): S18–S20.
48 Osofsky, S.A. (1997). A practical anesthesia monitoring protocol for free-ranging adult African elephants (*Loxodonta africana*). *Journal of Wildlife Diseases* 33 (1): 72–77.
49 Stegmann, G.F. (1999). Etorphine-halothane anaesthesia in two five-year-old African elephants (*Loxodonta africana*). *Journal of the South African Veterinary Association* 70 (4): 164–166.
50 Rubio-Martinez, L.M., Hendrickson, D.A., and Stetter, M. (2014). Laparoscopic vasectomy in African elephants (*Loxodonta africana*). *Veterinary Surgery* 43 (5): 507–514.
51 Cheeran, J.V., Chandresekharan, D., and Radhakrishnan, K. (1995). Principles and practice of fixing dose of drugs for elephants. In: *A Week with Elephants*, Proceedings of the International Seminar on Asian Elephants (ed. J.C. Daniel), 430–438. Bombay India: Oxford University Press.
52 Raath, J.P. (1999). Relocation of African elephants. In: *Zoo and Wild Animal Medicine, Current Therapy*, vol. 4 (ed. M.E. Fowler and R.E. Miller), 525–533. St. Louis, MO: Saunders/Elsevier.
53 Kock, M.D., Martin, R.B., and Kock, N. (1993). Chemical immobilization of free-ranging African elephants (*Loxodonta africana*) in Zimbabwe, using etorphine (M99) mixed with hyaluronidase, and evaluation of biological data collected soon after immobilization. *Journal of Zoo and Wildlife Medicine* 24 (1): 1–10.

54 Kock, R.A., Morkel, P., and Kock, M.D. (1993). Current immobilization procedures used in elephants. In: *Zoo and Wild Animal Medicine Current Therapy*, vol. 3 (ed. M.E. Fowler and R.E. Miller), 436–441. Philadelphia, PA: W.B. Saunders Company.
55 Schumacher, J., Heard, D.J., Caligiuri, R. et al. (1995). Comparative effects of etorphine and carfentanil on cardiopulmonary parameters in juvenile African elephants (*Loxodonta africana*). *Journal of Zoo and Wildlife Medicine* 26 (4): 503–507.
56 Smuts, G.L. (1975). An appraisal of naloxone hydrochloride as a narcotic antagonist in the capture and release of wild herbivores. *Journal of the American Veterinary Medical Association* 167 (7): 559–561.
57 Lance, W.R. (1991). New pharmaceutical tools for the 1990s. *Annual Proceedings of the American Association of Zoo Veterinarians*. 354–359.
58 Allen, J.L. (1986). Use of tolazoline as an antagonist to xylazine-ketamine-induced immobilization in African elephants. *American Journal of Veterinary Research* 47 (4): 781–783.
59 Abou-Madi, N., Kollias, G.V., Hackett, R.P. et al. (2004). Umbilical herniorrhaphy in a juvenile Asian elephant (*Elephas maximus*). *Journal of Zoo and Wildlife Medicine* 35 (2): 221–225.
60 Chandrasekharan, K. (1992). Prevalence of infectious diseases in elephants in Kerala and their treatment. In: The Asian Elephant: Ecology, Biology, Diseases, Conservation and Management. *Proceedings of the National Symposium on the Asian Elephant*, Trichur, India (ed. E.G. Silas, M.K. Nair, and G. Nirmalan). 148–155.
61 Chandrasekharan, K. (2002). Specific diseases of Asian elephants. *Journal of Indian Veterinary Association Kerala* 7 (3): 31–34.
62 Raman, M., Jayathagaraj, M.G., Rajavelu, G. et al. (2000). Strongylosis in captive elephants – a report. *Indian Journal of Animal Health* 39 (2): 85–86.
63 Rao, D.S.T., Yathiraj, S., Choudhuri, P.C. et al. (1992). Treatment of helminthiosis in elephants. *Indian Journal of Animal Science* 62 (12): 1155–1156.
64 Ripathy, S.B., Acharjyo, L.N.M., and Padhi, N.K. (1991). Use of Fenbendazole against murshidiasis in zoo elephant. *International Seminar on Veterinary Medicine in Wild and Captive Animals*. 29.
65 Roy, S. and Mazumdar, B.K. (1988). Anthelmintic activity of fenbendazole (Panacur) against *Murshidia murshida* in zoo elephants. *Indian Veterinary Journal* 65 (6): 531–532.
66 Wyatt, J. and DiVincenti, L. (2012). Eradication of elephant ear mites (*Loxoanoetus bassoni*) in two African elephants (*Loxodonta africana*). *Journal of Zoo and Wildlife Medicine* 43 (1): 141–143.
67 Stadler, C. and Burns, E. (2007). Treatment of a louse (*Haematomyzus elephantis*) infestation in a captive herd of African elephants (*Loxodonta africana*). *Annual Proceedings of the American Association of Zoo Veterinarians*. 152.
68 Chandrasekharan, K., Cheeran, J.V., Nair, K.N.M. et al. (1982). Comparative efficacy of 6 anti-helminthics against strongylosis in elephants. *Kerala Journal of Veterinary Science* 13: 15–20.
69 Carreno, R.A., Neimanis, A.S., Lindsjo, J. et al. (2001). Parasites found in faeces of Indian elephants (*Elephas maximus*) in Thailand following treatment with mebendazole. *Helminthologia* 38 (2): 75–79.
70 Schmitt, D.L. (2001). Riddle's Elephant and Wildlife Sanctuary Elephant Birth Protocol. https://www.yumpu.com/en/document/view/39936674/birth-protocol-elephant-care-international (accessed 26 November 2018).
71 Schaftenaar, W. (1996). Vaginal vestibulotomy in an Asian elephant (*Elephas maximus*). *Annual Proceedings of the American Association of Zoo Veterinarians*. 434–439.
72 Heard, D.J., Kollias, G.V., Webb, A.I. et al. (1988). Use of halothane to maintain anesthesia induced with etorphine in juvenile African elephants. *Journal of American Veterinary Medical Association* 193 (2): 254–256.

73 Ball, R. and Brown, J. (2006). Preliminary results of a cabergoline trial in captive elephants with hyperprolactinemia. *Annual Proceedings of the American Association of Zoo Veterinarians.* 174–176.

74 Van Sonsbeek, G.R., Van der Kolk, J.H., Van Leeuwen, J.P.T.M. et al. (2013). Effect of calcium and cholecalciferol supplementation on several parameters of calcium status in plasma and urine of captive Asian (*Elephas maximus*) and African elephants (*Loxodonta africana*). *Journal of Zoo and Wildlife Medicine* 44 (3): 529–540.

75 Cheeran, J.V., Chandrasekharan, K., and Radhakrishnan, K. (1992). A case of ochlophobia in a tusker. In: The Asian Elephant: Ecology, Biology, Diseases, Conservation and Management. *Proceedings of the National Symposium on the Asian Elephant*, Trichur, India. (ed. E.G. Silas, M.K. Nair, and G. Nirmalan). (January 1989). 176.

76 Pittsburgh Zoo & PPG Aquarium (2018). Personal communication.

77 Murray, S., Bush, M., and Tell, L.A. (1996). Medical management of postpartum problems in an Asian elephant (*Elephas maximus*) cow and calf. *Journal of Zoo and Wildlife Medicine* 27 (2): 255–258.

78 De Oliveira, C.A., West, G.D., Houck, R. et al. (2004). Control of musth in an Asian elephant bull (*Elephas maximus*) using leuprolide acetate. *Journal of Zoo and Wildlife Medicine* 35 (1): 70–76.

79 Schaftenaar, W., Hildebrandt, T.B., Flugger, M. et al. (2001). Guidelines for veterinary assistance during the reproduction process in female elephants. *Proceedings of the AAZV, AAWV, ARAV, and the NAZWV Joint Conference*. 348–355.

80 Isaza, R., Davis, R.D., Moore, S.M. et al. (2006). Results of vaccination of Asian elephants (*Elephas maximus*) with monovalent inactivated rabies vaccine. *American Journal of Veterinary Research* 67 (11): 1934–1936.

81 Miller, M.A. and Olea-Popelka, F. (2009). Serum antibody titers following routine rabies vaccination in African elephants. *Journal of the American Veterinary Medical Association* 235 (8): 978–981.

82 Lindsay, W.A., Wiedner, E., Isaza, R. et al. (2010). Immune responses of Asian elephants (*Elephas maximus*) to commercial tetanus toxoid vaccine. *Veterinary Immunology and Immunopathology* 133 (2–4): 287–289.

83 Dierenfeld, E.S. and Dolensek, E.P. (1988). Circulating levels of vitamin E in captive Asian elephants (*Elephas maximus*). *Zoo Biology* 7 (2): 165–172.

84 Dierenfeld, E.S. (1994). Vitamin E in exotics: effects, evaluation and ecology. *Journal of Nutrition* 124 (12s): 25795–25815.

85 Papas, A.M., Cambre, R.C., Citino, S.B. et al. (1991). Efficacy of absorption of various vitamin E forms by captive elephants and black rhinoceroses. *Journal of Zoo and Wildlife Medicine* 22 (3): 309–317.

86 Savage, A., Leong, K.M., Grobler, D. et al. (1999). Circulating levels of alpha-tocopherol and retinol in free-ranging African elephants (*Loxodonta africana*). *Zoo Biology* 18 (4): 319–323.

87 Shrestha, S.P., Ullrey, D.E., Bernard, J.B. et al. (1998). Plasma vitamin E and other analyte levels in Nepalese camp elephants (*Elephas maximus*). *Journal of Zoo and Wildlife Medicine* 29 (3): 269–278.

18

Hyraxes

Drug name	Drug dose	Species	Comments
Antimicrobials and Antifungals			
Amikacin	2–10 mg/kg SC IM or IV SID to TID [1]	Hyraxes	
Cefpodoxime proxetil	5–10 mg/kg PO SID for 7–10d [1]	Hyraxes	
Ceftazidime	40 mg/kg IM or IV TID [1]	Hyraxes	
Ceftiofur (Excede)	6.6 mg/kg IM q7d [1]	Hyraxes	
Ceftiofur (Excede)	8 mg/kg SC [2]	Rock hyraxes	n = 1, 8 yr old female with uterine adenomyosis with incision infection postoperatively that healed after treatment.
Chloramphenicol	30–50 mg/kg SC IM or IV BID to TID [1]	Hyraxes	
Ciprofloxacin	5–15 mg/kg PO BID [1]	Hyraxes	
Doxycycline	2.5–5 mg/kg PO BID [1]	Hyraxes	
Enrofloxacin	5–20 mg/kg PO SC IM or IV BID [1]	Hyraxes	
Gentamicin	2–4 mg/kg SC IM or IV SID to TID [1]	Hyraxes	
Metronidazole	20–40 mg/kg PO BID for 3–5d [1]	Hyraxes	
Oxytetracycline	10–15 mg/kg SC or IM SID [1]	Hyraxes	
Penicillin G procaine and benzathine	20 000–80 000 IU/kg IM or SC q48 hrs [1, 3]	Rock hyraxes	n = 3 (1.2) 4 mo old rock hyrax with generalized demodicosis, treated with penicillin prior to diagnosis due to clinical signs of severe generalized dermatitis.
Penicillin G Procaine	20 000–60 000 IU/kg SC or IM SID [1]	Hyraxes	
Tetracycline	50 mg/kg PO BID to TID [1]	Hyraxes	
Trimethoprim sulfadiazine	30 mg/kg SC SID to BID [1]	Hyraxes	
Trimethoprim sulfamethoxazole	15–30 mg/kg PO BID [1]	Hyraxes	

(*Continued*)

Zoo and Wild Mammal Formulary, First Edition. Alicia Hahn.

Drug name	Drug dose	Species	Comments
Analgesia			
Buprenorphine	0.02 mg/kg SC [2]	Rock hyraxes	n = 1, 8 yr old female with uterine adenomyosis, perioperative pain control,.
Meloxicam	0.2 mg/kg PO [2]	Rock hyraxes	n = 1, 8 yr old female with uterine adenomyosis, perioperative pain control,.
Anethesia and sedation			
Acepromazine + diazepam	A: 0.5–1 mg/kg + Dia: 1–5 mg/kg IM.; antagonize with flumazenil 0.01–0.2 mg/kg slow IV to effect [1].	Hyraxes	
Isoflurane or sevoflurane gas anesthesia	Chamber induction, face mask or endotracheal tube for maintenance [1, 4, 5]	Rock hyraxes	Recommended.
Ketamine	10 mg/kg IM [4, 5]	Rock hyraxes	1 mg/kg xylazine can be added but this combination has a narrow safety range.
	20–50 mg/kg IM [1]	Hyraxes	
Ketamine + acepromazine	K: 40 mg/kg + A: 0.5–1 mg/kg IM [1]	Hyraxes	
Ketamine + diazepam + isoflurane	K: 5–30 mg/kg + Dia: 1–3 mg/kg IM; antagonize with flumazenil 0.01–0.2 mg/kg IV slowly to effect [1].	Hyraxes	
Ketamine + medetomidine	K: 5 mg/kg + M: 0.35 mg/kg IM; antagonize with atipamezole at 5 × the total mg of medetomidine [1].	Hyraxes	
Ketamine + xylazine	K: 10 mg/kg + X: 2 mg/kg IM [4]	Rock hyraxes	Narrow range of safety compared to inhalant anesthesia.
	K: 30–40 mg/kg + X: 3–5 mg/kg IM; antagonize with yohimbine 0.2–1 mg/kg IM or IV [1].	Hyraxes	
Medetomidine	0.25 mg/kg IM; antagonize with atipamezole at 5 × the mg total of medetomidine [1].	Hyraxes	
Midazolam	1–2 mg/kg IM [1]	Hyraxes	Antagonize with 0.01–0.2 mg/kg.
Propofol	7.5–15 mg/kg IV slow bolus over 5 minutes [1]	Hyraxes	Give IV slowly to effect.
Telazol	3 mg/kg IM [5]	Rock hyraxes	
	2–4 mg/kg IM [4]	Rock hyraxes	
	5–25 mg/kg IM; antagonize with flumazenil 0.01–0.2 mg/kg IV slowly to effect [1].	Hyraxes	
Xylazine	1–5 mg/kg IM; antagonize with yohimbine 0.2–1 mg/kg IM or IV [1]	Hyraxes	

Drug name	Drug dose	Species	Comments
Antiparasitic			
Amprolium 9.6%	1 ml/7 kg SID PO [1]	Hyraxes	For the treatment of coccidia.
Carbaryl 5% powder	dust lightly once per week [1]	Hyraxes	For the treatment of ectoparasites.
Doramectin	0.2 mg/kg SC IM [1]	Hyraxes	For the treatment of ectoparasites.
	0.6 mg/kg SC q7d for 10–14 weeks [3]	Rock hyraxes	n = 3 (2.1) 4 mo old rock hyrax with generalized demodicosis, successfully treated with doramectin.
Fenbendazole	25–50 mg/kg PO SID for 3–5d [1]	Hyraxes	For the treatment of roundworms.
Ivermectin	0.2 mg/kg PO or SC every 14d [1]	Rock hyraxes	
Praziquantel	5–10 mg/kg PO, SC or IM, repeat in 10d [1].	Hyrax	For the treatment of tapeworms.
Pyrethrins	Apply to effect topical [1]	Hyraxes	For the treatment of fleas.
Sulfadimethoxine	25–50 mg/kg PO SID × 10d [1]	Hyraxes	For the treatment of coccidia.

Species	Weight
Procavia Spp.: Rock hyrax *(Procavia capensis, Procavia ruficeps, Procavia habessinica, and Procavia johnstoni)*	3–5.4 kg [5]
Bush hyrax *(Heterohyrax brucei)*	1.3–2.4 kg
Dendrohydrax spp.: Tree hyrax *(Dendrohydrax arboreus, Dendrohydrax validus, Dendrohydrax dorsalis)*	1.7–4.5 kg

References

1 Napier, J. (2015). Hyracoidea (hyrax). In: *Fowler's Zoo and Wild Animal Medicine*, vol. 8 (ed. R.E. Miller and M. Fowler), 532–538. St. Louis, MO: Elsevier Saunders.

2 Holman, H.J. and Gailbreath, K. (2016). Uterine adenomyosis and an endometrial polyp in a rock hyrax (*Procavia capensis*). *Journal of Zoo and Wildlife Medicine* 47 (4): 1114–1117.

3 Takle, G.L., Suedmeyer, W.K., Mertins, J.W. et al. (2010). Generalized demodecosis in three sibling, juvenile rock hyraxes (*Procavia capensis*). *Journal of Zoo and Wildlife Medicine* 41 (3): 496–502.

4 Horne, W.A. and Loomis, M.R. (2007). Elephants and hyrax. In: *Zoo Animal and Wild Immobilization and Anesthesia* (ed. G. West, D. Heard and N. Caulkett), 519. Ames, IA: Wiley Blackwell.

5 Kreeger, T.J. and Arnemo, J.M. (2012). *Handbook of Wildlife Chemical Immobilization*, 4e. China: Kreeger.

19

Nondomestic Equids

Drug name	Drug dose	Species	Comments
Antimicrobials and Antifungals			
Ampicillin sodium	16 mg/kg IV [1]	Somali wild asses	n = 1 animal with abdominal surgery to remove an enterolith and postoperative care.
Ceftiofur sodium	4.2 mg/kg IV [2]	Przewalski's horses	n = 1 captive animal with anaplasmosis. Later changed antibiotics to oxytetracycline when diagnosis was made.
Ceftiofur crystalline-free acid	2.3–6.6 mg/kg SC or IM [2]	Przewalski's horses	n = 2 captive animals with anaplasmosis.
Kanamycin + penicillin	K: 1.5 mg/kg + P: 6000 IU daily [3]	Przewalski's horses	n = 1 animal successfully treated for salmonellosis and subsequent exungulation.
Gentamicin sulfate	8 mg/kg IV [1]	Somali wild asses	n = 1 animal with abdominal surgery to remove an enterolith and postoperative care.
Minocycline	4.1–4.4 mg/kg PO BID × 14–28d [2]	Przewalski's horses	n = 4 cases of anaplasmosis treated initially with oxytetracycline IV or IM then started on minocycline PO. Doxycycline is used in horses, but due to manufacturer availability, was not used in these cases.
Oxytetracycline	Average of 10 mg/kg IV or IM initially then switched to oral minocycline or doxycycline [2]	Przewalski's horses	n = 4 cases of anaplasmosis treated initially with oxytetracycline IV or IM then started on minocycline PO. Doxycycline is used in horses, but due to manufacturer availability, was not used in these cases.
Trimethoprim sulfadiazine	30 mg/kg PO SID × 2 weeks [3]	Przewalski's horses	n = 1 animal successfully treated for salmonellosis and subsequent exungulation.

(*Continued*)

Zoo and Wild Mammal Formulary, First Edition. Alicia Hahn.

Drug name	Drug dose	Species	Comments
Analgesia			
Flunixin meglumine	1–1.6 mg/kg IV or 1.2 mg/kg IM [1]	Somali wild asses	n = 1 animal with abdominal surgery to remove an enterolith and postoperative care.
	1.1 mg/kg PO SID [3]	Przewalski's horses	n = 1 animal successfully treated for salmonellosis and subsequent exungulation.
Phenylbutazone	6 mg/kg PO SID × 5d [1]	Somali wild asses	n = 1 animal with abdominal surgery to remove an enterolith and postoperative care.
	1 g PO SID × 10 weeks [3]	Przewalski's horses	n = 1 animal successfully treated for salmonellosis and subsequent exungulation.
Anesthesia and Sedation			Naltrexone may be less likely than diprenorphine to result in renarcotization after etorphine in equids.
Acepromazine (Vetranquil 1% granules, Sedalin paste)	0.5–1.5 mg/kg PO [4, 5]	Non-domestic equids	Granules are mixed into moistened pelleted feed or as paste mixed into apples. Valuable for transport and preimmobilization sedation.
Acepromazine	0.15–0.25 mg/kg IM [5]	Non-domestic equids	Sedation
Carfentanil	C: 0.011 mg/kg IM; antagonize with 1 mg/kg naltrexone IV [4, 6, 7].	Mountain zebras	No renarcotization in 12 study animals.
Carfentanil	C: 0.02 mg/kg IM; antagonize with naltrexone at 50 : 1, IV [4, 6].	Mongolian wild horses	No renarcotization in 18 study animals.
	C: 0.055 mg/kg IM; antagonize with naltrexone 50 : 1, IV [4, 6].	Persian onagers	
	C: 0.044 mg/kg IM; antagonize with naltrexone 50 : 1, IV [4, 6].	Eastern kiangs	
	C: 0.046 mg/kg IM; antagonize with naltrexone 50 : 1, IV [4, 6].	Somali wild asses	
Carfentanil + detomidine	C: 12 mg + D: 13; antagonize with naltrexone 100 mg per 1 mg carfentanil [7]	Grévy's zebras	Repeated immobilizations of one female.
Detomidine + carfentanil	D: 13 mg IM, C: 12 mg 21 min. later; antagonize with naltrexone 600 mg IV and 510 mg IM [8]	Grévy's zebras	n = 1 animal immobilized 5 times over a 6-week period, for a traumatic carpal joint injury. Average time to recumbency post carfentanil was 13 min. Average time to standing after naltrexone was 4 min.
Detomidine + carfentanil + ketamine	D: 0.1–0.15 mg/kg IM then C: 0.098 mg/kg + K: 2 mg/kg IM 20 min. later [5]	Grévy's zebras	Significant hypertension noted. Etorphine combinations are preferred.

Drug name	Drug dose	Species	Comments
Detomidine	0.02–0.08 mg/kg IM [5]	Wild equids	Sedation. In contrast, medetomidine and romifidine should not be used alone as preanesthetics due to significant ataxia.
Detomidine + butorphanol	D: 0.1 mg/kg IM + B: 0.13 mg/kg IM 10 min. later; antagonized with atipamezole 2 mg/mg detomidine IV + naltrexone 0.1 mg/kg IV [9].	Grévy's and Burchell's zebras	Median doses for 70 standing sedation procedures. Some required supplemental etorphine (median 2.5 mg/kg) and acepromazine (median 10 mg/kg) IM.
	D: 0.1–0.17 mg/kg + B: 0.07–0.13 mg/kg IM; antagonized with atipamezole at 1.5 times the dose (in mg) of detomidine IV and/or IM [10].	Multiple species	n = 1 Przewalski's horse, 4 Onager, 3 Kiang, 4 Grévy's zebra, and 7 Somali wild ass. Sedation allowing for minor procedures.
Etorphine	3 mg; antagonize with diprenorphine ne 6 mg [7].	Kulans	
Etorphine + acepromazine	E: 0.0085–0.01 mg/kg + A: 0.035–0.04 mg/kg IM. Antagonize with diprenorphine 0.045 mg/kg IV [5].	Burchell's/ Plains zebras	n = 75 animals.
	E: 0.016 mg/kg + A: 0.067 mg/kg IM; antagonize with diprenorphine 0.042 mg/kg + nalorphine 0.4 mg/kg IM [5].	Kulans	n = 76 animals.
	E: 0.012 mg/kg + A: 0.05 mg/kg IM; antagonize with diprenorphine 0.025 mg/kg IM [5].	Kiangs	n = 36 animals. If not recumbent in 20 min, repeat full dose.
Etorphine + acepromazine	E: 0.017 mg/kg + A: 0.07 mg/kg; antagonize with diprenorphine 0.045 mg/kg IM [5].	Somali wild asses	n = 14 animals. If not recumbent in 20 min, repeat full dose.
	E: 0.02 mg/kg + A: 0.04 mg/kg IM; antagonize with diprenorphine 0.04 mg/kg IV and naltrexone 1 mg/kg IV [1].	Somali wild asses	n = 1 animal immobilized for surgery and postoperative evaluation.
Etorphine + detomidine	E: 0.02 mg/kg IM + D: 0.04–0.06 mg/kg IM; antagonize with naltrexone 1.45 mg/kg IV and yohimbine 0.1 mg/kg IV [1].	Somali wild asses	n = 1 animal immobilized for surgery and postoperative evaluation.
Etorphine + acepromazine	E: 6 mg + A: 25 mg; antagonize with diprenorphine 2 mg per mg Etorphine [7].	Grévy's zebras	If not recumbent in 20 min, repeat full dose.
	E: 5 mg IM initially, then A: 14 mg in 4 hrs, total 15 mg given; antagonize with diprenorphine 14 mg IV [4].	Grévy's zebras	Prolonged anesthesia for cesarean section.
Etorphine + acepromazine + detomidine	E: 4.6 mg + A: 10 mg + D: 15.2 mg IM [4]	Grévy's zebras	Mean values for 20 animals under cardiac evaluation. Supplements also given as needed.

(*Continued*)

Drug name	Drug dose	Species	Comments
	E: 0.01–0.017 mg/kg + A: 0.02–0.04 mg/kg + D: 0.03–0.04 mg/kg IM; antagonize with naltrexone 100:1 ratio with etorphine in mg [4].	Grévy's zebras	Used for free-ranging animals.
Etorphine + acepromazine + detomidine + butorphanol	E: 0.008 mg/kg + A: 0.033 mg/kg + D: 0.033 mg/kg + B: 0.033 mg/kg IM; antagonize with naltrexone 0.16 mg/kg + atipamezole 0.04 mg/kg IV [5].	Przewalski's horses	n = 34 wild animals.
Etorphine + acepromazine + xylazine	E: 0.018 mg/kg + A: 0.075 mg/kg + X: 0.16 mg/kg IM; antagonize with 0.045 mg/kg diprenorphine IV [5].	Przewalski's horses	n = 73 animals.
Etorphine + detomidine + butorphanol	E: 0.008 mg/kg + D: 0.033 mg/kg + B: 0.033 mg/kg; antagonize with 0.16 mg/kg naltrexone + 0.04 mg/kg atipamezole IV [7].	Przewalski's horses	
	E: 0.7–1.4 mg + B: 10 mg + D: 10 mg IM; antagonize with 150 mg naltrexone IV [11].	Przewalski's horses	n = 6 animals. Supplementation with guaifenesin-ketamine-xylazine needed for surgical plane of anesthesia.
Etorphine + acepromazine + xylazine	1.7 ml Large Animal Immobilon (LAI) + X: 30 mg. Supplement with 1 ml LAI as needed; antagonize with 2 mg diprenorphine per mg etorphine + 0.125 mg/kg yohimbine [5, 7].	Kulans	LAI is a combo of etorphine hydrochloride 2.45 mg/ml and acepromazine maleate 10 mg/ml.
	2.5 ml LAI + X: 50 mg xylazine; antagonize with 2 mg diprenorphine per mg etorphine + 0.125 mg/kg yohimbine [7].	Burchell's and Mountain zebras	LAI is a combo of etorphine hydrochloride 2.45 mg/ml and acepromazine maleate 10 mg/ml.
Etorphine + azaperone	E: 7 mg (male) or 6 mg (female) + A: 60 mg [7]	Burchell's zebras	Etorphine may be more effective than carfentanil in zebras; thiafentanil cannot be used in zebras. Equids tend to overheat easily.
	E: 6 mg (male), 4 mg (female) + A: 80 mg; antagonize with diprenorphine 2.4 mg per mg etorphine [5, 7].	Mountain zebras	If not recumbent in 20 min, repeat full dose.
Etorphine + acepromazine	E: 0.009–0.01 mg/kg + A: 0.037–0.044 mg/kg IM; antagonize with diprenorphine 0.045 mg/kg IV [5].	Mountain zebras	n = 122 animals.
Etorphine + butorphanol + detomidine	E: 4.4 mg + B: 10 mg + D: 10 mg total; antagonize with diprenorphine 6 or 200 mg naltrexone and 20 mg atipamezole [5].	Kulans	n = 17 wild animals.

Drug name	Drug dose	Species	Comments
	E: 2.3–3 mg + B: 10 mg + D: 10 mg IM [5]	Przewalski's horses	n = 14 wild captures and 35 semi-captive procedures. Initial effects within 3–5 min, with high-stepping gait and ataxia, lateral recumbency in 5–10 min, and procedures lasting 35 min. Smooth reversal following IV antagonist.
Etorphine + ketamine	E: 5.4 mg + K: 150 mg IM; antagonize with naltrexone 250 mg [5].	Kulans	n = 3 animals.
Etorphine + ketamine + detomidine	E: 3 mg + K: 150 mg + D: 10 mg IM; antagonize with 2 mg diprenorphine per mg etorphine + 50 mg atipamezole [7].	Burchell's zebras	If not recumbent in 20 min, repeat full dose.
Etorphine + medetomidine	E: 5 mg + M: 5 mg; antagonize with diprenorphine 10 mg and atipamezole 0.1 mg/kg IM [7].	Burchell's zebras	
Etorphine + xylazine	E: 6 mg + X: 100 mg; antagonize with diprenorphine 2 mg per mg etorphine + yohimbine 0.125 mg/kg IM [7].	Grévy's and Mountain zebras	
Etorphine + xylazine	E: 3 mg + X: 200 mg; antagonize with 2 mg diprenorphine per mg of etorphine used [7].	Wild asses	Supplement with 1.5 mg of etorphine.
Fluphenazine decanoate	0.1 mg/kg IM [12]	Persian onagers	n = 6 females treated to determine if fluphenazine decanoate would decrease stress levels during reproductive management. Overall there was no difference in peak estrogen or progesterone, mild to significant decreases in cortisol, and all animals ovulated during the normal time frame expected.
Guaifenesin + ketamine + xylazine	Solution of 1 l of 5% guaifenesin with added 1000 mg ketamine and 500 mg xylazine; antagonize with naltrexone 150 mg IV [5].	Przewalski's horses	An adult horse during a procedure had an average GKX rate of 12.6 ml/min. Despite oxygen supplementation, animals became slightly hypoxemic and hypercapnic. Approximately 10 min prior to the end of procedure, IV GKX should be stopped.
Haloperidol	20–40 mg, adults [7]	Burchell's/ Plains, Grévy's, and Mountain zebras	Long-acting tranquilizer.
	0.2–0.35 mg/kg IM [4]	Grévy's zebras, Przewalski's horses	8–18 hr duration.

(Continued)

Drug name	Drug dose	Species	Comments
Haloperidol (Haldol 5 mg/ml or 1 or 10 mg tablets)	0.3 mg/kg IM, IV, or PO [5]	Burchell's/ Plains zebras	Long-acting neuroleptic, onset in 5–10 min, duration of 8–18 hrs. Extrapyramidal symptoms (involuntary movements, tremors, changes in breathing and heart rate, and anorexia) have been reported. They can be treated with biperidine and diazepam.
	0.28–0.35 mg/kg [5]	Hartmann's zebras	See previous dose in Burchell's zebra for more information.
Haloperidol + perphenazine (Haldol 5 mg/ml or 1 or 10 mg tablets)	H: 0.2–0.3 mg/kg PO + P: 150–200 mg/adult IM [5]	Przewalski's horses	Give at least 12–24 hrs prior to transport. Onset of haloperidol is 5–10 min, with 8–18 hrs of sedation. Onset of perphenazine is 12–16 hrs with a duration of 10 days.
Haloperidol + perphenazine	H: 0.3 mg/kg PO + P: 0.5 mg/kg IM [13]	Przewalski's horses	n = 8 male animals attempting to form a bachelor herd in captivity. Perphenazine administered 48 hrs prior to introductions. Haloperidol administered 2 hrs prior to introductions. After 7–8d period of tranquilization, there was minimal aggression, excitement, and anxiety. Four months later the group was a successful, established bachelor herd.
Ketamine + medetomidine	K: 1.8–2.6 mg/kg + M: 0.07–0.1 mg/kg IM; antagonize with atipamezole 0.17–0.23 mg/kg [4, 5].	Przewalski's horses	n = 11/14 animals.
Naltrexone	20 mg per mg of etorphine [5]	Mixed species	Reversal of etorphine. Longer half-life than diprenorphine and reduces risk of renarcotization.
Perphenazine	100 mg adults [7]	Burchell's, Grévy's, and Mountain zebras	Long-acting tranquilizer.
	100–200 mg/adult IM [4, 5]	Burchell's zebras	Long-acting tranquilizer. Onset in 12–16 hours and duration of 10 days.
	200 mg/adult [5]	Hartmann's zebras	Long-acting tranquilizer. Onset in 12–16 hours and duration of 10 days.
Propofol (1%)	3–5 mg/kg IV to effect [4]		Supplemental drug to provide relaxation.

Drug name	Drug dose	Species	Comments
	1–1.5 mg/kg IV over 1–2 min [14]	Multiple species	n = 19 animals in 23 anesthetic events receiving supplemental IV propofol post-induction with carfentanil/etorphine/detomidine + butorphanol. Given as a CRI as 0.005–0.03 mg/kg/sec and provided 8–10 min of improved muscled relaxation and anesthesia. Well tolerated but apnea was seen and treated with doxapram 200–300 mg IV (4 animals), 5–8 min after propofol administration.
Telazol + detomidine	T: 5.5–8.3 mg/kg + D: 0.06–0.08 mg/kg IM [5]	Burchell's/ Plains zebras	n = 11 animals, prolonged recovery.
Telazol + romifidine	T: 1.8 mg/kg + R: 0.35 mg/kg IM; antagonize with tolazoline 2.5–3 mg/kg IV [5].	Mountain zebras	n = 9 animals.
	T: 3.3 mg/kg + R: 0.6 mg/kg IM; antagonize with tolazoline 2.5–3 mg/kg IV [5].	Przewalski's horses	n = 15 animals.
Zuclopenthixol	1 mg/kg [7]	Burchell's, Grévy's, and Mountain zebras	Long-acting tranquilizer.
	50–100 mg/adult [4, 5]	Burchell's zebras, Hartmann's zebras, and Przewalski's horses	Long-acting tranquilizer. Onset in 1 hr, duration of 3–4 days.
Other			
Altrenogest	19.8–39.8 mg PO SID [15]	Grant's zebras	n = 1 captive male treated for aggressive behavior against mares and humans; proved successful.
5-Fluorouracil (5-FU) ± allogenous vaccine (A)	5-FU: 4–5 ml infiltrated around a 5 cm sarcoid. A: 1 ml SC in neck [16].	Cape mountain zebras	n = 7 animals with sarcoids. Two treated with surgical excision, two with 5-FU, two with allogenous vaccine alone, and one with vaccine and 5-FU. One animal left untreated. At 2 yr recheck all but the untreated animal's sarcoids were successfully removed without regrowth.
Cloprostenol	25ug IM [17]	Persian onagers	Analogue of Prostaglandin F2alpha. Administered on day 11 (after giving long-acting progesterone and estradiol on day 1) to n = 6 adult, non-pregnant, non-lactating females for estrous cycle synchronization.

(Continued)

Drug name	Drug dose	Species	Comments
Doxapram	200–300 mg IV 5–8 min. after propofol administration [14]	Multiple species	n = 4 animals experienced apnea that improved post doxapram.
Estradiol (long-acting)	75 mg IM [17]	Persian onagers	n = 6 adult, non-pregnant, non-lactating females. Administered in combination with long-acting Progesterone for estrous cycle synchronization.
Gabapentin	2.5 mg/kg PO BID × 60d [18]	Burchell's/ Plains/ Common zebra	Analgesic and mild sedative treatment for an n = 1 postpartum female with a comminuted ischial fracture and resulting lameness. Response noted over a 4-month period.
Omeprazole	at equine doses [4]	Non-domestic Equids	During hospitalization, arrival into quarantine, or under short-term stress, may prevent gastric ulceration.
	2 mg/kg PO SID × 4 weeks [1]	Somali wild asses	Standard postoperative care of non-domestic equids after enterolith removal (n = 16 cases).
Pergolidemesylate	1 mg PO SID [19]	Chapman's zebras, Przewalski's horses	Treatment for pituitary pars intermedia dysfunction diagnosed with serum ACTH elevation along with increased weight gain, laminitis, and long hair coat.
Porcine Zona Pellucida Vaccine	Initial inoculation with Freund's Complete Adjuvant (FCA) followed by 1–2 subsequent inoculations with Freund's Incomplete Adjuvant over 6 wks [20].	Zebras	n = 29 animals: 4 first year failures (1 pregnant, 3 human error [HE]), 2 second-year failures (HE), and 1 third-year failure (contraceptive failure). Overall contraceptive success barring technical problems was 96%.
Progesterone (long-acting)	1500 mg IM [17]	Persian onagers	n = 6 adult, non-pregnant, non-lactating females. Administered in combination with long-acting estradiol for estrous cycle synchronization.
Vitamin E	8.7–12.6 IU/kg SC [2]	Przewalski's horses	n = 3 captive animals with anaplasmosis.

Species	Weight [4, 5, 7]
Burchell's/Plains zebra *(Equus burchelli)*	175–450 kg
Chapman's zebra *(Equus quagga chapmani)*	Female: 230–320 kg, Male: 270–360 kg
Grévy's zebra *(Equus grevyi)*	350–450 kg
Hartmann's zebra *(Equus hartmannae)*	200–260 kg

Species	Weight [4, 5, 7]
Kiang *(Equus kiang)*	250–400 kg
Kulan/Khulan/Asiatic wild ass *(Equus hemionus)*	180–250 kg
Mountain/Cape Mountain zebra *(Equus zebra)*	150–350 kg
Onager *(Equus onager)*	250–400 kg
Persian onagers *(Equus hemionus onager)*	200–260 kg
Przewalski's/Mongolian wild horse *(Equus przewalskii)*	250–375 kg
Somali wild ass *(Equus africanus somalicus)*	275 kg

References

1 Howard, L.L, Allen, J.L., Zuba, J.R. et al. (2004). Management of enterolithiasis in a Somali wild ass (*Equus africanus somalicus*) at the San Diego Wild Animal Park. *Proceedings of the American Association of Zoo Veterinarians.*

2 Sim, R.R., Joyner, P.H., Padilla, L.R. et al. (2017). Clinical disease associated with Anaplasma phagocytophilum infection in captive Przewalski's horses (*Equus przewalskii*). *Journal of Zoo and Wildlife Medicine* 48 (2): 497–505.

3 Vercammen, F., DeDeken, R., and Brandt, J. (2003). Salmonellosis and exungulation in a Przewalski horse (*Equus Przewalskii*). *Proceedings of the American Association of Zoo Veterinarians.*

4 Janssen, D.L. and Allen, J.L. (2015). Equidae. In: *Fowler's Zoo and Wild Animal Medicine*, vol. 8 (ed. R.E. Miller and M.E. Fowler), 559–567. St. Louis, MO: Elsevier Saunders.

5 Walzer, C. (2014). Anesthesia: nondomestic equids. In: *Zoo Animal and Wildlife Immobilization and Anesthesia*, 2e (ed. G. West, D. Heard and N. Caulkett), 719–728. Ames, IA: Wiley Blackwell.

6 Allen, J.L. (1997). Anesthesia of nondomestic horses with carfentanil and antagonism with naltrexone. *Proceedings of the American Association of Zoo Veterinarians.*

7 Kreeger, T.J. and Arnemo, J.M. (2012). *Handbook of Wildlife Chemical Immobilization.* China: Kreeger.

8 Renner, M.S. and Bryant, W. (1998). Detomidine and carfentanil immobilization of Grévy's zebra (*Equus grevyi*). *Proceedings of the American Association of Zoo Veterinarians.*

9 Hoyer, M., De Jong, S., Verstappen, F. et al. (2012). Standing sedation in captive zebra (*Equus grevyi* and *Equus burchellii*). *Journal of Zoo and Wildlife Medicine* 43 (1): 10–14.

10 Bouts, T., Dodds, J., Berry, K. et al. (2017). Detomidine and butorphanol for standing sedation in a range of zoo-kept ungulate species. *Journal of Zoo and Wildlife Medicine* 48 (3): 616–626.

11 Walzer, C., Stalder, G., Petit T. et al. (2009). Surgical field anesthesia in Przewalski's horses (*Equus przewalskii*) in Hortobagy National Park, Hungary. *Proceedings of the American Association of Zoo Veterinarians.*

12 Wagman, J.D., Wolf, B.A., and Schook, M.W. (2015). The effect of fluphenazine decanoate on glucocorticoid production, reproductive cyclicity, and the behavioral stress response in the Persian onager (*Equus hemionus onager*). *Zoo Biology* 34 (6): 525–534.

13 Atkinson, M.W. and Blumer, E.S. (1997). The use of a long-acting neuroleptic in the Mongolian wild horse (*Equus przewalskii przewalskii*) to facilitate the establishment of a bachelor herd. *Proceedings of the American Association of Zoo Veterinarians.*

14 Zuba, J.R. and Burns, R.P. (1998). The use of supplemental propofol in narcotic anesthetized non-domestic equids. *Proceedings of the American Association of Zoo Veterinarians.*

15 Zehnder, A.M., Ramer, J.C., and Proudfoot, J.S. (2006). The use of Altrenogest to control aggression in a male Grant's zebra (*Equus burchelli boehmi*). *Journal of Zoo and Wildlife Medicine* 37 (1): 61–63.
16 Marais, H.J. and Page, P.C. (2011). Treatment of equine sarcoid in seven Cape mountain zebra (*Equus zebra zebra*). *Journal of Wildlife Diseases* 47 (4): 917–924.
17 TerBeest, J.M. and Schook, M.W. (2016). Estrous cycle synchronization in the Persian onager (*Equus hemionus onager*). *Zoo Biology* 35 (2): 87–94.
18 Bronson, E., Wack, A., Johnson, R. et al. (2008). Use of oral gabapentin to aid healing of a periparturient pelvic fracture in a common zebra (*Equus burchelli*). *Proceedings of the American Association of Zoo Veterinarians*.
19 Shotton, J.C.R., Justice, W.S.M., Salguero, F.J. et al. (2018). Pituitary pars intermedia dysfunction (equine Cushing's disease) in nondomestic equids at Marwell wildlife: a case series. One Chapman's zebra (*Equus quagga chapmani*) and five Przewalski's horses (*Equus przewalskii*). *Journal of Zoo and Wildlife Medicine* 49 (2): 404–411.
20 Frank, K.M. and Kirkpatrick, J.F. (2002). Porcine zona pellucida immuno contraception in captive exotic species: species differences, adjuvant protocols, and technical problems. *Proceedings of the American Association of Zoo Veterinarians*.

20

Tapirs

Drug name	Drug dose	Species	Comments
Antimicrobials and Antifungals			
Ceftiofur (Naxcel)	1.2 mg/kg IM [1]	Malayan tapirs	n = 1 animal evaluated for oral mass.
Procaine and benzathine penicillin	20 mg/kg IM once daily [2]	Malayan tapirs	n = 1 abdominal abscess; therapy based on culture.
Trimethoprim sulfadimidine	5 mg/kg PO twice daily [2]	Malayan tapirs	n = 1 abdominal abscess; therapy based on culture.
Gentamicin	6.6 mg/kg IM once daily [2]	Malayan tapirs	n = 1 abdominal abscess; therapy based on culture.
Anesthesia and Sedation			
Acepromazine + butorphanol + detomidine + ketamine	Ace: 7.7 mg/kg + B: 0.13–0. 2 mg/kg + D: 0.065–0.13 mg/kg + K: 2.2 mg/kg IM [3]	Tapirs	
Azaperone	1 mg/kg IM [4]	Tapirs	Standing sedation for minor procedures or introductions.
Butorphanol + detomidine	B: 0.15 mg/kg + D: 0.05 mg/kg IM; antagonize with yohimbine 0.2–0.3 mg/kg IV + naltrexone/naloxone 0.2–0.3 mg/kg IV [3, 4, 5]	Malayan and Mountain tapirs	n = 19 animals, good relaxation seen at 10 min. If needed, ketamine 0.5 mg/kg IV can be given for supplementation.
	B: 0.15–0.2 mg/kg + D: 0.06 mg/kg IM [3, 5]	Tapirs	n = 11 males anesthetized for semen electroejaculation in three captive institutions, also used in females with same effects. Ketamine 1–2 mg/kg used to reach or maintain recumbency and light anesthesia. Boluses of propofol 0.2–2 mg/kg per bolus, IV used to effect as needed.
	B: 0.24 mg/kg + D: 0.035 mg/kg IM; antagonize with naltrexone 0.6 mg/kg IM and tolazoline 4.1 mg/kg IM [1].	Malayan tapirs	n = 1 animal evaluated for oral mass, then immobilized with same protocol 4 times total for intralesional chemotherapy.

(*Continued*)

Zoo and Wild Mammal Formulary, First Edition. Alicia Hahn.

Drug name	Drug dose	Species	Comments
	B: 10 mg + D: 5 mg IM hand injection [3]	Malayan tapirs	Animal was ill, debilitated.
Butorphanol + detomidine + ketamine	B: 0.22 mg/kg + D: 0.13 mg/kg + K: 2.2 mg/kg IM [6]	Tapirs	Rapid and smooth recovery; sufficient arterial pressure; hypoventilation occurs. An addition of 1.5 mg/kg of ketamine IV for endotracheal intubation. Wait 30 minutes after ketamine before reversal.
Butorphanol + medetomidine	B: 0.15 mg/kg + M: 0.03 mg/kg IM; antagonize with atipamezole 0.06 mg/kg and naltrexone 0.6 mg/kg IV [3, 5].	Lowland tapirs	Capture of free-ranging animals in pens or pitfall for radiocollaring and biologic sampling. Average induction time 10 min.
Butorphanol + xylazine	B: 0.15 mg/kg + X: 0.3 mg/kg IM; antagonize with yohimbine 0.2–0.3 mg/kg IV + naltrexone/naloxone [3, 5, 7]	Malayan and Mountain tapirs	n = 19 animals, good relaxation seen at 10 min, if needed ketamine 0.5 mg/kg IV can be given for supplementation.
	B: 0.15–0.25 mg/kg + X: 0.3–0.5 mg/kg IM [3, 5]	Tapirs	
Butorphanol + xylazine	B: 50 mg + X: 100 mg IM, supplement with propofol 100–200 µg/kg/min IV CRI or ketamine 0.3–0.4 mg/kg IV [8]	Baird's tapirs	n = 6 animals in a study of blood pressure.
	B: 0.24 mg/kg + X: 0.35 mg/kg IM; antagonize with naltrexone 0.6 mg/kg IM and tolazoline 4.1 mg/kg IM [1, 3, 5]	Malayan tapirs	n = 1 animal evaluated for oral mass.
	B: 40–50 mg + X: 100 mg per animal IM; antagonize with naltrexone 50 mg IM and tolazoline 1200 mg IM [3, 5].	Baird's tapirs	Capture of free-ranging animals at a bait station. Supplemental drugs included either ketamine 146–228 mg or CRI of propofol 50–200 µg/kg/min, IV. Wait to antagonize at least 30 min after last ketamine dose. Average time to sternal recumbency 11 min, and 12 min to stand after reversal.
Carfentanil	C: 0.02 mg/kg IM [4]	Tapirs	
Carfentanil + ketamine + xylazine	C: 0.0054 mg/kg + K: 0.26 mg/kg + X: 0.1 3 mg/kg IM; antagonize with yohimbine 0.2 mg/kg, naltrexone 100–200 mg/kg, half IV half SC [3, 5].	Mountain tapirs	n = 6 animals anesthetized for footwork, GI endoscopy or reproductive surgery.

Drug name	Drug dose	Species	Comments
Detomidine + butorphanol	D: 0.065–0.13 mg/kg + B: 0.13–0.2 mg/kg IM [9]	Baird's tapirs	n = 1 animal immobilized twice. At the second immobilization, ketamine 2.2 mg/kg IV was given to fully induce and 20 min later another 1.5 mg/kg IV given to facilitate endotracheal intubation. No antagonists were given, and the animal's recovery was rapid and smooth.
Detomidine + carfentanil	D: 0.14–0.2 mg/kg PO, 20 min later C: 6–9.7 mg/kg PO (OR D: 0.03 mg/kg PO, followed 20 min later by C: 1.85 μg/kg PO); antagonize with yohimbine 0.2 mg/kg IV and naltrexone 100–200 mg half IV and half SC [3, 5, 10]	Baird's tapirs	n = 1 animal immobilized 8 times successfully for short medical procedures with protocol. At 10–15 min animal was reversed.
Etorphine	E: 0.01 mg/kg IM [4]	Tapirs	
Etorphine + acepromazine	E: 1.88 mg + A: 7.7 mg per animal IM; antagonize with diprenorphine hydrochloride at 3 × total etorphine dose [3].	Baird's tapirs	Capture of free-ranging animals attracted to bait stations with ripe bananas.
	E: 1.96 mg + A: 5.9 mg IM per animal via dart; antagonize with diprenorphine hydrochloride 5.88 mg [3]	Baird's tapirs	Capture of free-ranging animals on a slope of greater than 60° with minimized induction times to reduce injury.
Etorphine + acepromazine + guaifenesin	E: 2.45 mg + A: 10 mg Total IM, then G: IV until intubation was possible, then maintenance with isoflurane [3]	Malayan tapirs	n = 1, 18 mo female for diagnosis and surgical management of abdominal abscess.
Ketamine + medetomidine	K: 0.62–0.42 mg/kg + M: 0.004–0.006 mg/kg IM; antagonize with atipamezole 0.06 mg/kg ± atropine in original dart 0.025–0.04 mg/kg [3, 5]	Mountain and Lowland tapirs	Capture of free-ranging animals with average induction time 5 min, good muscle relaxation and stable cardiopulmonary parameters.
Ketamine + xylazine	K: 3.5–4 mg/kg + X: 2–2.2 mg/kg IM. Supplement with 1.4 mg/kg ketamine as needed; antagonize with tolazoline 4 mg/kg IM [3, 5].	Lowland tapirs	Capture of free-ranging animals via dart or IV induction.
Ketamine + dexmedetomidine + midazolam	K: 4 mg/kg, Dx: 0.015 mg/kg + M: 0.1 mg/kg IM [11]	Lowland tapirs	n = 2 corneal ulceration.
Telazol	1–2 mg/kg [4]	Tapirs	n = 2 animals as of 1996.

(*Continued*)

Drug name	Drug dose	Species	Comments
Telazol	T: 2.5–2.8 mg/kg IM supplemented with ketamine as needed 1.2–1.5 mg/kg IM; antagonize with tolazoline 4 mg/kg IM [3]	Lowland tapirs	Capture of free-ranging animals via dart or IV.
Xylazine + azaperone	X: 0.8 mg/kg + A: 0.8 mg/kg IM, followed by ketamine 0.5–1 mg/kg IV [4, 12]	Tapirs	Azaperone has caused adverse reactions in horses (CNS excitement) and some caution may be indicated in tapirs.
Analgesia			
Meloxicam	0.5 mg/kg PO [13]	Lowland tapirs	
Flunixin meglumine (Banamine)	1.1 mg/kg every 24 h IM, PO [14]	Baird's tapirs	Do not exceed a week of treatment.
Tramadol	2 mg/kg PO every 12 hrs [14]	Baird's tapirs	
Phenylbutazone	4–8 mg/kg 24 h IM [14]	Baird's tapirs	
Antiparasitic			
Ivermectin	0.2 mg/kg IM, SC, PO [15]	Tapirs	
Cambendazole	20 mg/kg PO [16]	Tapirs	
Mebendazole	8.8 mg/kg topically [16]	Tapirs	
Tetramisole	9 mg/kg PO [16]	Tapirs	
Thiabendazole	44 mg/kg PO [16]	Tapirs	
Toxaphene	1 gal copper tox in 150 gal water used as a topical spray	Tapirs	For sarcoptic mange: two spray applications two weeks apart.
Griseofulvin	10 mg/kg PO q24 hr × 50d [14]		Animal with alopecia caused by Microsporum canis responded well to the long treatment of course of griseofulvin.
Levamisole	10 mg/kg PO once [14]		
Other			
Altrenogest (Rgumate)	0.044 mg/kg/day PO [5, 17]	Tapirs	Effective contraception.
Deslorelin	Implant [5, 17]	Tapirs	Effective contraception.
Equine colostrum	DO NOT USE as Colostrum replacer for perinatal calves	Baird's tapirs	DO NOT USE – 2 confirmed cases of neonatal isoerythrolysis [18].
Fluorouracil	25 mg injections bilaterally, five injections over 17 weeks [19]	Malayan tapirs	n = 1 animal with bilateral corneal papillomas that resolved with treatment.
	1.47 mg/kg or 500 mg intralesional [1]	Malayan tapirs	n = 1 animal with oral squamous cell carcinoma that was treated with intralesional fluorouracil 5 occasions over 17 weeks and was full resolved without recurrence for at least 15 mo afterward.

Drug name	Drug dose	Species	Comments
Iron dextran	10 mg/kg IM [20]	Malayan tapirs	n = 2 calves with anemia due to iron deficiency, two injections given, and animals appeared to be improving. Unfortunately, both died later of septicemia.
Medroxyprogesterone acetate (Depo-Provera)	2.5–5 mg/kg injection [4]	Tapirs	For contraception.
	5 mg/kg q3 mo [5, 17]	Tapirs	For contraception, commonly used. Could also use implants instead.
Porcine Zona Pellucida Vaccine (PZP)		Tapirs [5, 17]	Can use in consecutive years for up to 3 and after stopping could regain fertility in 1–4 yrs. If continue every other year for 5–7 years may induce permanent infertility.
Tuberculosis testing	0.1 ml purified protein derivative (PPD) of Mycobacterium bovis		0.1 ml PPD of Mycobacterium bovis in regions where the skin is thin and pliable such as the inguinal area near the nipples, the axillary area, or perineum [5].
Rabies			
Equine encephalomyelitis virus			
Tetanus			
Other clostridial disease			
West Nile Virus [5]			

Species	Weight [3, 5]
Baird's tapir *(Tapirus bairdii)*	Females: 180–270, Males: 225–340
Lowland tapir *(Tapirus terrestri)*	Females: 160–250, Males: 180–295
Malayan tapir *(Tapirus indicus)*	Females: 195–385, Males: 340–430
Mountain tapir *(Tapirus pinchaque)*	Females: 135–225, Males: 160–250

References

1 Miller, C.L., Templeton, R.S., and Karpinski, L. (2000). Successful treatment of oral squamous cell carcinoma with intralesional fluorouracil in a Malayan tapir (*Tapirus indicus*). *Journal of Zoo and Wildlife Medicine* (2): 262–264.

2 Lambeth, R.R., Dart, A.J., Vogelnest, L. et al. (1998). Surgical management of an abdominal abscess in a Malayan tapir. *Australian Veterinary Journal* 76 (10): 664–666.

3 Hernandez, S.M., Bailey, J., and Padilal, L.R. (2014). Tapirs. In: *Zoo Animal and Wild Immobilization and Anesthesia* (ed. G. West, D. Heard and N. Caulkett), 729–740. Ames, IA: Wiley Blackwell.

4 Janssen, D.L. (2003). Tapiridae. In: *Zoo and Wild Animal Medicine: Current Therapy*, 5e (ed. M.E. Fowler and R.E. Miller), 569–577. Philadelphia: W.B. Saunders.

5 Zimmerman, D.M. and Sonia Hernandez, S. (2015). Tapiridae. In: *Fowler's Zoo and Wild Animal Medicine*, vol. 8 (ed. R.E. Miller and M. Fowler), 555. St. Louis, MO: Elsevier Saunders.

6 Nunes, L.A.V., Mangini, P.R., and Ferreira, J.R.V. (2001). Order Perissodactyla, family Tapiridae (tapirs): capture and medicine. In: *Biology, Medicine and Surgery of South American Wild Animals* (ed. M. Fowler and S.K. Mikota), 367–376. Ames, IA: Wiley-Blackwell.

7 Hernandez-Divers, S.M., Aguilar, R., Leandro-Loria, D. et al. (2005). Health evaluation of a radio-collared population of free-ranging Baird's tapirs (*Tapirus bairdii*) in Costa Rica. *Journal of Zoo and Wildlife Medicine* 36 (2): 176–187.

8 Bailey, J.E., Foerster, S.H., and Foerster, C.R. (2001). Evaluation of oscillometric blood pressure monitoring during immobilization of free-ranging Baird's tapirs (*Tapirus bairdii*) in Costa Rica. *Veterinary Anesthesia and Analgesia* 28 (2): 61–108.

9 Trim, C.M., Lamberski, N., Kissel, D.I. et al. (1998). Anesthesia in a Baird's tapir (*Tapirus bairdii*). *Journal of Zoo and Wildlife Medicine* 29 (2): 195–198.

10 Pollock, C.G. and Ramsay, E.C. (2003). Serial immobilization of a Brazilian tapir (*Tapirus terrestrus*) with oral detomidine and oral carfentanil. *Journal of Zoo and Wildlife Medicine* 34 (4): 408–410.

11 Da Silva1, M.O., Hermoza, C., Rojas, G. et al. (2013). Identifying an effective treatment for corneal ulceration in captive tapirs. *Conservation Medicine* 22 (31): 12–14.

12 Janssen, D.L., Rideout, B.A., and Edwards, M.S. (1999). Tapir medicine. In: *Zoo and Wild Animal Medicine: Current Therapy IV* (ed. R.E. Miller and M.E. Fowler), 562–568. Philadelphia: Saunders.

13 Simpson, E.L. (2017). First reported caesarean section performed under light anaesthesia in a lowland tapir. *The Veterinary Record* 5: e000435. https://doi.org/10.1136/vetreccr-2017–000435.

14 Quse, V. and Fernandes-Santos, R.C (2014). Tapir Veterinary Manual. IUCN/SSC Tapir specialist group.

15 Danek, J., Routa, V., Sevcik, B. et al. (1985). Ivermectin treatment for mange and helminthoses in ruminants and south American tapirs. *Biologizace a Chemizace Zivocisne Vyroby-Veterinaria* 21 (2): 183–192.

16 Kuehn, G. (1986). Tapiridae. In: *Zoo and Wild Animal Medicine* (ed. M.E. Fowler), 931–933. Philadelphia: Saunders.

17 AZA Reproductive Management Center (2018). Personal communication.

18 Wack, R., DVM, DACZM (2018). Personal communication.

19 Karpinski, L.G. and Miller, C.L. (2002). Fluorouracil as a treatment for corneal papilloma in a Malayan tapir. *Veterinary Ophthalmology* 5 (3): 241–243.

20 Helmick, K.E. and Milne, V.E. (2012). Iron deficiency anemia in captive Malayan tapir calves (*Tapirus indicus*). *Journal of Zoo and Wildlife Medicine* 43 (4): 876–884.

21

Rhinoceroses

Drug name	Drug dose	Species	Comments
Antimicrobials and Antifungals			
Amikacin	5 mg/kg IV or SC BID × 6d [1]	White rhinos	n = 1, 3-day-old calf with apparent septicemia and hypoglycemia.
Ceftiofur Crystalline Free Acid (Excede)	6.6 mg/kg SC × 2 doses [2]	White rhinos	n = 1 calf with repaired patent urachus.
Enrofloxacin	5 mg/kg PO SID [3]	Black and White rhinos	n = 2 Black rhinos with 25 prescriptions and 5 White rhinos with 10 prescriptions and no adverse effects noted.
	8.75 mg/kg PO SID × 60d [4]	Eastern black rhinos	n = 1 animal with osteomyelitis.
Metronidazole	55 mg/kg PO BID × 7 wks [5]	Eastern black rhinos	n = 1 animal, assumed 455 kg, with necrotic laminar disease that was treated chronically and successfully.
Procaine penicillin G with benzathine	30 000 IU/kg IM [2]	White rhinos	n = 1 calf with repaired patent urachus.
Sodium benzyl penicillin	22 000 IU/kg IV [6]	White rhinos	n = 1 animal, captive, 2 yr old male, with an osteochondroma of the distal third metacarpal bone removed successfully. Antibiotic given perioperatively.
Trimethoprim sulfadiazine	20 mg/kg PO SID × 14d [4]	Eastern black rhinos	n = 1 animal with osteomyelitis.
	34 mg/kg PO BID × 7 wks [5]	Eastern black rhinos	n = 1 animal, assumed 455 kg, with necrotic laminar disease that was treated chronically and successfully.
	20 mg/kg PO BID × 10d [1]	White rhinos	n = 1, 3-day-old rhino with dermatitis and wounds.

(*Continued*)

Drug name	Drug dose	Species	Comments
	25–30 mg/kg PO SID [3]	Black rhinos	n = 5 animals, 15 prescriptions, tablets crushed and misted grain lightly with water then coat with powder from crushed tablets. One adverse reaction: some skin sloughing on medial aspect of hind limbs, resolved with discontinuation of medication.
	25–30 mg/kg PO SID [3]	White rhinos	n = 11 animals with 41 prescriptions, no adverse effects noted.
	33 mg/kg PO SID × 7d [7]	Black rhinos	n = 1 calf, 2–3 mo old, with diarrhea with positive salmonella culture, successfully treated.
Analgesia			
Butorphanol	0.05–1 mg/kg PO BID [8]	White and Black rhinos	n = Retrospective results of 3/33 institutions contacted regarding analgesic use in Rhinos: 3/3 institutions felt this provided good to excellent analgesia subjectively. Sedation, and anorexia (at highest dose) noted.
Carprofen	1 mg/kg IM once [9]	White rhinos	Pharmacokinetic, not dynamic, study of 6 White Rhino – resulted in serum levels that may be effective for up to 48 hrs in most animals.
Firocoxib	Reaction noted: 0.06 mg/kg PO SID × 6d then 0.03 mg/kg PO SID × 14d, then a few yrs later 0.06 mg/kg PO SID × 12d [10, 11]	White rhinos	Resulted in generalized vesiculobullous dermatitis coinciding with 2nd treatment of firocoxib.
	0.088–0.1 mg/kg PO SID [8]	White rhinos	n = Retrospective results of 4/33 institutions contacted regarding analgesic use in Rhinos: 4/4 institutions felt this provided good to excellent analgesia subjectively. No adverse effects were reported.
Flunixin meglumine	0.2–1.6 mg/kg PO SID or EOD [8]	White, Black, Indian, and Sumatran rhinos	n = Retrospective results of 24/33 institutions contacted regarding analgesic use in Rhinos: 20/24 institutions felt this provided good to excellent analgesia subjectively. Taste aversion was noted with some animals.
Flunixin meglumine	1.1 mg/kg PO SID × 2d [7]	Black rhinos	n = 1 calf, 2–3 mo old, with diarrhea with positive salmonella culture, successfully treated.
Flunixin meglumine (Finadyne)	1.1 mg/kg IV BID × 3d [12]	White rhinos	n = 1, 10 mo old, 580 kg juvenile, with colonic impaction and celiotomy.

Drug name	Drug dose	Species	Comments
Gabapentin	1–8.5 mg/kg PO BID [3]	Black rhinos	n = 1 animal, under treatment for chronic foot abscess, started low and increased until pain control perceived without sedation, used with and without phenylbutazone, used continuously for >3 yrs, no adverse effects noted.
	2.5–5 mg/kg PO SID [8]	Black rhinos	n = Retrospective results of 4/33 institutions contacted regarding analgesic use in Rhinos: 2/4 institutions felt this provided fair to good analgesia subjectively.
Glucosamine Chondroitin	1.1–4 mg/kg PO SID to BID [8]	White and Indian rhinos	n = Retrospective results of 7/33 institutions contacted regarding analgesic use in Rhinos: 4/7 institutions felt this provided fair to good analgesia subjectively.
Ketoprofen	0.5 mg/kg PO SID to BID [8]	White and Black rhinos	n = Retrospective results of 3/33 institutions contacted regarding analgesic use in Rhinos: 2/3 institutions felt this provided good to excellent analgesia subjectively.
Lidocaine	IV regional perfusion 2%: 30 ml Given IV after tourniquet placed on foot. Then L: 50 ml + 50 ml of 0.75% bupivicaine given topically into the wound [4]	Eastern black rhinos	n = 1 animal with osteomyelitis and digit amputation.
Meloxicam	0.2 mg/kg PO BID × 4d [12]	White rhinos	n = 1, 10 mo old, 580 kg, juvenile with colonic impaction and celiotomy.
	0.6 mg/kg IV [6]	White rhinos	n = 1 animal, captive, 2 yr old male, with an osteochondroma of the distal third metacarpal bone removed successfully. meloxicam given perioperatively.
Phenylbutazone	2–4 mg/kg PO or IV SID [3]	Black rhinos	n = 2 animals, with 66 total prescriptions, one on long-term treatment for chronic foot abscesses with fecal occult blood check every other month with no adverse effects noted.
	2–4 mg/kg PO or IV SID [3]	White rhinos	n = 9 animals, with 28 prescriptions, no adverse effects noted.

(Continued)

Drug name	Drug dose	Species	Comments
	3–10 mg/kg PO SID to BID (>4 mg/kg not given for more than 3 d) [8]	White, Black, and Indian rhinos	n = Retrospective results of 25/33 institutions contacted regarding analgesic use in Rhinos: 21/25 institutions felt this provided good to excellent analgesia subjectively. Taste aversion was noted with some animals.
	6 g PO SID × 5d [5]	Eastern black rhinos	n = 1 animal with necrotic laminal disease that required chronic foot trimming and after each immobilization and trim was started on phenylbutazone for 5 days. Assumed 1000 lb animal.
	4.7 mg/kg PO EOD × 28 doses [4]	Eastern black rhinos	n = 1 animal with osteomyelitis.
Tramadol	0.8–3 mg/kg PO BID [8]	White and Black rhinos	n = Retrospective results of 4/33 institutions contacted regarding analgesic use in Rhinos: 3/4 institutions felt this provided good to excellent analgesia subjectively. Mild to moderate sedation was noted.
Anesthesia and Sedation			
Azaperone	A: 80–200 mg IM [10]	Rhinos	Sedation for 2–4 hrs.
	100–250 mg IM q6 hrs [13]	Black rhinos	To facilitate transport.
Butorphanol	Calf 66–159 kg: 10–20 mg butorphanol IV or 0.13–0.15 mg/kg IV [14]	White rhino calves (likely Greater one-horned rhino calves, too)	Captive calves. Antagonize with naltrexone at 5 mg per mg butorphanol.
	B: 25 mg IV for a 500 kg subadult calf [14]	Black rhinos	Captive calves, heavy standing sedation. Antagonize with naltrexone at 5 mg per mg butorphanol.
	B: 25–40 mg IM [10]	Greater one-horned rhinos	Standing sedation, captive animals.
	B: 25–50 mg IV or IM; antagonize with 2.5 mg naltrexone per mg butorphanol IM or IV [10, 14]	Black rhinos	Standing sedation, captive animals.
	B: 25–40 mg IM; antagonize with 2.5 mg naltrexone per mg butorphanol IM or IV [14]	Sumatran rhinos	Captive animals, Standing sedation. May be able to train with food to crate without any medication.

Drug name	Drug dose	Species	Comments
Butorphanol + azaperone	B: 30–50 mg + A: 50–60 mg IM; antagonize with 2.5 mg naltrexone per mg butorphanol IM or IV [10, 14]	Sumatran rhinos	Captive animals, Higher doses for recumbency.
Butorphanol + azaperone	B: 80 mg + A: 80 mg total IM; antagonize with 2.5 mg naltrexone per mg butorphanol given [13].	Sumatran rhinos	
	B: 50–70 mg + A: 100 mg IM [10, 13, 14]	White rhinos	Captive animals, Standing sedation or for transport of calm, captive rhinos. Use a CRI of drug combo for long procedures.
	B: 70–120 mg + A: 100–160 mg IM; antagonize with 2.5 mg naltrexone per mg butorphanol IM or IV [10, 14]	White and Black rhinos	For recumbency, captive animals.
	B: 80 mg + A: 80 mg IM; antagonize with 2.5 mg naltrexone per mg butorphanol, IV or IM [14].	Sumatran rhinos	Wild animals, if can approach give 25–40 mg IV butorphanol instead.
	B: 100 mg + A: 100 mg IM; antagonize with 2.5 mg naltrexone per mg butorphanol IM or IV [10, 14].	Greater one-horned rhinos	Standing sedation. Captive animals.
Butorphanol + detomidine	B: 0.015 mg/kg + D: 0.015 mg/kg IM [15]	White and Greater one-horned rhinos	n = 12 White and 4 Indian rhinoceros, captive animals, standing sedation.
	Calf: 69–122 kg: B: 2.5–5 mg + D: 1.5–1.8 mg IM (B: 0.03 mg/kg + D: 0.07 mg/kg) [14]	White rhinos	Captive calves. Surgical anesthesia. Antagonize with naltrexone at 4 mg per mg butorphanol, and yohimbine 0.125 mg/kg.
	B: 20–30 mg + D: 20–50 mg IM [10]	Black rhinos	Standing sedation, captive animals.
	B: 120 mg + D: 80 mg IM [10]	Greater one-horned rhinos	Immobilization of captive animals.
Butorphanol + detomidine + etorphine + acepromazine	Initial dart B: 10 mg + D: 10 mg-wait 20 min, then give E: 1.2 mg + Ace: 5 mg IM via 2nd dart [10, 14]	Sumatran rhinos	Captive animals, antagonize with naltrexone 150 mg IV and atipamezole 20 mg IV, use 50 mg ketamine boluses to extend anesthesia.
	E: 1.1 mg + Ace: 5 mg + B: 15 mg + D: 15 mg [10]	White rhinos	Standing sedation, captive animals.

(*Continued*)

Drug name	Drug dose	Species	Comments
Butorphanol + medetomidine	B: 120–150 mg + M: 5–7 mg IM via dart; then give 1–2 mg nalorphine IV to keep standing [10, 14]	White, Black, and Greater one-horned rhinos	Captive animals, standing sedation. Antagonize with naltrexone 1 mg per mg butorphanol, and atipamezole 5 mg per mg medetomidine.
	B: 120–150 mg + M: 5–7 mg IM via dart; ± 5% guaifenesin drip [10, 14]	White rhinos	Captive animals, recumbency in 20 min. Improved analgesia for surgery. Antagonize with naltrexone 1 mg per mg butorphanol, and atipamezole 5 mg per mg medetomidine.
	B: 160 mg + M: 10 mg; ketamine 200–400 mg IV can induce recumbency if still standing; antagonize with IV naltrexone and atipamezole [16]	White rhinos	Adult and compromised adult animals, standing sedation at 6–8 min, recumbency in 12–15 min.
Butorphanol + midazolam + propofol + sevoflurane	B: 0.04 mg/kg + Mid: 0.1 mg/kg IM, 30 min later induced with P: 4 mg/kg IV and maintained with S [17].	Black rhinos	n = 1, 53 kg, 30-day-old calf anesthetized 3 times successfully for MRI and evaluation.
Carfentanil	C: 0.7–1 mg IM; antagonize with 100 mg naltrexone per mg carfentanil [10, 14]	Greater one-horned rhinos	For wild animals, immobilization, induction times longer for breeding males.
	C: 1.2 mg IM; antagonize with naltrexone 100 mg per mg carfentanil [10, 14]	White rhinos	Recumbency.
	C: 3 mg total IM; antagonize with naltrexone 300 mg [13]	Black rhinos	Add 5000 IU hyaluronidase to hasten induction. Consider supplemental oxygen 15–30 l/min or doxapram 200 mg IV.
Carfentanil + azaperone	C: 0.001 mg/kg + A: 0.1 mg/kg IM; antagonize with naltrexone 0.1 mg/kg [13]	White rhinos	
Carfentanil + midazolam	C: 0.7–1.2 mg ± Mid: 10 mg [10]	Black rhinos	Immobilization of captive animals.
Diazepam	5–20 mg IV (or the same mg midazolam IV) [14]	White rhinos	To decrease muscle tremors.
Diazepam or midazolam	D: 10–30 mg IM or Mid: 5–50 mg IM [10]	Rhinos	Sedation for 2–6 hrs.

Drug name	Drug dose	Species	Comments
Etorphine + butorphanol	Newborn or very small: B: 20 mg IM, For older calves: E: 0.1 mg for every month of age up to one yr, combined with IM butorphanol at 10–20× E dose in mg [16].	White rhinos	Calves, dart cow 2–3 min prior to calf, do not calf once cow is recumbent.
Etorphine	Calf: 0.1–1 mg; Juvenile: 1–2.5 mg; Subadult: 2.5–3.5 mg; once recumbent give butorphanol 10–20 mg/mg etorphine for respiratory support [14].	White rhinos	Antagonize with diprenorphine 2.5 mg IV per mg etorphine for transport. Full reversal 40 mg naltrexone per mg etorphine. Always dart mother 30–60 sec prior to calf – most important for black rhino calves.
	Calf: E: 0.1–1 mg; Subadult: E: 2.5–3.5 mg; antagonize with 40 mg naltrexone per mg etorphine, IV [14]	Black rhinos	Wild calves.
	Adult: E: 0.5–0.85 mg IM [10]	Black rhinos	Standing sedation. Doses as low as 0.25 mg etorphine have been used to walk animal into a crate.
	Adult: E: 0.5–1.5 mg IM [10]	Greater one-horned rhinos	Standing sedation. Captive animals.
	Adult: E: 0.8–1.5 mg IM [10]	White and Greater one-horned rhinos	Standing sedation. Captive animals.
	Adult 1.5 mg; Sub-adults 3 mg; Juveniles 2 mg; Calves 1 mg IM [13]	White rhinos	Calm captive animals may require less etorphine than wild/free-ranging.
Etorphine	E: 0.8–1.5 mg IM; antagonize with naltrexone at 40 mg per mg etorphine [14]	White rhinos	Captive animals, standing sedation.
Etorphine hydrochloride + acepromazine maleate (Large Animal Immobilon)	Drug solution is E: 2.45 mg/ml + A: 10 mg/ml) Give 1.6 ml IM; antagonize with 2 mg diprenorphine per mg of etorphine given [13]	White rhinos	

(Continued)

Drug name	Drug dose	Species	Comments
Etorphine + acepromazine	E: 2.25 mg + Ace: 10 mg total; antagonize with 2 mg diprenorphine per mg etorphine given [10, 13].	Indian rhinos	Supplement with 2 mg etorphine as needed, for wild animals.
Etorphine + azaperone	Calf: E: 0.1–1 mg + A: 5–20 mg; Subadult: E: 2.5–3.5 mg + A: 30–60 mg [14]	White rhinos	Wild calves, antagonize with diprenorphine 3 mg IV per mg etorphine.
	Calf: E: 0.1–1 mg + A: 10–50 mg; Subadult: E: 1.75–3.5 mg + A: 100 mg [14]	Black rhinos	Wild calves, antagonize with diprenorphine 3 mg IV per mg etorphine. Always dart mother 30–60 seconds prior to calf. Could add 5 mg butorphanol or nalorphine IV, titrate to effect to prevent arousal, for respiratory support.
	Calf: E: 0.5–1 mg + A: 5 mg; Subadult: E: 2–2.5 mg + A: 10 mg [14]	Black rhinos	Wild calves, antagonize with diprenorphine 2.5 mg IV per mg etorphine. For subadults, use adult doses.
	E: 1–1.5 mg + A: 60 mg IM; antagonize with 50 mg naltrexone per mg etorphine half IV and half IM [10, 14]	Sumatran rhinos	Captive animals, recumbency.
	E: 1–1.5 mg + A: 100 mg IM; antagonize with 50 mg naltrexone per mg etorphine half IV and half IM [14]	Black rhinos	Recumbency, lower doses can be used for hand injections.
	E: 2–3 mg + A: 20–40 mg IM; antagonize with naltrexone at 40 mg per mg etorphine [10, 14]	White rhinos	Recumbency, captive animals.
	E: 2 mg + A: 80 mg + 5000 IU hyaluronidase; antagonize with 50 mg naltrexone per mg etorphine given [13, 14].	Sumatran rhinos	
	E: 2.5–3 mg + A: 60 mg IM; antagonize with 20–40 mg naltrexone per mg etorphine [10, 14].	Black rhinos	Recumbency, captive animals.
	E: 4 mg + A: 250 mg total; antagonize with naltrexone 160 mg IV [13]	Black rhinos	If no signs of drug effect develop in 6 min, repeat full dose. Add 5000 IU hyaluronidase to hasten induction. Consider supplemental oxygen 15–30 l/min or doxapram 200 mg IV. In captive Rhinos may be able to use 1–1.5 mg etorphine.

Drug name	Drug dose	Species	Comments
Etorphine + azaperone or detomidine ± midazolam	E: 3–4.5 mg + A: 40–60 mg if transporting. If not transporting substitute 20 mg Det for azaperone. Consider 5–20 mg Mid IV slowly for muscle relaxation [14]	White rhinos	Wild/Free-ranging animals, standard translocation protocol. For crate reversal: 2–4 mg diprenorphine per mg etorphine plus 1–2 mg naltrexone IV if pushing. For Full reversal 40 mg naltrexone per mg etorphine IV. For respiratory support, butorphanol 20 mg per mg etorphine (or reduce to 10–15× etorphine if animal is light) or could be used instead 20–30 mg nalorphine IV OR 20–40 mg nalbuphine IV, and/or 1 mg diprenorphine.
	E: 4 mg + A: 40–60 mg (or Det: 10 mg or xylazine 100 mg) + 5000 IU hyaluronidase [14].	Black rhinos	Wild/Free-ranging animals. Could increase azaperone to 200 mg for a quicker induction if not transporting or could combine with the alpha-2 agonists. For crate reversal: 20 mg butorphanol per mg etorphine, or 5–20 mg nalorphine per mg etorphine or 1–1.8 mg diprenorphine IV. For field or boma reversal: naltrexone 40 mg per mg etorphine IV (full reversal).
Etorphine + butorphanol + midazolam	E: 2–3.5 mg + B: 40–90 mg + Mid: 25–50 mg IM; antagonize with 40 mg naltrexone per mg etorphine (full reversal) or 2–2.5 mg diprenorphine per mg etorphine, IV [14].	White rhinos	Wild/Free-ranging animals. Avoid butorphanol in combination with etorphine in rough terrain where a quick induction is preferred. Produces respiratory depression, hypoxia, tachycardia, muscle rigidity, and tremors, but with slower induction and animal may stay on its feed.
Etorphine + detomidine	Female: E: 3 mg + D: 12 mg IM; Male: E: 4 mg + D: 20 mg IM; antagonize with naltrexone 150 mg and atipamezole 60 mg [13]	White rhinos	If no signs of drug effect develops in 6 min, repeat full dose.
Etorphine + detomidine + butorphanol	E: 2–2.5 mg + D: 10 mg + B: 15 mg IM [14]	Black rhinos	Standing sedation. Captive animals. Antagonize with 40 mg naltrexone per mg etorphine and 5 mg atipamezole per mg detomidine.
Etorphine + detomidine + butorphanol + acepromazine + ketamine	E: 2.5–3.7 mg + D: 8–12 mg + B: 10 mg + A: 10–15 mg IM and as needed K: 200–400 mg IV [18]	White rhinos	n = 20 events with 11 animals for reproductive evaluation, xylazine 20–40 mg IV allowed for semen collection. Duration of 28–124 min.; antagonized with naltrexone 250 mg and atipamezole 20 mg IV. Smooth reversal, all standing and alert within 2 min.

(*Continued*)

Drug name	Drug dose	Species	Comments
Etorphine + detomidine + ketamine	E: 3.5–3.8 mg + D: 14 mg + K 400 mg; antagonize with naltrexone 150–300 mg half IV and half IM. No reversal for detomidine [10, 13, 14].	Indian and Greater one-horned rhinos	Recumbency, captive animals.
Etorphine + medetomidine	E: 1.5–2 mg + M: 2–3 mg total IM; then give 1–2 mg nalorphine IV to keep standing [10, 14]	Black rhinos	Standing sedation, captive animals, antagonize with 30 mg naltrexone per mg etorphine, and 5 mg atipamezole per mg medetomidine.
Etorphine + medetomidine	E: 1.5–2 mg + M: 2–3 mg total IM; antagonize with 30 mg naltrexone per mg etorphine, and 5 mg atipamezole per mg medetomidine [14].	Black rhinos	Captive animals, recumbency in 15 min, enhanced analgesia for dental surgery.
Etorphine + medetomidine + ketamine + guaifenesin	E: 1.5–2 mg + M: 2–3 mg + 1 g/l ketamine in a 5% guaifenesin bag as CRI [10]	Black rhinos	Recumbency and maintenance as CRI.
Etorphine + Thiafentanil	E: 2.5 mg + T: 2.5 mg total IM; antagonize with naltrexone 100 mg IV [13, 14]	Black rhinos	In captive rhino may be able to use 1–1.5 mg etorphine. Add 5000 IU hyaluronidase to hasten induction. Consider supplemental oxygen 15–30 l/min or doxapram 200 mg IV. In wild animals could use thiafentanil alone, up to 5 mg, but watch respirations.
Etorphine + xylazine	E: 4 mg + X: 100 mg; antagonize with naltrexone 160 mg IV [13]	Black rhinos	Add 5000 IU hyaluronidase to hasten induction. Consider supplemental oxygen 15–30 l/min or doxapram 200 mg IV.
Ketamine + diazepam (+ CRI ketamine + medetomidine)	K: 0.5 mg/kg + D: 0.05 mg/kg IV in 3 aliquots at 3 min intervals given IV. Total of K: 300 mg, D: 30 mg. Two additional boluses of K: 100 mg and D: 10 mg were required in addition to isoflurane 5% and a CRI of K: 1.6 mg/kg/hr + M: 0.016 mg/kg/hr [12]	White rhinos	n = 1, 10 mo old 580 kg juvenile with colonic impaction and celiotomy.

Drug name	Drug dose	Species	Comments
Perphenazine (Trilafon-LA)	100–200 mg IM [10]	Rhinos	Onset in 12–18 hrs duration of 7–10 days.
Perphenazine	Adult 300 mg; Subadult 100 mg; Juveniles 50 mg [13]	Black and White rhinoceroses	
Zuclopenthixol	60–200 mg [10]	Rhinoceroses	Sedation for up to 3 d.
	300 mg Adults [13]	Black and White rhinoceroses	
Antiparasitic			
Praziquantel	3 mg/kg PO [19]	Sumatran rhinoceroses	Slight decrease in Fasciola eggs in feces.
Other			
Diphenhydramine	2 mg/kg PO TID [1]	White rhinos	n = 1 calf, treated for urticaria of unknown cause.
Di-Tri-octahedral smectite (Equine Biosponge)	PO BID [1]	White rhinos	n = 1 calf treated for diarrhea in conjunction with probiotic PO SID.
Dobutamine	0.7 μg/kg/min or 10 ml/kg/hr, then increased up to 22 ml/kg/hr [20]	White rhinos	n = 1, 10 mo old 580 kg juvenile with colonic impaction and celiotomy. Used in an attempt to maintain a MAP of 8 kPa–9.33 kPa. Phenylephrine also used.
Fractionated vegetable fat (Manna Pro's Cool Calories Equine Fat Supplement)	30 g per animal sprinkled on food SID [3]	Black rhinos	Used for assistance with weight gain in thin animals. Start at 10 g for 3–5 days then 20 g for 3–5 days then full 30 g/day to prevent diarrhea.
GnRF vaccination (Improvac Zoetis)	Vaccinated at 0,4,16 wks and q6–8 months [20]	White and Greater one-horned rhinos	n = 4 White and 3 Greater one-horned rhino females with repro tract tumors that decreased by approx 50% in size after 3 months post vaccine.
Hydroxyzine pamoate	Initially 0.5 mg/kg PO BID × 3d, then 0.75 mg/kg PO BID × 3d then 1 mg/kg PO BID continuously [21]	Black rhinos	n = 2 animals with chronic eosinophilic granulomas managed successfully with chronic or continuous hydroxyzine.
Monosodium phosphate (equine powdered product 26%)	12 g powder PO SID [3]	Black rhinos	n = 2 animals with 23 prescriptions, for hypophosphatemia, no adverse effects noted, treated until phosphorus levels were again within normal limits.
Omeprazole	2 mg/kg PO SID × 3–5d [3]	Black rhinos	n = 1 animal with 13 prescriptions, no adverse effects noted.
Oxytocin	100 IU [10]	Rhinos	Captive species with dystocia, given if no signs of labor for 4–6 hrs after rupture of fetal membranes.

(Continued)

Drug name	Drug dose	Species	Comments
Phenylephrine	10 mg added to a fluid bag for dilution of 33 μg/ml [20]	White rhinos	n = 1, 10 mo old 580, kg juvenile with colonic impaction and celiotomy. Resulted in increased heart rate from 50 to 65 beats per minute.
Phosphorus (Equiphos)	1–4 oz per day PO [19]	Sumatran rhinos	n = 1, 30 yr old male with renal disease, azotemia, hypercalcemia, and hypophosphatemia. Fed daily, increased by 1–2 oz per day when Ca:Phos ratio exceeded 5:1, managed for 5 yrs thus.
Reported Toxicities			
Kale		Hemolysis	
Onions		Hemolysis	
Red maple		Hemolysis	
Brassica plants		Hemolysis	
Creosote		Causes liver dysfunction [10]	

Species	Weight [1, 20]
Rhinoceros, Black *(Diceros bicornis)*	800–1400 kg
Rhinoceros, Indian *(Rhinoceros unicornis)*	1600–2200 kg
Rhinoceros, Sumatran *(Dicerorhinus sumatrensis)*	800–1000 kg
Rhinoceros, White *(Ceratotherium simum)*	Female: 1400–1700 kg; Male: 2000–2300 kg

References

1 Warren, J.D., Aitken-Palmer, C., and Citino, C.B. (2014). Critical care for a hypothermic and hypoglycemic white rhinoceros (*Ceratotherium simum simum*) calf. *Journal of Zoo and Wildlife Medicine* 45 (3): 650–653.

2 Bloch, R.A., Haefele, H., and Stephens, L. (2014). Medical management of a patent urachus in a southern White rhinoceros (*Ceratotherium simum simum*) calf. *Journal of Zoo and Wildlife Medicine* 45 (2): 420–422.

3 Swenson, J., DVM DACZM (2018). Fossil Rim Wildlife Center, Personal communication.

4 Harrison, T.M., Stanley, B.J., Sikarskie, J.G. et al. (2011). Surgical amputation of a digit and vacuum-assisted-closure (VAC) management in a case of osteomyelitis and wound care in an eastern black rhinoceros (*Diceros bicornis michaeli*). *Journal of Zoo and Wildlife Medicine* 42 (2): 317–321.

5 Nance, M.B. (1998). Clinical Management of Severe Necrotic Laminar Disease in an Eastern Black Rhinoceros (*Diceros bicornis michaeli*) associated with an undetermined etiology. *Proceedings of the American Association of Zoo Veterinarians.*

6 Smit, Y., Steyl, J., and Marais, J. (2016). Solitary Osteochondroma of the distal third metacarpal bone in a two-year-old white rhinoceros (*Ceratotherium simum*). *Journal of Zoo and Wildlife Medicine* 47 (4): 1086–1089.

7 Love, D., Madrigal, R., Cerveny, S. et al. (2017). Case series: clinical salmonellosis in four black rhinoceros (*Diceros bicornis*) calves. *Journal of Zoo and Wildlife Medicine* 48 (2): 466–475.
8 Kottwitz, J., Boothe, M., Harmon, R. et al. (2016). Results of the megavertebrate analgesia survey: elephants and rhino. *Journal of Zoo and Wildlife Medicine* 47 (1): 301–310.
9 Leiberich, M., Krebber, R., Hewetson, M. et al. A study of the pharmacokinetics and thromboxane inhibitory activity of a single intramuscular dose of Carprofen as a means to establish its potential use as an analgesic drug in white rhinoceros. *Journal of Veterinary Pharmacology* 41 (4): 605–613.
10 Miller, M.A. and Buss, P.E. (2015). Rhinoceridae (Rhinoceroses). In: *Fowler's Zoo and Wild Animal Medicine*, vol. 8 (ed. R.E. Miller and M. Fowler), 568–583. St. Louis, MO: Elsevier Saunders.
11 Stringer, E.M., DeVoe, R.S., Linder, K. et al. (2012). Vesiculobullous skin reaction temporally related to firocoxib treatment in a white rhinoceros (*Ceratotherium simum*). *Journal of Zoo and Wildlife Medicine* 43 (1): 186–189.
12 Zeiler, G.E. and Stegmann, G.F. (2012). Anaesthetic management of a 10-month-old white rhinoceros (*Ceratotherium simum*) calf for emergency exploratory celiotomy. *Journal of the South African Veterinary Association* 83 (1): 1–5.
13 Kreeger, T.J. and Arnemo, J.M. (2012). *Handbook of Wildlife Chemical Immobilization*, 4e. China: Kreeger.
14 Radcliff, R.W. and Morkel, P.V. (2014). Rhinoceroses. In: *Zoo Animal and Wildlife Immobilization and Anesthesia*, 2e (ed. G. West, D. Heard and N. Caulkett), 741–772. Ames, IA: Wiley Blackwell.
15 Bouts, T., Dodds, J., Berry, K. et al. (2017). Detomidine and butorphanol for standing sedation in a range of zoo-kept ungulate species. *Journal of Zoo and Wildlife Medicine* 48 (3): 616–626.
16 Morkel, P. and Nel, P. (2018). Updates in African rhinoceros field immobilization and translocation. In: *Fowler's Zoo and Wild Animal Medicine Current Therapy*, vol. 9 (ed. R.E. Miller, N. Lamberski and P.P. Calle), 692–698. St. Louis, MO: Elsevier Saunders.
17 Ratliff, C., Sayre, R.S., and Leipz, M. (2016). Anesthesia in a captive juvenile black rhinoceros (*Diceros bicornis*) for magnetic resonance imaging and computed tomography. *Journal of Zoo and Wildlife Medicine* 47 (3): 872–875.
18 Walzer, C., Goritz, F., Pucher, H. et al. (2000). Chemical restraint and anesthesia in White rhinoceros (*Ceratotherium simum*) for Reproductive evaluation, Semen collection, and Artificial insemination. *Proceedings of International Association for Aquatic Animal Medicine*.
19 Radcliff, R.W. and Khairani, K.O. (2018). Health of the Forest rhinoceros of Southeast Asia: Sumatran and Javan rhinoceros. In: *Fowler's Zoo and Wild Animal Medicine Current Therapy*, vol. 9 (ed. R.E. Miller, N. Lamberski and P.P. Calle), 707–715. St. Louis, MO: Elsevier Saunders.
20 Hermes, R., Schwarzenberger, F., Goritz, F. et al. (2016). Ovarian down regulation by GnRF vaccination decreases reproductive tract tumour size in female white and greater one-horned rhinoceroses. *PLoS One* 11 (7): e0157963.
21 Bishop, G.T., Zuba, J.R., Pessier, A.P. et al. (2016). Medical management of recurrent eosinophilic granuloma in two black rhinoceros (*Diceros bicornis*). *Journal of Zoo and Wildlife Medicine* 47 (3): 855–861.

22

Nondomestic Pigs

Drug name	Drug dose	Species	Comments
Antimicrobials and Antifungals			
Ampicillin sodium	10–20 mg/kg IV q6–8 hrs [1]	Domestic pigs	
Amoxicillin	10–22 mg/kg PO SID to BID [1, 2]	Miniature pigs	Also used in Visayan warty pigs 15 mg/kg PO BID.
Amoxicillin trihydrate	6.6–22 mg/kg IM q8, 12, or 24 hrs [1]	Domestic pigs	
Amoxicillin/clavulanate (Clavamox)	12.8–15 mg/kg PO BID × 8–18d [2, 3]	African warthogs, Visayan warty pigs	n = 2 Visayan warty pigs at 15 mg/kg PO BID.
	11–13 mg/kg PO SID [4]	Domestic pigs	
Ampicillin	6.5 mg/kg IM SID [4]	Domestic pigs	
Cefpodoxime	5–10 mg/kg PO SID × 19d [2, 5]	Babirusas	n = 1 female post parturition with toxic mastitis.
Cephalexin	10–15 mg/kg PO BID [2]	Babirusas	
Ceftiofur hydrochloride (Excenel)	4 mg/kg IM SID × 5d [2, 5]	Babirusas	n = 1 female post parturition with toxic mastitis.
Ceftiofur	3–10 mg/kg IM SID [4]	Domestic pigs	
Danofloxacin	6.75 mg/kg SC [5]	Babirusas	n = 1 female post parturition with Toxic mastitis.
Doxycycline	0.3 mg/kg PO BID × 30d on, 30d off, 1–8 cycles [6]	Chacoan peccaries	n = 1 animal with low-dose doxycycline given in a pulsatile fashion to treat periodontal disease.
Enrofloxacin	5 mg/kg SC or PO [5]	Babirusas	n = 1 female post parturition with toxic mastitis.
Erythromycin	2–20 mg/kg SID to BID [4]	Domestic Pigs	

(*Continued*)

Zoo and Wild Mammal Formulary, First Edition. Alicia Hahn.

Drug name	Drug dose	Species	Comments
Florfenicol	15 mg/kg IM SID [2, 4]	Domestic pigs	n = 1 Warty pig at 20 mg/kg.
Gentamicin	5 mg/kg PO SID [4]	Domestic pigs	
Lincomycin	10–11 mg/kg IM SID [1, 4]	Domestic pigs	
Penicillin G potassium or sodium	20 000 IU/kg IV or IM q6 hrs [1]	Domestic pigs	
Penicillin benzathine/procaine	30 000 IU/kg IM [3]	African warthogs	n = 1 ovariohysterectomy with perioperative antibiotics.
Procaine penicillin G	20–60 000 IU/kg IM SID [4]	Domestic pigs	
Oxytetracycline LA 200	20 mg/kg IM [1]	Domestic pigs	
Tetracycline	10–20 mg/kg IM or PO SID [4]	Domestic pigs	
Tetracycline (long-acting)	20 mg/kg IM q48 hr [4]	Domestic pigs	
Trimethoprim sulfadoxine	16 mg/kg IM BID [4]	Domestic pigs	
Tulathromycin	2.5 mg/kg IM SID [4]	Domestic pigs	
Tylosin	8.8–9 mg/kg IM SID to BID [1, 4]	Domestic pigs	
Analgesia			
Buprenorphine sustained release	0.18 mg/kg SC [7]	Göttingen minipigs	n = 5 plasma concentrations >0.1 ng/ml – hypothesized therapeutic threshold for 10 days. High individual variability, injection site reactions with firm SC nodules in 4/5.
Buprenorphine	0.002–0.006 mg/kg SC or IM [2]	Babirusas	n = 3 postop analgesia.
Buprenorphine transdermal	30 μg/hr (1 of each 20 μg/hr and 10 μg/hr patches) [7]	Göttingen minipigs	n = 5 shaved dorsal trunk between 12th rib and 2nd lumbar vertebrae. Plasma concentrations >0.1 ng/ml – hypothesized therapeutic threshold – in 12–24 hrs and lasted up to 72 hrs. 1/5 did not develop plasma concentrations and 1/5 had a mild dermal reaction of erythema with a few papules.

Drug name	Drug dose	Species	Comments
Butorphanol	0.05–0.1 mg/kg IM or SC [2]	Babirusas	Analgesia
Carprofen	1–3 mg/kg PO SID or 1–2 mg/kg PO BID [2]	Babirusas	Used frequently in exotic suids with osteoarthritis with perceived efficacy.
Gabapentin	9–20 mg/kg PO BID [2]	Babirusas, Visayan warty pigs	Used frequently in exotic suids with osteoarthritis with perceived efficacy.
Meloxicam	0.2 mg/kg SC; 0.15 mg/kg PO SID × 5d [3]	African warthogs	n = 1 animal pre and postoperative ovariohysterectomy.
	0.2–0.38 mg/kg SC SID; 0.28 mg/kg PO SID [2, 5]	Babirusas	n = 1 female post parturition with toxic mastitis. Also used in a private zoo collection in a number of exotic suids 0.1–0.4 mg/kg PO/SC/IM SID with perceived efficacy.
Tramadol	2–5 mg/kg PO SID or BID [2]	Babirusas, Visayan warty pigs	Variable compliance due to taste aversion.
Anesthesia and Sedation			
Alpha-chloralose	2.2 g/40 kg of body weight; (maximum safe dose is 2.2 g/10 kg of body weight) [8]	Feral pigs	To capture wild pigs by adding to baited food such as corn.
Alprazolam (Xanax)	0.15 mg/kg PO [9]	Domestic and Pot-bellied pigs	For mild sedation, for transport or for introductions.
Atropine	0.04 mg/kg IM as adjunct to premedication [8]	Vietnamese Potbellied pigs and domestic pigs	Anticholinergic decreases likelihood of bradycardia, avoids bronchoconstriction, minimizes airway secretions, and decreases salivation. Caution when giving with drugs that can cause peripheral hypertension such as alpha-2 agonists.
Azaperone	1–2 mg/kg IM [10]	Non domestic suids	To facilitate animal introductions.
	0.25–2 mg/kg IM [8]	Potbellied pigs	Sedation

(*Continued*)

Drug name	Drug dose	Species	Comments
	0.5–1.5 mg/kg IM [10]	Non domestic suids	Has been administered prior to recovery to prevent excitability or violent recovery.
	2–8 mg/kg IM [8]	Potbellied pigs	Immobilization. However, at higher doses prolonged recoveries can be seen.
Butorphanol + detomidine + midazolam	B: 0.3–0.4 mg/kg + D: 0.06–0.125 mg/kg + Mid: 0.3–0.4 mg/kg IM; antagonize with naltrexone 5 mg/kg + yohimbine 0.3 mg/kg IM [8, 10, 11]	European wild, Wart, and Red River hogs, Vietnamese potbellied and Bearded pigs, Babirusas	Rapid, smooth induction with excellent relaxation. Could replace detomidine with xylazine 2–3 mg/kg. Wild hog and Warthogs consistently easy to arouse so the additional of Telazol is preferred for these species.
Butorphanol + detomidine + Telazol	B: 0.3–0.4 mg/kg + D: 0.06–0.125 mg/kg + T: 0.6 mg/kg IM [8]	Multiple species	Smaller induction volume than But+ Det+ Mid. Red River hogs, Babirusa, and Potbellied pigs may consider using lower end of dose range, while higher should be used for Bearded pigs, Eurasian boars, and Warthogs.
Butorphanol + medetomidine + midazolam	B: 0.15 mg/kg + M: 0.04 mg/kg + Mid: 0.08 mg/kg IM [8]	Babirusas, Red River hogs, and Warthogs	
	B: 0.08–0.3 mg/kg + M: 0.04–0.07 mg/kg + Mid: 0.08–0.3 mg/kg IM [10, 11]	Chacoan, Collared and White-lipped peccaries	Antagonize with naltrexone 3 mg/kg + atipamezole 0.35 mg/kg IM; flumazenil in a 1:10–1:20 ratio with midazolam IM will counteract resedation or can be used with previous 2 at conclusion of procedure. Bradycardia, hypoxemia reported. Lower dose range used in calm, captive individuals.

Drug name	Drug dose	Species	Comments
	B: 0.15–0.3 mg/kg + M: 0.04–0.07 mg/kg + Mid: 0.08–0.3 mg/kg IM; antagonize with atipamezole and naltrexone [8]	Multiple species	Preferred combination can be used in all species. Lower dose range used in calm, captive individuals; Med or Mid can be administered as premedication and B 10–15 min later or all concurrently. Significant bradycardia and hypoxemia are common, and unexplained severe hypoglycemia in fasted and unfasted animals.
Butorphanol + medetomidine + Telazol	B: 0.2 mg/kg + M: 0.05 mg/kg + T: 3 mg/kg IM; antagonize with atipamezole 0.25 mg/kg IM [12]	European wild hogs	n = 8 animals, smooth and rapid induction with rough and prolonged recoveries with paddling and ataxia.
	B: 0.33–0.57 mg/kg + M: 0.08–0.11 mg/kg + T: 0.66–1.1 mg/kg IM [13].	Visayan warty pigs	n = 4 males anesthetized for evaluation for urolithiasis.
Butorphanol + midazolam + ketamine	B: 0.25 mg/kg + Mid: 0.1 mg/kg + K: 0.5 mg/kg IM; antagonize with naltrexone 2.5 mg/kg IM [5]	Babirusas	n = 1 female post parturition with toxic mastitis.
Butorphanol + midazolam + xylazine	B: 0.3–0.4 mg/kg + Mid: 0.3–0.4 mg/kg + X: 2–3 mg/kg IM [8, 10]	Multiple species	Antagonize with yohimbine or atipamezole and naltrexone; xylazine or midazolam can be administered as premedication with remaining 10–15 min later, or all drugs concurrently.
Butorphanol + xylazine	B: 0.3 mg/kg + X: 0.1–2 mg/kg IM [14]	Potbellied pigs	n = 2 animals, captive, butorphanol produced profound sedation.
Butorphanol + xylazine + midazolam	B: 0.3 mg/kg + X: 0.1–2 mg/kg + Mid: 0.3 mg/kg IM; antagonize with yohimbine 0.3 mg/kg and naltrexone 50 mg IM [14].	Potbellied pigs	n = 2 animals, Complete immobility with relaxation and analgesia, 2 castrations with intratesticular lidocaine performed. Recovery was rapid and smooth.

(*Continued*)

Drug name	Drug dose	Species	Comments
Butorphanol + xylazine + Telazol	B: 0.3–0.4 mg/kg + X: 2–3 mg/kg + T 0.6 mg/kg IM [8]	Multiple species	
Diazepam + amitriptyline	D: 0.5 mg/kg each PO BID [10]	Non domestic suids	To help reduce excitability during shipment or other relocation events.
Detomidine + butorphanol + midazolam	D: 0.06–0.125 mg/kg + B: 0.3–0.4 mg/kg + Mid: 0.3–0.4 mg/kg IM [8]	Multiple species	Antagonize with yohimbine or atipamezole and naltrexone; animals may resedate within hours of antagonism; can give detomidine or midazolam as premedication and butorphanol 10–15 min later or all concurrently.
Detomidine + butorphanol + Telazol	D: 0.12 mg/kg + B: 0.3 mg/kg + T: 0.6 mg/kg IM [10]	Multiple species	
Etorphine + acepromazine	E: 0.022 mg/kg + A: 0.11 mg/kg IM [11]	European wild hogs	Monitor carefully as hogs can readily overheat. Antagonize with diprenorphine 0.044 mg/kg.
Etorphine + azaperone + butorphanol	E: 0.035 mg/kg + azaperone 0.4 mg/kg IM in single dart, then when can approach give butorphanol IV; antagonize with naltrexone 20× etorphine dose in mg, IV [15]	Warthogs	Butorphanol dose is same number of mg of etorphine used total. Be careful with higher doses as may cause premature rousing. Very rapid recovery.
Etorphine + xylazine	E: 4 mg + X: 20 mg; antagonize with 8 mg diprenorphine + yohimbine 0.125 mg/kg [11]	Warthogs	Respiratory depression can be severe with opiods. Highly susceptible to overheating. Use low impact darting systems with enough pressure to penetrate tough skin. Do not stress prior to induction and keep cool during recovery.

Drug name	Drug dose	Species	Comments
Glycopyrrolate	0.005–0.02 mg/kg IM, as an adjunct to premedication [8]	Vietnamese Potbellied and Domestic pigs	Anticholinergic decrease likelihood of bradycardia, avoid bronchoconstriction, minimize airway secretions, and decrease salivation. Caution when giving with drugs that can cause peripheral hypertension such as alpha-2 agonists.
Ketamine	20 mg/kg IM [8, 10]	Collared peccaries	NOT recommended as first choice for immobilization: recoveries may be violent and prolonged >120 min, and fatalities reported associated with ambient temperature. Muscle rigidity precludes endotracheal intubation.
Ketamine + medetomidine	K: 5 mg/kg + M: 0.2 mg/kg IM; supplement with K: 2 mg/kg IM as needed; antagonize with atipamezole 0.5 mg/kg IM [11]	European wild hogs	
	K: 200 mg + M: 2 mg IM total [11]	Warthogs	Ketamine and Telazol combinations may result in light anesthesia, poor analgesia, and muscle spasms.
Ketamine + medetomidine + butorphanol	K: 0.6–1.1 mg/kg + M: 0.06–0.1 mg/kg + B: 0.3–0.4 mg/kg IM [8]	Bearded pigs	
Ketamine + Telazol + medetomidine	K: 3.9 mg/kg + T: 0.63 mg/kg + M: 0.03 mg/kg IM [8, 10]	Chacoan peccaries	Prolonged recoveries despite antagonizing with atipamezole, residual ataxia.
Ketamine + xylazine	K: 3.5 mg/kg + X: 0.2 mg/kg IM [11]	Warthogs	Ketamine and Telazol combinations may result in light anesthesia, poor analgesia, and muscle spasms.

(*Continued*)

Drug name	Drug dose	Species	Comments
	K: 7.7 mg/kg + X: 4.3 mg/kg IM [8]	White-lipped peccaries	n = 17 free-range animals immobilized for field collaring, recoveries were prolonged 1–3 hrs without antagonism.
Ketamine + xylazine	K: 8 mg/kg + X: 10 mg/kg IM [11]	Collared peccaries	
	K: 10 mg/kg + X: 0.5 mg/kg IM [11]	European wild hogs	Monitor carefully as hogs can readily overheat.
Midazolam	2 mg/kg IN or IM [9]	Domestic and Pot-bellied pigs	For mild sedation, anti-anxiety.
Perphenazine	30–50 mg/animal [8]	Warthogs	Long-acting tranquilizer. 2 animals that received 5 mg/kg died within 3 days.
Propofol	5 mg/kg IV [16]	Collared peccaries	n = 9 animals, received either propofol or Telazol 2 mg/kg IV for electroejaculation. Propofol resulted in 8/9 successful collections with improved sperm motility and rapid recoveries.
Telazol	T: 2.2 mg/kg IM; supplement with ketamine 2.2 mg/kg as needed [8, 10, 11]	Chacoan peccaries	Prolonged recoveries 90–240 min, poor relaxation. Doses of up to 3.2 mg/kg resulted in recoveries of >8 hrs.
	T: 3 mg/kg IM; supplement with ketamine 2 mg/kg IM as needed [11]	Warthogs	Ketamine and Telazol combinations may result in light anesthesia, poor analgesia, and muscle spasms.
	T: 2–5 mg/kg IM [8, 10]	Multiple species	Smooth induction, poor muscle relaxation, prolonged recoveries and may be rough. Duration of recovery is dose dependent.
Telazol + butorphanol	T: 1.26 + B: 0.36 mg/kg IM [10]	Babirusas	Antagonize with naltrexone, poor overall relaxation.

Drug name	Drug dose	Species	Comments
	T: 1.5 mg/kg + B: 0.14 mg/kg IM [8, 10, 11]	White-lipped peccaries	If not recumbent in 15 min after administration, repeat full doses of T + B. Similar doses were ineffective for Collared peccaries.
Telazol + romifidine	T: 3–6 mg/kg + R: 0.1 mg/kg [8, 10]	Wild pigs	
Telazol + medetomidine	T: 5 mg/kg + M: 0.1 mg/kg IM; antagonize with atipamezole 0.5 mg/kg IM [11, 12]	European wild hogs	Studied in juveniles, smooth and rapid induction, rough recoveries with paddling and ataxia.
Telazol + xylazine	T: 1.8–3.3 mg/kg + X: 1.2–2.1 mg/kg IM. Give xylazine as premedicant, then 20 min later Telazol [8, 10, 17]	Babirusas	n = 12 Babirusa 8.4-anesthetized 30 times over 4 yrs. Bradycardia seen in some cases; antagonize with yohimbine 0.14 mg/kg and flumazenil 1 mg per 20 mg zolazepam.
	T: 1.25 mg/kg + X: 1.25 mg/kg IM [8, 10, 11]	White-lipped peccaries	1.51 mg of each for Collared peccaries was not successful.
	T: 2.35 mg/kg + X: 2.35 mg/kg [8, 10]	Collared peccaries	n = 107 animals, prolonged recoveries but study did not antagonize xylazine. One fatality was associated with double dose.
	T: 3 mg/kg + X: 0.5 mg/kg IM [8, 10]	Warthogs	Recoveries >90 min.
	T: 3.3 mg/kg + X: 1.6 mg/kg IM [8, 10]	Feral pigs	Animals recovered and released within 120 min of initial injection.
	T: 4.4 mg/kg + X: 2.2 mg/kg IM; antagonize with yohimbine 0.15 mg/kg IM [11]	Collared peccaries	If not recumbent in 15 min after administration, repeat full doses of T + X.
Telazol + xylazine	T: 4.4 mg/kg + X: 2.2 mg/kg IM; antagonize with yohimbine 0.15 mg/kg IM [11]	European wild hogs	

(Continued)

Drug name	Drug dose	Species	Comments
Telazol + butorphanol + medetomidine + ketamine	T: 0.69 mg/kg + B: 0.26 mg/kg + M: 0.07 mg/kg + K: 1.43 mg/kg (single dart) [15]	Warthogs	Free ranging, Usually recumbent in 5–6 min, and walking in 7 min; antagonize with naltrexone 2 × butorphanol dose in mg, and atipamezole 5 × medetomidine dose in mg IV.
Antiparasitic			
Dichlorvos	11.2–21.6 mg/kg in feed with 1/3 ration [18]	Common swine	
Doramectin	300 μg/kg IM [18]	Common swine	
Fenbendazole	9 mg/kg PO over 3–12d via feed [18]	Common swine	
Ivermectin	300 μg/kg SQ; or 100 μg/kg PO For 7d via feed [18]	Common swine	
	500 μg/kg PO q7d [10]	Red River hogs	Resolved cases of sarcoptic mange over a 6-month period.
Levamisole	8 mg/kg PO [2]	Babirusas	Use with caution during pregnancy, may cause abortion.
Piperazine	275–400 mg/kg in feed or water [18]	Common swine	
Pyrantel tartrate	22 mg/kg PO once or 96 g/ton of feed as prophylactic dose [18].	Common swine	
Other			
Calcium gluconate	115 mg/kg SC once [5]	Babirusas	n = 1 female post parturition with toxic mastitis.
Dexamethasone SP	0.2–0.25 mg/kg IM [5]	Babirusas	n = 1 female post parturition with toxic mastitis.
Famotidine	0.2–0.3 mg/kg PO SID [2]	Babirusas, Visayan warty pigs	
Metoclopramide	0.2 mg/kg PO BID × 12d [3]	African warthogs	n = 1 postoperative for ovariohysterectomy, with attempted prevention and treatment for postoperative ileus.

Drug name	Drug dose	Species	Comments
Metoclopramide	0.2–0.5 mg/kg PO IM or IV TID to QID [3]	Potbellied pigs	
Ranitidine	1.47 mg/kg PO BID × 28d [3]	African warthogs	n = 1 animal, postoperative for ovariohysterectomy, with attempted prevention and treatment for postoperative ileus.

Species	Weight
Buru babirusa *(Babyrousa babyrussa)*	40–100 kg
Bola Batu babirusa *(Babrousa bolabatensis)*	up to 90 kg
Malenge babirusa *(Babyrousa togeanesis)*	up to 90 kg
Northwest Sulawesi babirusa *(Babyrousa celebensis)*	up to 90 kg
Bearded pig *(Sus barbatus)*	100–200 kg
Bush pig *(Potamochoerus larvatus)*	50–120 kg
Chacoan peccary *(Catagonus wagneri)*	30–45 kg
Common warthog *(Phacochoerus africanus)*	50–150 kg
Collared peccary *(Tayassu tajacu)*	15–35 kg
Desert warthog *(Phacochoerus aethiopicus)*	45–140 kg
European wild hog/boar *(Sus scrofa)*	40–300 kg
Giant Forest hog *(Hylochoerus meinertzhagen)*	100–275 kg
Javan warty pig *(Sus verrocosus)*	35–185 kg
Pygmy hog *(Porcula salvanius)*	6–10 kg
Red River hog *(Potamochoerus porcus)*	50–120 kg
Sulawesi warty *(Sus celebensis)*	40–70 kg
Vietnamese potbellied pig	32–100 kg
Visayan warty pig *(Sus cebifrons)*	20–80 kg
White-lipped peccary *(Tayassu pecari)*	20–50 kg

References

1 Howard, J.L. (1999). Antimicrobial use in food animals. In: *Current Veterinary Therapy 4: Food Animal Practice*, vol. 5 (ed. D.E. Anderson and D.M. Rings). Ithica, NY: Saunders Elsevier.
2 Padilla, L., DVM, DACZM, (2018). St. Louis Zoo, Personal communication.
3 Thompson, K.A., Niehaus, A., Shellabarger, W. et al. (2015). Antemortem diagnosis of cystic endometrial hyperplasia and successful ovariohysterectomy in an African warthog (*Phacochoeru safricanus*). *Journal of Zoo and Wildlife Medicine* 46 (4): 904–908.
4 Friendship, R.M. (2006). Antimicrobial drug use in swine. In: *Antimicrobial Therapy in Veterinary Medicine* (ed. S. Giguere), 535–543. Ames, IA: Wiley Blackwell.

5 Alexander, A.B., Hanley, C.S., Fischer, M.T. et al. (2015). Management of toxic mastitis in a babirusa (*Babyrousa celebensis*). *Journal of Zoo and Wildlife Medicine* 46 (4): 949–952.
6 Bicknese, B., Fagan, D.A., and Lamberski, N. (2008). "Cyclic" regimen of Low-dose doxycycline to treat periodontal disease in a Chacoan peccary (*Catagonus wagneri*), Red Pandas (*Ailurus fulgens*), and Bat-eared foxes (*Otocyon megalotis megalotis*). *Proceedings of the American Association of Zoo Veterinarians*. 167–168.
7 Emerson, J.A. and Guzman, D.S. (2018). Sustained-release and long-acting opiod formulations of interest in zoological medicine. In: *Fowler's Zoo and Wild Animal Medicine Current Therapy*, vol. 9 (ed. R.E. Miller, N. Lamberski and P.P. Calle), 151–163. St. Louis, MO: Elsevier Saunders.
8 Padilla, L.R. and Ko, J.C. (2014). Nondomestic suids. In: *Zoo Animal and Wildlife Immobilization and Anesthesia*, 2e (ed. G. West, D. Heard and N. Caulkett), 773–785. Ames, IA: Wiley Blackwell.
9 Petritz, O., DVM, DACZM, (2018). North Carolina University, Personal communication.
10 Sutherland-Smith, M. (2016). Suids and Tayassuidae. In: *Fowler's Zoo and Wild Animal Medicine*, vol. 8 (ed. R.E. Miller and M. Fowler), 568–583. St. Louis, MO: Elsevier Saunders.
11 Kreeger, T.J. and Arnemo, J.M. (2012). *Handbook of Wildlife Chemical Immobilization*, 4e. China: Kreeger.
12 Enqvist, K.E., Arnemo, J.M., Lemel, J.P., et al. (2000). Medetomidine/Tiletamine-Zolazepam and Medetomidine/Butorphanol/Tiletamine-Zolazepam: A comparison of two anesthetic regimens for surgical implantation of intraperitoneal radiotransmitters in free-ranging juvenile, European Wild boars (*Sus scrofa scrofa*). *Annual Proceedings of the International Association of Aquatic Animal Medicine*.
13 Chatterton, J., Unwin, S., Lopez, J. et al. (2017). Urolithiasis in a group of Visayan warty pigs (*Sus cebifrons negrinus*). *Journal of Zoo and Wildlife Medicine* 48 (3): 842–850.
14 Morris, P.J., Bicknese, B., Janssen, D.L. et al. (1999). Chemical Immobilization of Exotic Swine at the San Diego Zoo. *Proceedings of the American Association of Zoo Veterinarians*. 150–153.
15 Miller, M.A., DVM, MPH, PhD, DECZM (ZHM), (2018). Stellenbosch University, Personal communication.
16 Souza, A.L., Castelo, T.S., Queiroz, J.P. et al. (2009). Evaluation of anesthetic protocol for the collection of semen from captive collared peccaries (*Tayassuta jacu*) by electroejaculation. *Animal Reproduction Science* 116 (3–4): 370–375.
17 James, S.B., Cook, R.A., Raphael, B.L. et al. (1999). Immobilization of babirusa (*Babyrousa babyrussa*) with Xylazine and Tiletamine/Zolazepam and reversal with yohimbine and flumazenil. *Journal of Zoo and Wildlife Medicine* 30 (4): 521–525.
18 Zimmerman, J., Karriker, L.A., Ramirez, A. et al. (2012). *Diseases of Swine, Drug Pharmacology, Therapy, and Prophylaxis*. West Sussex, UK: Wiley-Blackwell.

23

Hippopotamuses

Drug name	Drug dose	Species	Comments
Antimicrobials and Antifungals			
Amoxicillin	20 mg/kg PO BID [1]	Hippos	n = 1, 59 yr old female captive hippopotamus with bacterial dermatitis that over a 12-week period finally cleared after being treated with amoxicillin, sulfamethoxazole and trimethoprim, and pentoxifylline orally.
Trimethoprim sulfadimethoxazole	30 mg/kg PO SID [1]	Hippos	n = 1, 59 yr old female captive hippopotamus with bacterial dermatitis that over a 12-week period finally cleared after being treated with amoxicillin, sulfamethoxazole and trimethoprim, and pentoxifylline orally.
	20 mg/kg PO BID [2]	Pygmy hippos	n = 1, 25 yr old male with a benign osteoma removed and treated with postoperative antibiotics and phenylbutazone.
Analgesia			
Butorphanol	0.02 mg/kg PO SID [3]	Hippos	Megavertebrate analgesia study: 1 institution used this medication at this dose with a report of good perceived efficacy.
Etodolac	5–10 mg/kg PO SID [3]	Hippos	Megavertebrate analgesia study: 3 institutions used this medication at this dose with 2 reporting good perceived efficacy and 1 reporting fair.
Flunixin meglumine	0.3–1.3 mg/kg PO SID or BID [3]	Hippos	Megavertebrate analgesia study: 9 institutions used this medication at this dose with 2 reporting excellent, 4 good, 1 fair, 1 poor and 1 no response reported.

(*Continued*)

Drug name	Drug dose	Species	Comments
	1.1 mg/kg IM SID [3]	Hippos	Megavertebrate analgesia study: 2 institutions used this medication at this dose with 1 reporting good perceived efficacy and 1 without effect noted or difficult to discern.
Gabapentin	1.5 mg/kg PO BID [3]	Hippos	Megavertebrate analgesia study: 1 institution used this medication at this dose with a report of fair perceived efficacy.
Ketoprofen	0.8–2 mg/kg PO SID [3]	Hippos	Megavertebrate analgesia study: 2 institutions used this medication at this dose with 1 reporting good perceived efficacy and 1 without effect noted.
Meloxicam	0.1–0.15 mg/kg PO SID [3]	Hippos	Megavertebrate analgesia study: 4 institutions used this medication at this dose and 3/4 reported excellent results. 1 did not respond with regard to perceived efficacy. One institution used 2.17 mg/kg IM SID and reported good efficacy.
Phenylbutazone	1.5 mg/kg PO BID [2]	Pygmy hippos	n = 1, 25 yr old male with a benign osteoma removed and treated with postoperative antibiotics and phenylbutazone.
Phenylbutazone	2–6.8 mg/kg PO every other day or BID [3]	Hippos	Megavertebrate analgesia study: 12 institutions used this medication at this dose with 2 reporting excellent, 8 good, 1 fair, and 1 poor. One animal had ulcerative gastritis identified postmortem. One animal had positive fecal occult blood while receiving medication.
Tramadol	3 mg/kg PO SID [3]	Hippos	Megavertebrate analgesia study: 1 institution used this medication at this dose with a report of excellent perceived efficacy.
Anesthesia and Sedation			Fasting of at least 12 but ideally 24–48 hrs with water withheld for 12–24 hrs prior to anesthesia is preferred to reduce gut volume and pressure on diaphragm [4]. Injections should be given IM in cervical region caudal to the ear. Use long 6–9 cm darts. If not given IM, may result in prolonged induction. Minimize immobilization times (<30 min best). Hippos are very sensitive to opioids and if not dosed correctly can result in respiratory arrest [5].
Acepromazine	0.2 mg/kg PO [4]	Hippos	Mild sedation.
Azaperone	400–800 mg/kg IM [4]	Hippos	Sedation only.

Drug name	Drug dose	Species	Comments
Butorphanol + azaperone + medetomidine	B: 0.12 mg/kg + A: 0.05–0.1 mg/kg + M: 0.05 mg/kg IM; antagonize with naltrexone 0.24 mg/kg + atipamezole 0.1 mg/kg IM [4–6]	Hippos	n = 13 hippo, 3 captive, 10 wild, resulted in 8 min induction times and appeared safer than other protocols. Initial dart was 2.2 × 60 mm needle, antagonist given by hand injection with 3.5″ 18ga spinal needle in the neck or tongue. Transient apnea self-limited breath holding for 4–7 min, metabolic acidosis.
	B: 0.04 mg/kg + A: 0.05–0.1 mg/kg + M: 0.06–0.08 mg/kg IM; antagonize with atipamezole at 3–5 times mg dosage of medetomidine [7].	Hippos	Supplement with ketamine 1 mg/kg as needed.
	M: 0.04–0.05 mg/kg + A: 0.05 mg/kg (max 125 mg) + B: 0.05–0.1 mg/kg IM; antagonize with naltrexone 0.12 mg/kg + atipamezole 0.36 mg/kg IM. In captive hippo if the animal is not standing in 45–60 min give additional doses of both by dart [7].		n = 20 wild and 5 captive common hippopotamus. An additional dose of 1–2 mg/kg may provide additional analgesia and safety. Procedures were successful for up to 3 hrs.
Butorphanol + Detomidine	B: 0.06–0.2 mg/kg + D: 0.02–0.06 mg/kg IM; antagonize with naltrexone at a 20:1 ratio of butorphanol in mg, or 0.4–0.6 mg/kg IM. Atipamezole at five times the mg dose of detomidine or medetomidine IM [4, 7].	Hippos	Initial effects may be observed in 10–20 min with recumbency in 20–30 min, but full effect may take longer and stimulation may cause arousal. Supplemental doses can be administered in a ratio of 1:3 detomidine:butorphanol based on effect. Invasive, painful, or prolonged procedures should be supplemented with ketamine 0.1–1 mg/kg IM, propofol (0.5 mg/kg or 50–100 μg/kg/min as CRI), low dose etorphine, or supplemental detomidine/medetomidine or butorphanol.
Butorphanol + detomidine	B: 0.1–0.2 mg/kg + detomidine or medetomidine 0.04–0.06 mg/kg IM [4, 7].	Pygmy hippos	Anesthesia can be extended with supplemental doses of ketamine or gas anesthesia. For prolonged, painful or invasive procedures it is recommended to intubate and maintain on isoflurane.
Butorphanol + medetomidine	B: 0.2 mg/kg + M: 0.035 mg/kg; antagonize with atipamezole at 5 × the mg dose of medetomidine and naltrexone at 5–16 × the dosage of opioid [4, 7].	Pygmy hippos	Recovery times were reported as mild sedation at 2–17 min post antagonist administration.

(*Continued*)

Drug name	Drug dose	Species	Comments
Carfentanil + xylazine	C: 0.0075 mg/kg (total dose 1.5 mg) + X: 0.05 mg/kg (total dose 10 mg) IM [4].	Pygmy hippos	Antagonize with naltrexone 100 × carfentanil dose and yohimbine 0.1–0.3 mg/kg IM.
Diazepam	0.2 mg/kg PO [4]	Hippos	Mild sedation.
	0.5 mg/kg PO prior to induction [5, 7]	Hippos	Sensitive to diazepam and good sedation can be obtained with 10 mg increments. For oral premedication prior to immobilization with alpha-2 agonist + butorphanol. No overt drug response noted but procedure did go well.
Diazepam + detomidine	Dia: 0.5 mg/kg + Det: 0.044 mg/kg PO; antagonize with yohimbine 0.11 mg/kg IM [4].	Pygmy hippos	As premedication.
Detomidine + butorphanol + ketamine	D: 0.07–0.08 mg/kg + B: 0.15–0.2 mg/kg + K: 0.8–2 mg/kg IM; antagonize with atipamezole at 5 × the mg dose of detomidine and naltrexone at 5–16 × the dosage of opioid [7].	Pygmy hippos	Recovery times were reported as mild sedation at 2–17 min post antagonist administration.
Etorphine	0.001–0.005 mg/kg IM (total 2–6 mg) [4]	Hippos	Fatal complications with high doses of etorphine in the 7–12 mg total range.
Etorphine + azaperone + succinylcholine	E: 2 mg + A: 200 mg + S: 250 mg IM; antagonize with naltrexone 200 mg [5].	Hippos	
Etorphine + xylazine	E: 0.001–0.005 (2–6 mg total) + X: 0.067–0.083 (100–150 mg total) IM [4].	Hippos	Fatal complications with high doses of etorphine in the 7–12 mg total range. Antagonize with naltrexone at 100 × etorphine dose and yohimbine at 0.1–0.3 mg/kg IM.
	E: 2.5 mg + X: 100–150 mg IM. Antagonize with diprenorphine 5 mg + 0.1–0.3 mg/kg yohimbine [4, 5].	Pygmy hippos	Supplement as needed with 1.5 mg etorphine.
	E: 0.011–0.017 mg/kg + X: 0.046–0.2 mg/kg IM. Total doses max of 2–3 mg and 10 mg respectively; antagonize with diprenorphine 2–3 × etorphine dose [4].	Pygmy hippos	
	E: 0.7 ml + X: 8 mg; antagonize with naloxone 85 mg [5].	Hippos	

Drug name	Drug dose	Species	Comments
Etorphine + xylazine	E: 0.25 ml; antagonize with 2 mg diprenorphine per mg etorphine given [5].	Pygmy hippos	
Ketamine + medetomidine	K: 1 mg/kg + M: 0.06–0.08 mg/kg IM; antagonize with atipamezole 0.3 mg/kg half IV and half IM [4, 7–9].	Hippos	n = 10 adult male hippo undergoing castration. Complete immobilization with surgical anesthesia plane in 16–39 min post injection. Anesthesia was maintained for between 57 and 188 min with 1–5 additional injections of 0.1–0.4 mg/kg ketamine. 5 animals exhibited transitory apnea for 1–9 min but other parameters did not change so this was characterized as a "self-limiting dive response". Post reversal animals were standing within 5–7 minutes.
	K: 1.2 mg/kg + M: 0.08 mg/kg [4, 10]	Pygmy hippos	Maintain with isoflurane.
Midazolam	0.1 mg/kg IM [4, 7]	Pygmy hippos	Has shown promising results for minor sedation or adjunct for induction. Could also try oral detomidine or diazepam.
Telazol	2.2–3.5 mg/kg IM [7]	Pygmy hippos	
Telazol + ketamine	T: 3 mg/kg + K: 1 mg/kg [7]	Hippos	Profound sedation.
Other			
Depo-Provera (Medroxyprogesterone acetate)	800 mg IM every 6 weeks [7, 11, 12]	Hippos	n = 3 cases of captive female hippopotamus of 2.5–3.5 yrs of age, who at the onset of puberty were given Depo-Provera and this resulted in a shortened luteal phase measured by fecal samples and prevented normal cyclicity for 100 days. Note that this dose is hampered by the lack of body weight measures for individual animals.
MGA grain (medroxyprogesterone acetate)	2–3 mg/animal/day [7, 11]	Hippo females	Contraception.
Mitomycin and cisplatin intralesional chemotherapy	M: 0.4 mg/cm3 of tumor and C: 1 mg/cm3 of tumor [13].	Pygmy hippos	n = 1 case of oral anaplastic sarcoma with intralesional injection of two chemotherapeutic agents post debulking surgically.
Pentoxifylline	4 mg/kg PO BID [1]	Hippos	n = 1, 59 yr old female captive hippopotamus with bacterial dermatitis that over a 12-week period finally cleared after being treated with amoxicillin, sulfamethoxazole and trimethoprim, and pentoxifylline orally.
Salt bath	2–3 g/l of water [14]	Hippos	n = 2 treatment of ulcerative skin lesions in 2 captive females, commercial cattle food-grade salt used and after 4 months complete healing of all skin lesions.

Species	Weight [5, 7]
Nile hippopotamus *(Hippopotamus amphibius)*	1000–2000 kg
Pygmy hippopotamus *(Choeropsis liberiensis)*	160–270 kg

References

1 Spriggs, M. and Reeder, C. (2012). Treatment of vasculitis and dermatitis in a 59-yr-old Nile hippopotamus (*Hippopotamus amphibius*). *Journal of Zoo and Wildlife Medicine* 43 (3): 652–656.
2 Weston, H.S., Fagella, A.M., Burt, L. et al. (1996). Immobilization of a Pygmy Hippopotamus (*Choeropsis liberiensis*) for the removal of an oral mass. *Annual Proceedings of the American Association of Zoo Veterinarians.*
3 Kottwitz, J., Boothe, M., Harmon, R. et al. (2016). Results of the megavertebrate analgesia survey: elephants and rhino. *Journal of Zoo and Wildlife Medicine* 47 (1): 301–310.
4 Walzer, C. and Stalder, G. (2015). Hippopotamidae (*Hippopotamus*). In: *Fowler's Zoo and Wild Animal Medicine*, vol. 8 (ed. R.E. Miller and M. Fowler), 584–591. St. Louis, MO: Elsevier Saunders.
5 Kreeger, T.J., Arnemo, J.M., and Raath, J.P. (2002). *Handbook of Wildlife Chemical Immobilization.* Fort Collins, Colorado: Wildlife Pharmaceuticals Inc.
6 Fleming, G.J., Citino, S.B., Hofmeyer, M. et al. (2010). Reversible chemical restraint of Nile Hippopotamus (*Hippopotamus amphibius spp.*) *Annual Proceedings of the American Association of Zoo Veterinarians.*
7 Miller, M., Fleming, G.J., Citino, S.B. et al. (2014). Hippopotamidae. In: *Zoo Animal and Wild Immobilization and Anesthesia* (ed. G. West, D. Heard and N. Caulkett), 787–796. Ames, IA: Wiley Blackwell.
8 Fleming, G.J. and Walzer, C. (2012). Compare and contrast two successful anesthetic protocols in the Nile Hippopotamus (*Hippopotamus amphibius spp.*) *Annual Proceedings of the American Association of Zoo Veterinarians.*
9 Stalder, G.L., Petit, T., Horowitz, I. et al. (2012). Use of a Medetomidine-ketamine combination for anesthesia in captive common hippopotami (*Hippopotamus amphibius*). *Journal of the American Veterinary Medical Association* 241 (1): 110–116.
10 Bouts, T., Hermes, R., Gasthuys, F. et al. (2012). Medetomidine-ketamine-isoflurane anesthesia in pygmy hippopotami (*Choeropsis liberiensis*) – a case series. *Veterinary Anesthesia and Analgesia* 39: 111–118.
11 AZA Reproduction Management Center (2018). Contraception recommendations for artiodactyls. http://stlzoo.org/animals/scienceresearch/reproductivemanagementcenter/contraceptionrecommendatio/contraception-methods/artiodactyls (accessed 26 November 2018).
12 Graham, L.H., Webster, T., Richards, M. et al. (2002). Ovarian function in the Nile hippopotamus and the effects of Depo-Provera administration. *Reproduction* 60: 65–70.
13 Franklinos, L.H., Masters, N., Feltrer, Y. et al. (2017). The management of an oral anaplastic sarcoma in a pygmy hippopotamus (*Choeropsis liberiensis*) using intralesional chemotherapy. *Journal of Zoo and Wildlife Medicine* 48 (1): 260–264.
14 Helmick, K.E. (2017). Salt bath as a treatment for idiopathic dermatitis in a captive Nile hippopotamus (*Hippopotamus amphibius*). *Journal of Zoo and Wildlife Medicine* 48 (3): 915–917.

24

Camelids: Alpacas, Camels, Guanacos, and Llamas

Drug name	Drug dose	Species	Comments
Antimicrobials and Antifungals			
Amikacin	4.4–6.6 mg/kg SC, IV SID for MAX 5d [1]	Camelids	Due to renal toxicity potential only give for 5 days maximum. gentamicin considered more toxic than Amikacin. Give with IV fluids.
Ampicillin sodium (for IV use)	11 mg/kg IV TID to QID [1]	Camelids	For treatment of listeriosis. Considered safe in many species, no studies performed in camelids.
Amoxicillin-clavulanate (Clavamox)	20 mg/kg IV q6 hrs [2]	Alpacas	n = 1 alpaca cria with surgical removal of a brain abscess, treated peri- and postoperatively.
Ampicillin (Polyflex)	22 mg/kg SC BID [1]	Camelids	Considered reasonably safe in many species.
Ceftazidime	10 mg/kg IM recommended BID [3]	Dromedary camels	n = 8 healthy adult camels, given IV and IM dosing-IM was cleared slower. Distribution from plasma to milk was rapid and extensive and thus may be a useful treatment for camels with mastitis.
Ceftiofur	2–2.2 mg/kg IV [4]	Llamas, Alpacas	Ceftiofur was given in 70 cases/123 of which 58 were IV, and 12 were given SC. 53% SID, 41% BID and 6% EOD. for a range of 2–20 days. Tooth root abscesses were reviewed in 123 cases presented to a university. The most commonly isolated bacterial organisms were Actinomyces spp (n = 49 isolates), unidentified anaerobes (26), Actinobacillus spp (6), and Escherichia coli (2). All bacteria were susceptible to Ceftiofur.
Ceftiofur (Naxcel or Excenel)	4.4 mg/kg SC or IV, SID to BID [1]	Camelids	Commonly used to treat neonatal sepsis, upper respiratory infection, retained placenta, and uterine infections. Naxcel can be used IV or SC, but IV must be given BID. Excenel given SC only.

(Continued)

Drug name	Drug dose	Species	Comments
Ceftiofur	2 mg/kg SQ SID [2]	Alpacas	n = 1 alpaca cria with surgical removal of a brain abscess, treated perioperatively.
Ceftiofur crystalline Free Acid (Excede)	6.6 mg/kg SC [1, 5, 6]	Alpacas, Dromedary camels	n = 6 adult alpacas pharmacokinetic study, 1 Dromedary camel treated for leptospirosis – successful. Has been suggested to repeat on day 4. Injection site reaction noted occasionally.
Ceftiofur hydrochloride	2.5 mg/kg IM BID [7]	Dromedary camels	12 wk old female with Streptococcus pleuropneumonia and peritonitis. Treated with IV antibiotics and thoracocentesis, then IM antibiotics for home care.
Ceftiofur sodium (Excenel)	1.05 mg/kg IV SID × 4.5 wks [8]	Bactrian camels	n = 1 animal with surgical lengthening of the mandible, given postoperative antibiotics and pain control.
	5 mg/kg IV q6 hrs [7]	Dromedary camels	n = 1, 12 wk old female with Streptococcus pleuropneumonia and peritonitis. Treated with IV antibiotics and thoracocentesis.
Chlortetracycline	Added to feed 22 mg/kg feed [9]	Camelids	To treat herd-level enterotoxemias.
Enrofloxacin (Baytril 100 mg/ml)	5 mg/kg SC, IV SID to BID (IV route) [1]	Camelids	To treat neonatal sepsis, upper respiratory infection, pneumonia and uterine infections. Not to be used as "first choice". A Guanaco with 26-day treatment became blind. Unknown if cartilage damage occurs in crias.
Florfenicol	20 mg/kg SC EOD for 1 wk [4]	Llamas, Alpacas	n = 6 cases of a retrospective review of 123 cases of tooth root abscesses in Llamas and Alpacas presenting to a university.
Florfenicol (Nuflor)	19.8 mg/kg IM or SC SID [1]	Camelids	Commonly used to treat upper respiratory infection, pneumonia, and tooth rot. Based on studies at Oregon State University in alpacas, best given SID IM. Due to liver metabolism do not give to crias/juveniles less than 3 months old. Contraindicated to use with other antibiotics. Can cause anorexia in some animals.
Florfenicol-flunixin meglumine	80 mg/kg IM [2]	Alpacas	n = 1 alpaca cria treated for suspected bacterial infection.
Gentamycin	4.4–6.6 mg/kg SC, IV SID [1]	Llamas, Alpacas	Amikacin recommended over gentamycin; due to renal toxicity potential only give for 5 days maximum. Gentamicin considered more toxic than Amikacin. Give with IV fluids.

Drug name	Drug dose	Species	Comments
Iodine 2%	Topical application daily for 2 weeks [9]	Camelids	To treat dermatophytosis or ringworm.
Isoniazid	5–10 mg/kg PO SID: SEE COMMENT [9]		For mycobacterial infections, treatment is not allowed in the US unless special permission is granted for valuable zoo artidactylids.
	10 mg/kg PO SID 15–30d [4]	Llamas, Alpacas	n = 13
	11 mg/kg PO SID × 30d [1]	Camelids	For use in combination with antibiotics for chronic infections. Most commonly used to treat tooth root abscesses or lumpy jaw. Helps antibiotics penetrate abscess capsule. Needs to be used long term.
Metronidazole	15 mg/kg IV q8 hrs [2]	Alpacas	n = 1 alpaca cria with surgical removal of a brain abscess, treated peri- and postoperatively.
Oxytetracycline (Terramycin LA)	8 g IM once (15.2 mg/kg) [10]	Dromedary camels	n = 1 8 yr old 525 kg male with urethral obstruction relieved with urethrostomy and given antibiotics post.
Oxytetracycline (Biomycin 200 LA 200, Duramycin 300 or Noromycn 300)	19.8 mg/kg SC [1]	Camelids	Used for mycoplasma haemolamae in camelids. Very irritating IM, give SC carefully. Biomcyin 200 or LA 200 is less irritating and preferred. Give every 3 days for 5 treatments. If still anemic further treatments may be needed. If used IV give SID.
Penicillin Procaine	22 000 U/kg SC BID [7]	Dromedary camels	n = 1, 12 wk old female with Streptococcus pleuropneumonia and peritonitis. Treated with IV antibiotics and thoracocentesis.
Tulathromycin (Draxxin)	2.4 mg/kg SC, can be repeated in 10d if no improvement [1]	Llamas, Alpacas	Big gun, should only be used after other treatment tried.
Procaine penicillin G	22 222 U/kg IM SID × 6d [11]	Dromedary camels	n = 1 calf undergoing surgery for polydactyly and receiving peri- and postoperative antibiotics.
Procaine penicillin G (300 000 IU/ml)	22 046 IU/kg SC BID or 44 092 IU/kg SC SID [1]	Camelids	Do not use benzathine form. Occasionally anaphylactic shock can occur and should be treated with Epinephrine 0.45 ml/kg IM immediately and do not use Penicillins again in that animal. Commonly used for skin, foot pad, umbilical, follow up treatment for listeriosis, and best choice for clostridial infection. Not good for respiratory infections.

(*Continued*)

Drug name	Drug dose	Species	Comments
Procaine penicillin	200 000–40 000 U/kg [4]	Llamas, Alpacas	n = 47 cases of a retrospective review of 123 cases of tooth root abscesses in Llamas and Alpacas presenting to a university. 79% gave SID and 21% BID dosing. For a range of 3–30 days.
Sulfadimethoxine	15–20 mg/kg IV and PO [12]	Dromedary camels	n = 6 pregnant females; was not sufficient at achieving therapeutic levels.
Analgesia			
Buprenorphine sustained release	B: 0.12 mg/kg SC [13, 14]	Alpacas	n = 6 animals in a study, only 2/6 had detectable plasma concentrations at 8 hrs post injection.
Butorphanol	B: 0.5 mg/kg IM BID × 3d [8]	Bactrian camels	n = 1 animal with surgical lengthening of the mandible, given postoperative antibiotics and pain control.
Etogesic (Etodolac)	10 mg/kg PO SID [4]	Llamas	n = 6 cases of a retrospective review of 123 cases of tooth root abscesses in Llamas and Alpacas presenting to a university.
	9.9 mg/kg PO SID × 7d then decrease to EOD [1]	Camelids	Primarily for pain of bone origin. No formal research in camelids. Due to potential concern for ulcers in compartment 3, use SID for 7 days then EOD for 2–3 weeks, then twice weekly if long-term medication is needed.
Fentanyl patch	300 μg/h (4 of the 75 μg/hr patches) [14, 15]	Llamas	n = 9 animals, 3 receiving 300 μg/hr – resulted in 12–72 hrs of 0.22–0.38 ng/ml, no sedation, Placed on medial antebrachium with stapled corners and adhesive bandage placed.
Fentanyl	2 μg/kg IV or 2 μg/kg/hr [14, 15]	Alpacas	n = 6 animals, received fentanyl IV once or patch in place for 72 hrs. No significant changes in heart rate or respiratory rate, peak plasma concentrations of 1.2 ng/ml at 24 hrs.
Flunixin meglumine	F: 1.1 mg/kg IV SID [9]	Llamas	Effective for colicky pain.
Flunixin meglumine	0.5–1.1 mg/kg IV, IM, SC SID to BID [1]	Camelids	May lead to ulcers in third compartment if used long term. Use with caution in dehydrated animals to prevent renal damage. Not effective orally. Use SID, unless painful again at 12 hrs, then BID.
	F: 1 mg/kg IV once, then 0.5 mg/kg IV BID [7]	Dromedary camels	12 wk old female with Streptococcus pleuropneumonia and peritonitis.

Drug name	Drug dose	Species	Comments
	F: 1 mg/kg IV q8 hrs × 5d [2]	Alpacas	n = 1 alpaca cria with surgical removal of a brain abscess, treated peri- and postoperatively.
	F: 1.1–2.2 mg/kg IV for 1–6d [4]	Llamas, Alpacas	n = 73 cases of a retrospective review of 123 cases of tooth root abscesses in Llamas and Alpacas presenting to a university. 1/3 of cases were given SID and the remaining 2/3 BID.
Lidocaine HCl (without epinephrine) (2%)	L: 1–5 ml used epidurally [9]	Llamas	Onset within 5 min, and persisted as long as 5 hrs. Higher doses may result in paralysis of hind limbs.
Lidocaine (2%)	2 ml topical on arytenoid cartilage [9]	Camelids	Prior to intubation.
Lidocaine (2%)	12–15 ml as per a caudal epidural injection [16]	Camels	Provided anesthesia of the perineum, scrotum or udder for 1–2 hrs without influencing motor control.
Lidocaine ± xylazine	L: 0.22 mg/kg ± X: 0.17 mg/kg Caudal epidural [16]	Llamas, Alpacas	Lidocaine alone onset in 3–4 min, for duration of 1 hour. Lidocaine + xylazine onset in 3–4 min, duration of 6 hrs, xylazine alone onset in 20 min and duration 3 hrs. In Alpacas both doses combined were best but many animals had incomplete block of spermatic cord. Mild sedation occurred with the xylazine group.
Meloxicam	1 mg/kg PO q3d [1, 17]	Llamas	
Morphine	M: 0.25 mg/kg IV q4 hrs [18]	Llamas	n = 6 healthy llamas. Large apparent volume of distribution and high systemic clearance.
Phenylbutazone	P: 2–4 mg/kg PO or IV SID [9]	Camelids	Perivascular injection can cause phlebitis and adjacent skin sloughing, Can be ulcergenic in horses.
	P: 5 mg/kg PO SID for 1–5d [4]	Llamas, Alpacas	n = 12 cases of a retrospective review of 123 cases of tooth root abscesses in Llamas and Alpacas presenting to a university.
	2 mg/kg BID PO × 3d [19]	Juvenile camels	n = 1, post casting of displaced comminuted radial fracture.
Anesthesia and Sedation			
Acepromazine	A: 0.05–0.1 mg/kg IM [9, 16, 20]	Camelids, Camels	Onset in 5–15 min, duration 1–4 hrs.
Atipamezole	0.3–0.5 mg/kg [9]	Camelids	Reversal for alpha-2 agonists.
Atracurium	Atr: Initial bolus of 0.15 mg/kg IV, then IV drip set of 0.4 mg/kg/hr [9, 16]	Camelids	Onset 1 min, duration 7 min, for obtaining muscular relaxation in an animal under anesthesia. Applications in orthopedic and ocular surgeries.

(*Continued*)

Drug name	Drug dose	Species	Comments
Butorphanol tartrate	B: 0.05–0.1 mg/kg IM [20]	Camelids	Antagonize with naloxone 0.1–0.25 mg/kg IV and 0.04–0.07 mg/kg SC.
Butorphanol	B: 0.05–0.1 mg/kg IV [16]	Neonatal domesticated camelids	Sedation. Onset 30–60 sec, duration 10–20 min.
	0.02–0.1 mg/kg IV, IM, SC [9]	Camelids	
Butorphanol + Lidocaine	B: 0.1 mg/kg IM, and L: 2–5 ml 2% intratesticular block/testicle [16]	Llamas	n = 100 animals for standing sedation and castration.
Chlorpromazine	2.2 mg/kg q6 hr [9]	Llamas	n = 1 sedation.
Detomidine	Det: 0.03–0.06 mg/kg for immobilization [9]	Camels	Antagonize with atipamezole.
Detomidine + butorphanol	D: 0.04–0.06 mg/kg and B: 0.03–0.06 mg/kg [21]	Bactrian camels	n = 6 animals, standing sedation.
Diazepam	D: 0.05–0.2 mg/kg IV [16]	Neonatal domesticated camelids	Sedation. Onset 30–60 sec, duration 10–20 min.
	D: 0.05–0.3 mg/kg IM [20]	Camelids	Antagonize with flumazenil 1–2 mg/kg IM.
	0.1–0.5 mg/kg IV, IM [9]	Camelids	Onset within 1–2 min IV, 15–30 min IM; clinical effects gone in 60–90 min; antagonize with flumazenil.
	0.2–0.4 mg/kg IV [9]	Camelids	Sedation prior to induction.
Diazepam + propofol	D: 0.05–0.1 mg/kg + P: 1–2 mg/kg IV [16]	Neonatal domesticated camelids	Onset 30–45 sec after administration, duration 5–15 min, recovery in 20–30 min.
Diprenorphine HCl	Double the dose in mg of etorphine [9]	Camels	Reversal for narcotics.
Etorphine	0.007 mg/kg [22]	Guanacos	
Etorphine + acepromazine	E: 3 mg + A: 0.1 mg/kg [22]	Camelids	
Etorphine + butorphanol + detomidine	E: 4.4 mg + B: 10 mg + D: 15 mg IM [16, 23]	Wild adult camels and Bactrian camels	Recommended over the etorphine, butorphanol, detomidine, Telazol combination; antagonize with naltrexone 200 mg and atipamezole 25 mg.
Etorphine + butorphanol + detomidine + Telazol	E: 4.4 mg + B: 10 mg + D: 13 mg + T: 160 mg [16]	Camels	n = 3 animals 1.2, due to cold ambient temperature propylene glycol was added to combination. An additional 10 animals were anesthetized with this combination and 1 of 10 died of unknown cause, but was an older animal. Antagonize with naltrexone 200 mg IV and atipamezole 25 mg IV. See E + B + D protocol above.

Drug name	Drug dose	Species	Comments
Etorphine + xylazine	E: 4.4 mg + X: 600 mg IM; antagonize with 6.6 mg diprenorphine [10]	Dromedary Camel	n = 1, 8 yr old, 525 kg male, with urethral obstruction sedated for urethrostomy.
Flumazenil	F: 10 × dose of diazepam in mg [9]	Camelids	Reversal for benzodiazepines.
Isoflurane	1–3% by mask to recumbency [16]	Neonatal domesticated camelids	Onset variable but within 5 min, recovery 15–30 min after discontinuation.
Isoflurane	Maintenance 1–2% inhaled [16] 4.5% for induction then 1–1.5% for maintenance [9]	Domesticated Camelids	Recovery 20–60 min after discontinuing.
Ketamine + detomidine	K: 2–4 mg/kg + Det: 0.02–0.04 mg/kg IM [9]	New World camelids	Antagonize with atipamezole.
Ketamine + diazepam	K: 1–2 mg/kg + D: 0.05–0.1 mg/kg IV [16]	Neonatal domesticated camelids	Onset 30–45 sec after administration, duration 10–20 min, recovery in 30 min.
	K: 3–5 mg/kg + D: 0.1–0.2 mg/kg IV; K: 5–8 mg/kg + D: 0.2–0.3 mg/kg IM [9]	New World camelids	
	K: 4 mg/kg + D: 0.1 mg/kg IV (After giving xylazine 0.3 mg/kg and butorphanol 0.1 mg/kg IM 15 min prior) [24]	Alpacas	Study of six alpaca with 3 IV anesthesia protocols. Propofol 4 mg/kg IV or ketamine 2 mg/kg + 2 mg/kg propofol IV both were also successful, all these protocols had similar duration of effect and hypoxemia.
	K: 5–6 mg/kg + D: 0.2–0.3 mg/kg IM [20]	Camelids	Antagonize with flumazenil.
	K: 5–8 mg/kg + D: 0.2–0.3 mg/kg IM [9]	Camelids	Antagonize with flumazenil.
Ketamine + medetomidine	K: 0.6 mg/kg + M: 0.05 mg/kg IV or K: 1 mg/kg + M: 0.05 mg/kg IM [25]	Dromedary camels	Antagonize with atipamezole 0.15 mg/kg IV.
	K: 2.5 mg/kg + M: 0.22 mg/kg [23]	Dromedary camels	Antagonize with atipamezole 0.66 mg/kg.
	K: 1 mg/kg + M: 0.05 mg/kg [23]	Alpacas, calm Llamas, Vicunas	Supplement with K: 1 mg/kg as needed. Antagonize with atipamezole 0.25 mg/kg.
	K: 2 mg/kg + M: 0.07 mg/kg [23]	Llamas	Supplement with K: 1 mg/kg as needed. Antagonize with atipamezole 0.35 mg/kg.
	K: 2–4 mg/kg + M: 0.06–0.08 mg/kg IM [9]	New World camelids	Antagonize with atipamezole 0.1–0.15 mg/kg or 1–5 × dose of medetomidine IV.

(*Continued*)

Drug name	Drug dose	Species	Comments
	K: 2 mg/kg + M: 0.1 mg/kg [23]	Guanacos	Supplement with K: 1 mg/kg as needed. Antagonize with atipamezole 0.5 mg/kg 1/2 IV and 1/2 IM.
	K: 2–4 mg/kg + M: 0.06–0.08 mg/kg IM [9, 20]	All camelids	Antagonize with atipamezole 4–5 × dose of medetomidine in mg, with 0.1–0.15 mg/kg IV and rest SC.
	K: 1.5–4 mg/kg + M: 0.12–0.3 mg/kg IM [26]	Dromedary camels	n = 27 animals, free-ranging, with 11 min to recumbency, and 5 min to recovery. Antagonize with atipamezole 0.1–0.36 mg/kg.
	K: 1–2 mg/kg + M: 0.06–0.1 mg/kg [22]	Camelids	
Ketamine + medetomidine + butorphanol	K: 1.5–2.9 mg/kg + M: 0.06–0.23 mg/kg + B: 0.02–0.11 mg/kg [26]	Dromedary camels	n = 29 animals, free-range, with 8.5 min to recumbency and 6 min to recovery. Antagonize with atipamezole 0.1–0.36 mg/kg + naltrexone 0.13–0.29 mg//kg.
Ketamine + medetomidine + butorphanol	K: 2.4–3 mg/kg + M: 0.08–0.1 mg/kg + B: 0.3 mg/kg [27]	Guanacos	n = 7 adult male animals, Smooth and rapid induction 1.5–4.5 min to initial effect, recumbency in 2–8 min, excellent muscle relaxation, 6/7 hypoxemic without oxygen supplementation, duration of 20–27 min, and standing within 8–18 min. Antagonize with atipamezole 0.4–0.5 mg/kg and naltrexone 2.5–3 mg/kg.
Ketamine + medetomidine + butorphanol	K: 3 mg/kg + M: 0.1 mg/kg + B: 0.3 mg/kg [23]	Guanacos	Antagonize with atipamezole 0.5 mg/kg and naltrexone 3 mg/kg.
Ketamine + xylazine	K: 0.6–1 mg/kg + X: 0.4–0.7 mg/kg [25]	Dromedary camels	When ketamine was given after xylazine it induced recumbency in 7 animals at 2–30 min post xylazine and in 6 animals at 15–35 min post xylazine. Antagonism with tolazoline 1–4 mg/kg resulted in standing n = 10, but lower dose ended up returning to recumbency multiple times, while higher dose kept standing but had residual salivation, drooping lips and soft stool.
	K: 1–3 mg/kg + X: 0.25–1 mg/kg [9]	Camels	Antagonize with tolazoline.
	K: 2–3 mg/kg + X: 0.25–0.4 mg/kg IM; antagonize with tolazoline [20]	Camelids	
	K: 2–3 mg/kg + X: 0.1–0.2 mg/kg IM [16]	Domesticated camelids	Onset recumbency 5–10 min, duration 10–20 min, Recovery 45 min to 2 hr.

Drug name	Drug dose	Species	Comments
	K: 2 mg/kg + X: 2 mg/kg [23]	Bactrian and Dromedary camels	Supplement with K: 1 mg/kg as needed. Antagonize with yohimbine 0.125 mg/kg or 0.2 mg/kg atipamezole.
	K: 2.5 mg/kg + X: 0.15 mg/kg IM [28]	Dromedary camels	n = 10 Study evaluating xylazine or ketamine alone or together: the combination of both resulted in fewer cardiorespiratory effects, better muscle relaxation less central nervous system irritability, and shorter recovery times.
	K: 5 mg/kg + X: 0.4 mg/kg; IM antagonize with tolazoline 0.5–1.5 mg/kg [9]	New World camelids	
	K: 3–5 mg/kg + X: 0.25 mg/kg IV; antagonize with tolazoline 0.5–1.5 mg/kg [9]	New World camelids	
	K: 2.22 mg/kg + X: 0.11 mg/kg [11]	Dromedary camel calves	n = 1
	K: 2–5 mg/kg + X: 0.25–0.5 mg/kg [22]	Camelids	
	K: 1 mg/kg + X: 0.5 mg/kg; one additional dose of ketamine at the same dosage [19]	Juvenile camels	n = 1 anesthesia for casting of a displaced comminuted radial fracture.
Ketamine + xylazine + butorphanol	K: 2–3 mg/kg + X: 0.1 mg/kg + B: 0.05–0.1 mg/kg IM [9, 20]	All camelids	Antagonize with tolazoline and naltrexone.
Ketamine + xylazine + butorphanol	K: 2–4 mg/kg + X: 0.03–0.05 mg/kg + B: 0.3–0.5 mg/kg IM [16]	Domesticated camelids	Onset recumbency 5–10 min, duration 10–20 min, recovery 20–60 min.
Ketamine + xylazine + butorphanol	K: 3–4 mg/kg + X: 0.03–0.04 mg/kg + B: 0.3–0.4 mg/kg IM [16]	Llamas, Alpacas	n = 7 male Llamas and 7 male Alpacas. Llama were recumbent in 4.3 min and Alpacas in 6.7 min. Induction was good, some ataxia before, Llamas were more deeply anesthetized and stood in 63 min, whereas Alpacas stood in 22 min.
	K: 4 mg/kg + X: 0.04 mg/kg + B: 0.4 mg/kg [23]	Alpacas, Llamas	Antagonize with yohimbine 0.125 mg/kg.
Ketamine + xylazine + diazepam	Give X: 0.1–0.2 mg/kg IM, then K: 1–2 mg/kg IV with D: 0.1–0.25 mg IV [16]	Domesticated camelids	Onset recumbency 45 sec after diazepam and ketamine, duration 10–20 min, recovery 45 min to 2 hr.

(*Continued*)

Drug name	Drug dose	Species	Comments
Ketamine + xylazine + guaifenesin	Give X: 0.1–0.2 mg/kg IM, then K: 1–2 mg/kg IV with G: 50–100 mg/kg IV [16]	Domesticated camelids	Onset recumbency 45 sec after guaifenesin and ketamine, duration 10–20 min, recovery 45 min to 2 hr.
Ketamine + xylazine + midazolam	K: 8 mg/kg + X: 1.2 mg/kg + M: 0.35 mg/kg [23]	Guanacos, Vicunas	Antagonize with atipamezole 0.1 mg/kg.
Ketamine + xylazine + midazolam + atropine	K: 7.8 mg/kg + X: 1.2 mg/kg ± Mid: 0.35 mg/kg + A: 0.07 mg/kg [16]	Vicunas	Wild animals, to collect semen via electroejaculation.
Ketamine + propofol	K: 2 mg/kg + P: 2 mg/kg IV (After giving xylazine 0.3 mg/kg and butorphanol 0.1 mg/kg IM 15 min prior) [24]	Alpacas	Study of six Alpacas with 3 IV anesthesia protocols. Ketamine 4 mg/kg + diazepam 0.1 mg/kg or 4 mg/kg propofol IV both were also successful, all three protocols had similar duration of effect and hypoxemia.
Medetomidine	M: 0.03 mg/kg IM [29]	Llamas	n = 15 healthy Llamas, medetomidine induced deep sedation with a short period of analgesia. Rapidly reversed and soon able to stand. Antagonize with atipamezole 0.125 mg/kg IV.
	M: 0.01 mg/kg sedation, 0.02–0.03 mg/kg [9]	Camels	Immobilization; antagonize with atipamezole.
Midazolam	M: 0.5 mg/kg IM or IV [30]	Alpacas	Moderate sedation at 15 min post IM injection, significantly greater and faster sedation after IV administration.
	0.1–0.2 IV [9]	Camelids	Sedation for induction and intubation.
Nalmefene	10 × dose of etorphine [9]	Camels	Reversal for narcotics.
Nalorphine HCl	0.006 mg/kg [9]	Camels	Reversal for narcotics.
Naltrexone HCl	100 × dose of carfentanil [9]	Camels	Reversal for narcotics.
Propionylpromazine	P: 0.03–0.2 mg/kg IM [20]	Camelids	
Propofol	P: 4 mg/kg IV (After giving xylazine 0.3 mg/kg and butorphanol 0.1 mg/kg IM 15 min prior) [24]	Alpacas	Study of six Alpacas with 3 IV anesthesia protocols. Ketamine 4 mg/kg + diazepam 0.1 mg/kg or ketamine 2 mg/kg + 2 mg/kg propofol IV both were also successful, all three protocols had similar duration of effect and hypoxemia.
Propofol	0.4 mg/kg/hr (After 2 mg/kg induction dose) [16]	Llamas	Dyspnea in 3 Llamas.
Propofol	1 mg/kg IV [9]	Camelids	After sedation with benzodiazepine for intubation/induction.

Drug name	Drug dose	Species	Comments
Sevoflurane	2–4% by mask to recumbency [16]	Neonatal domesticated camelids	Variable but induction within 5 min, recovery 15–30 min after discontinuation.
	Maintenance 2–3% inhaled [16]	Domesticated camelids	Recovery 20–60 min after discontinuing.
Telazol	T: 2–3 mg/kg [20]	Camelids	Antagonize with flumazenil.
	T: 4 mg/kg [23]	Alpacas, Llamas, Vicunas	
	T: 6 mg/kg [23]	Guanacos	
	T: 4–6 mg/kg [9]	New World camelids	Recumbency at 7 min, lasts 15 min.
	2.2–15 mg/kg [22]	Camelids	
Telazol + xylazine	T: 2 mg/kg + X: 0.2–0.4 mg/kg IM [31]	Llamas	n = 8, intact male Llamas, Given various doses of xylazine with Telazol to evaluate antinociception duration. 0.2 and 0.4 mg/kg resulted in increased duration.
Tolazoline HCl	0.5–5.0 mg/kg [9]	Camelids	Reversal for alpha-2 agonists.
Xylazine	X: 0.1–0.4 mg/kg IM [20]	Camelids	Antagonize with yohimbine 0.125–0.25 mg/kg, or tolazoline 0.5–5 mg/kg.
	X: 1.5 mg/kg [23]	Bactrian camels	
	X: 0.25–0.3 mg/kg IM sedation; 1–2 mg/kg Immobilization [9]	New world camelids	Antagonize with yohimbine 0.125–0.25 mg/kg or tolazoline 0.5–1.5 mg/kg.
	X: 0.25–0.5 mg/kg IM sedation; 1–2 mg/kg immobilization [9]	Old world camelids	Antagonize with yohimbine 0.125–0.25 mg/kg or tolazoline 0.5–1.5 mg/kg.
	X: 0.25 mg/kg IM; 0.1–0.2 mg/kg IV [16]	Domesticated camelids	Onset in 15 minutes IM and 5 minutes IV, duration 1–4 hrs.
	X: 0.4–0.7 mg/kg IM or IV [25]	Camels	n = 15 animals, sedation, 0.7 mg/kg induced recumbency in 2 animals.
	0.5 mg/kg [19]	Juvenile camels	n = 1 sedation for radiographs of displaced fracture.
Xylazine + butorphanol	X: 0.2 mg/kg + B: 0.05 mg/kg IM [9, 20]	Camelids	Sedation; antagonize with tolazoline 0.5–5 mg/kg.
	X: 0.3 mg/kg + B: 0.1 mg/kg [24]	Alpacas	Sedation or pre-medication.
Xylazine + butorphanol + diazepam	X: 0.1 mg/kg + B: 0.05 mg/kg + D: 0.2 mg/kg [9]	Camels	Antagonize with tolazoline, flumazenil and naltrexone.
Xylazine + diazepam + propofol	X: 0.1–0.25 mg/kg IV+ D: 0.25 mg/kg IV + P: 2 mg/kg IV [16]	Domesticated camelids	Onset of recumbency 1 min after propofol, duration 10–20 min, recovery 45 min to 2 hrs.
Yohimbine HCl	0.125–0.25 mg/kg [9]	Camelids	Reversal for alpha-2 agonists.

(*Continued*)

Drug name	Drug dose	Species	Comments
Antiparasitic			
Albendazole (Valbazen)	19.8 mg/kg PO once, only repeat in 5–7d for severe infections [1] See comments.	Camelids	Narrow margin of safety, should not be used in young crias <6 mo of age – fatalities due to liver failure. DO NOT USE in pregnant females as it leads to facial deformities in crias.
Albendazole	10 mg/kg PO [32, 33]	New World camelids	For Fasciola hepatica, Moniezia, Gastrointestinal nematodes, and lungworms. DO NOT use in pregnant animals.
Albendazole	5–7.5 mg/kg PO [33]	Camels	
Amprolium (Corid)	1 oz./5 gal of water SID × 5d [1]	Camelids	To be used for severe coccidiosis/diarrhea in adults only. Only give this as water source. Not to be used to have completely negative fecal of coccidia, only treat clinical cases. Not suitable for crias as they do not consume enough water. Give fresh daily. Overdose and prolonged use can result in Polioencephalomalacia that is thiamin-responsive.
Amprolium	5 mg/kg PO × 21d [32, 33]	New World camelids	Prevention, anticoccidial.
Clorsulon	7 mg/kg PO × 2 doses at 40–60 day intervals if needed [32, 33]	New World camelids	For treatment of Fasciola hepatica.
Decoquinate	0.5 mg/kg PO × 28d [32, 33]	New World camelids	Prevention, anticoccidial.
Doramectin (Dectomax)	2.5 ml/100 lb SC every 45–60d [1]	Camelids	Used for meningeal worm prevention, longer duration of action and need higher doses than other species. Stings/burns after administration therefore should change needle after drawing up drug.
Doramectin	0.2 mg/kg SC, IM [33]	Camelids	
Fenbendazole	20 mg/kg PO once, then 10 mg/kg PO twice at 3-week intervals [34]	Dromedary camels	n = 3 animals clinically affected with a Trichuris/whipworm infection. The two 3–4 yr old males survived, the adult male died 2 days after treatment.
	20–50 mg/kg PO SID to BID for 3–5d [1]	Camelids	Wide range of safety, can be used at higher doses, but 50 mg/kg usually for 5 days for Giardia diarrhea, safe for pregnant females. 50 mg/kg PO SID × 5–10 days for meningeal worm.
	10–20 mg/kg PO × 3d [32]	New World camelids	For gastrointestinal nematodes, lungworms, whipworms.

Drug name	Drug dose	Species	Comments
	20–50 mg/kg PO × 5d [32]	New World camelids	20 mg/kg for Nematodirus, 50 mg/kg for Moniezia.
	5–10 mg/kg PO [33]	New World camelids	15 mg/kg PO for Trichuris.
Ivermectin	0.2 mg/kg SC [35]	Llamas	Undetectable in plasma samples drawn up to 4 weeks after injection.
	0.2 mg/kg oral or SC [32]	New World camelids	For gastrointestinal nematodes, lungworms, sarcoptic mange, sucking lice.
Ivermectin	0.2 mg/kg SC cervical region [36]	Dromedary camels	n = 3 adult females between 4–8 yrs of age. Peak plasma concentration was lower than that for cows and sheep, and time to reach cMax was longer, and so there was a slower rate of absorption. Anecdotal evidence suggests it is still effective clinically, perhaps due to longer duration of action.
	0.4–0.6 mg/kg PO or SC [32]	New World camelids	For whipworms and Cephenemyia.
	0.2 mg/kg SC, PO [33]	Camels, Llamas	For sucking lice (ineffective for biting lice), Oestrus ovis, camel nasal bots, spinose eartick (larvae and nymph), sarcoptic mange.
	0.2 mg/kg SC every 16d for 2 doses [37]	Dromedary camels	Sarcoptic mange.
	0.44 mg/kg SC every 30–45d [1]		Meningeal worm prevention, stings when administered therefore change the needle after drawing up drug.
Levamisole (Levasole)	8.8 mg/kg PO once, repeat in ~10d [1].	Camelids	Paralyzes parasite and then expelled alive. Not effective for Trichuris spp. or lungworms. The injectable form or high oral doses may result in neurologic side effects. Narrow margin of safety and should not be used in debilitated animals. Only use as a last resort when other anthelmintics have failed. May cause coughing after oral administration.
	5–8 mg/kg PO or 6 mg/kg SC [32, 33]	New World camelids	For gastrointestinal nematodes and lungworms. Accurate weights are critical to proper dosing. Not recommended in lactating animals.
Levamisole	7.5 mg/kg PO [33]	Camels	
Mebendazole	22 mg/kg PO × 3d [32, 33]	New World camelids	For gastrointestinal nematodes.
	5 mg/kg PO × 3d [33]	Camels	
Metronidazole	51 mg/kg PO BID for 5–8d [1]	Camelids	For use in young crias <2 mo of age to treat Giardia diarrhea.

(*Continued*)

Drug name	Drug dose	Species	Comments
	25 mg/kg PO BID × 5d [33]	New World Camelids	
Moxidectin (Cydectin)	0.4 mg/kg PO once [1, 32, 33] See comments.	Camelids	Comes in three forms: oral, injectable, and topical. Topical does not work in camelids. Oral form is recommended at sheep doses. Should be reserved for benzimidazole-resistant parasites. Moderate degree of safety but dosing at 2 × label dosing resulted in seizures that may not resolve. Use in crias 4 months or older. No safety information regarding pregnant animals. Quest gel equine product is concentrated so be careful of overdosing. Not advised unless resistant nematodes are documented in the herd.
Oxfenbendazole	5 mg/kg PO [33]	Camelids	
Paromomycin sulfate (Humatin)	24–48.5 mg/kg PO BID for 5–10d [1]	Camelids	To treat cryptosporidium diarrhea in young crias. If severe case, may double dose and length of treatment. Comes as a capsule to open and mix powder with water. Human drug and is expensive but quite effective.
Ponazuril (Marquis)	19.8 mg/kg PO SID for 3–5d [1]	Camelids	To treat Eimeria macusaniensis infection. Preferred drug of choice for adults with coccidia. May work on Cryptosporidium diarrhea. Intended for horses and too concentrated for alpacas – mix 40 ml with 20 ml distilled water to create 100 mg/ml suspension.
Ponazuril	10–20 mg/kg PO SID × 3d [32]	New World camelids	Anticoccidial.
Praziquantel	50 mg/kg PO [32]	New World camelids	To treat Dicrocoelium dendriticum.
Pyrantel pamoate (Strongid)	8.5 mg/kg PO [32]	New World camelids	For gastrointestinal nematodes.
	18 mg/kg PO × 3d [32, 33]	New World camelids	For gastrointestinal nematodes and cestodes.
Pyrantel pamoate	25 mg/kg PO SID × 3d [33]	Camels	
Pyrantel pamoate (Strongid)	13–18 mg/kg PO once, then repeat in 7–10d [1]	Camelids	Works by paralyzing parasite. Minimal research in camelids but anecdotally used often and appears effective. Should be held as a second line drug. Moderate margin of safety. Do not use concurrently with levamisole.
Sulfadimethoxine (Albon)	55 mg/kg PO SID once, then 28.7 mg/kg PO SID × 4d [1]	Camelids	

Drug name	Drug dose	Species	Comments
Sulfadimethoxine	55 mg/kg SC once, then 22.5 mg/kg SC SID × 4d [32]	New World camelids	Anticoccidial.
Thiabendazole	50–100 mg/kg PO 1–3d [32] 100 mg/kg PO SID for 1–3d [33] 100–150 mg/kg PO SID for 1–3d [33] 2–4% topical ointment q3d [33]	New World camelids New World camelids Camels Ringworm treatment	For gastrointestinal nematodes and lungworms.
Toltrazuril (Baycox)	19.8 mg/kg PO once [1]	Camelids	Related to ponazuril, used for treatment of E. macusaniensis. May work in camelids, little research done.
Other			
Atropine (large animal 2 mg/ml)	0.04 mg/kg [9]	Camelids	
Calcium gluconate (23%)	0.7 mEq/ml [9]	Camelids	
Cimetidine	9.9 mg/kg IV, SC BID to QID [1]	Camelids	Blocks cells producing acid in the third compartment, thus increasing pH and allowing ulcerated tissue to heal. Give 1–2 hrs after Carafate/sucralfate if using together.
Clostridium type C, D &T toxoid	Day 2 of age 2 ml SC, then at day 30, 60, 6 months and yearly 3 ml. Dams give 3 ml, 2 days after giving birth [1].	New world camelids	Most commonly used vaccine in camelids. Used to prevent tetanus. No research on best technique. Doses listed are anecdotal.
Dexamethasone	2 mg/kg [9]	Camelids	Shock
Diazepam	0.1–0.5 mg/kg [9]	Camelids	For seizures.
Doxopram	0.1 mg/kg [9]	Camelids	
Dobutamine	4–8 μg/kg/min [16]	Alpacas	
Epinephrine (1:1000)	0.01 mg/kg [9]	Camelids	
Immodium	Young crias 3 ml, Older crias 4–5 ml, Yearlings 5–7 ml, Adults 7–10 ml; PO SID to BID as needed [1]	Camelids	To help control severe diarrhea in crias and adults, to be used with kaolin, estimated doses, base dose on what animal needs.
Iron dextran	300 mg Alpaca adult, 500 mg Llama adult SC every 3d for 3 treatments [1]	Alpacas, Llamas	To treat anemia, can be used in conjunction with Vit B 12. Very irritating so only give SC. Can dilute in equal parts saline to make less irritating. Can cross placenta so do not use in pregnant animals. Oral supplementation alone is not effective for iron deficiency anemia. No specific studies, doses based on anecdotal use.

(*Continued*)

Drug name	Drug dose	Species	Comments
Kaolin pectate	Young crias 5–7 ml, Older crias 7–10 ml, Yearlings 12–15 ml, Adults 20–30 ml; PO SID to BID as needed [1]	Camelids	To control moderate diarrhea, estimated doses, each animal needs to be monitored for what works for them.
Lactated Ringer's solution + 1% dextrose	2.5 ml/kg/hr[7]	Dromedary camels	Calf
Lidocaine 2%	0.5 mg/kg [9]	Camelids	Ventricular arrhythmias.
Magnesium sulfate	0.5 g/kg PO once, given in 1 l water [7]	Dromedary camels	12 wk old female with Streptococcus pleuropneumonia and peritonitis. Developed decreased fecal output and given as a laxative.
Norepinephrine	0.3–1 μg/kg/min [16]	Alpacas	Effective at the lower dosage.
Omeprazole	0.44–0.88 mg/kg IV QID [1]	Camelids	DOES NOT WORK orally in camelids that are old enough to ruminate if given orally (Gastroguard product). Instead in older animals give IV form.
Pantoprazole (Protonix)	2.2 mg/kg IV, SC SID [1]	Alpacas	Blocks acid secretion in third compartment, increasing pH and allowing ulcerated tissue to heal. Unknown how it will interact with Carafate/sucralfate.
Pantoprazole	0.65 mg/kg IV SID [7]	Dromedary Camels	12 wk old female with Streptococcus pleuropneumonia and peritonitis. Pantoprazole was given to prevent/treat compartment 3 ulceration.
Sodium Bicarbonate	0.5 mEq/ml [9]	Camelids	
Sucralfate (Carafate)	1 g/50 lb PO BID to QID [1]	Camelids	Binds to ulcerated tissue in third compartment. If used with cimetidine, Carafate must be given 1–2 hrs before cimetidine.
Tetanus toxoid	33 IU/kg [11]	Camels	n = 1 calf, no pharmacokinetics.
Tetanus antitoxin	225 U/kg IV ½ and ½ IM [9]	Llamas	Caution for anaphylactic shock.
Vitamin A &D	2204 IU/kg SC q60d or 33 000 IU PO q2 weeks [1].	Camelids	Used in crias to prevent rickets and angular limb deformities. Injectable form more consistently absorbed, but both are effective. Do NOT USE both forms. Calculate the dose based on the Vit D component.
Vitamin B 1 (thiamine)	20–40 mg/kg SC SID to QID [1]	Camelids	To treat polioencephalomalacia and other neurologic disorders. Can cause neuro signs if given IV too rapidly (seizures). Start with lower dose and only increase if the animal is not responding (still depressed and blind).

Drug name	Drug dose	Species	Comments
Vitamin B12	30000 μg Adult alpaca, 5000 μg Adult Llama, SC daily × 7d then 3 times weekly for 3 weeks [1].	Alpacas, Llamas	For use in anemic camelids. Can be used with Iron dextran as B12 helps absorption of iron. No labeled dose for camelids, doses listed used for years anecdotally with no reported issues.
Vitamin E & selenium (Bo-se)	0.055 mg/kg SC [1]	Camelids	Used in crias to prevent white muscle disease and stimulate the immune system. Anaphylactic reactions have been reported so monitor animal closely.

Species	Weight
Alpaca *(Vicugna pacos)*	40–90 kg
Camel, Bactrian *(Camelus bactrianus)*	300–690 kg
Camel, Dromedary *(Camelus dromedarius)*	300–690 kg
Guanaco *(Lama guanicoe)*	100–120 kg
Llama *(Lama glama)*	113–250 kg
Vicuna *(Vivugna vicugna)*	38–42 kg

References

1 Walker, P.G. Medications for Camelids. (Ohio State University) International Camelid Institute. www.icinfo.org (accessed 19 August 2018).

2 Talbot, C.E., Mueller, K., Granger, N. et al. (2007). Diagnosis and surgical removal of brain abscesses in a juvenile alpaca. *Journal of the American Veterinary Medical Association* 231 (10): 1558–1561.

3 Goudah, A.M. and Hasabelnaby, S.M. (2013). Pharmacokinetics and distribution of ceftazidime to milk after intravenous and intramuscular administration to lactating female dromedary camels (*Camelus dromedarius*). *Journal of the American Veterinary Medical Association* 243 (3): 424–429.

4 Niehaus, A.J. and Anderson, D.E. (2007). Tooth root abscesses in llamas and alpacas:123 cases (1994–2005). *Journal of the American Veterinary Medical Association* 231 (2): 284–289.

5 Dechant, J.E., Rowe, J.D., Rowe, B.A. et al. (2013). Pharmacokinetics of ceftiofur crystalline free acid after single and multiple subcutaneous administrations in healthy alpacas (*Vicugna pacos*). *Journal of Veterinary Pharmacology and Therapeutics* 36 (2): 122–129.

6 Gyimesi, Z.S., Burns, R.B., and Bolin, S.R. (2015). Acute clinical leptospirosis (*Grippo typhosa serovar*) in an adult dromedary camel (*Camelus dromedarius*). *Journal of Zoo and Wildlife Medicine* 46 (3): 605–608.

7 Stoughton, W.B. and Gold, J. (2015). Stretococcus equi subsp Zooepidemicus pleuropneumonia and peritonitis in a dromedary camel (*Camelus dromedarius*) calf in North America. *Journal of the American Veterinary Medical Association* 247 (3): 300–303.

8 Crawshaw, G., Mehren, K.G., Whiteside, D. et al. (2000). Surgical lengthening of the mandible of a Bactrian camel by distraction osteogenesis. *Annual Proceedings of the American Association of Zoo Veterinarians* 68–70.

9 Fowler, M.E. (2010). Anesthesia. In: *Medicine and Surgery of Camelids* (ed. M.E. Fowler with P.W. Bravo), 111–128. Ames, IA: Wiley Blackwell.

10 Kock, R.A. (1985). Obstructive urethral calculi in the male camel: report of two cases. *Veterinary Record* 117 (19): 494–496.

11 Bani-Ismail, Z., Hawkins, J.F., and Siems, J.J. (1999). Surgical correction of polydactyly in a camel (*Camelus dromedarius*). *Journal of Zoo and Wildlife Medicine* 30 (2): 301–304.

12 Chatfield, J., Jensen, J., Boothe, D. et al. (2001). Disposition of sulfadimethoxine in camels (*Camelus dromedarius*) following single intravenous and oral doses. *Journal of Zoo and Wildlife Medicine* 32 (4): 430–435.

13 Dooley, S.B., Aarnes, T.K., Lakritz, J. et al. (2017). Pharmacokinetics and pharmacodynamics of buprenorphine and sustained-release buprenorphine after administration to adult alpacas. *American Journal of Veterinary Research* 78 (3): 321–329.

14 Emerson, J.A. and Guzman, D.S. (2018). Sustained-release and long-acting opiod formulations of interest in zoological medicine. In: *Fowler's Zoo and Wild Animal Medicine Current Therapy*, vol. 9 (ed. R.E. Miller, N. Lamberski and P.P. Calle), 151–163. St. Louis, MO: Elsevier Saunders.

15 Grubb, T.L., Gold, J.R., Schlipf, J.W. et al. (2005). Assessment of serum concentrations and sedative effects of fentanyl after transdermal administration at three dosages in healthy llamas. *American Journal of Veterinary Research* 66 (5): 907–909.

16 Mama, K.R. and Walzer, C. (2014). Camelids. In: *Zoo Animal and Wildlife Immobilization and Anesthesia*, 2e (ed. G. West, D. Heard and N. Caulkett), 592–610. Ames, IA: Wiley Blackwell.

17 Kreuder, A.J., Coetzee, J.F., Wulf, L.W. et al. (2012). Bioavailability and pharmacokinetics of oral meloxicam in llamas. *BMC Veterinary Research* 8 (85).

18 Uhrig, S.R., Papich, M.G., KuKanich, B. et al. (2007). Pharmacokinetics and pharmacodynamics of morphine in llamas. *American Journal of Veterinary Research* 68 (1): 25–34.

19 Squire, K.R.E. and Boehm, P.N. (1991). External fixation repair of a displaced comminuted radial fracture in a juvenile camel. *Journal of the American Veterinary Medical Association* 199 (6): 769–771.

20 Brave, P.W. (2015). Camelids. In: *Fowler's Zoo and Wild Animal Medicine Current Therapy*, vol. 9 (ed. R.E. Miller, N. Lamberski and P.P. Calle), 592–601. St. Louis, MO: Elsevier Saunders.

21 Bouts, T., Dodds, J., Berry, K. et al. (2017). Detomidine and butorphanol for standing sedation in a range of zoo-kept ungulate species. *Journal of Zoo and Wildlife Medicine* 48 (3): 616–626.

22 Nielsen, L. (1999). *Chemical Immobilization of Wild and Exotic Animals*. Ames, IA: Wiley Blackwell.

23 Kreeger, T.J. and Arnemo, J.M. (2018). *Handbook of Wildlife Chemical Immobilization*. China: Kreeger.

24 Taylor, S.D., Baird, A.N., Weil, A.B. et al. (2017). Evaluation of three intravenous injectable anaesthesia protocols in healthy adult male alpacas. *Veterinary Record* 181 (12): 322.

25 deMaar, T.W., von Bolhuis, H., and Mugo, M.J. (1998). Field anesthesia of camels (*Camelus dromedarius*) and the use of Medetomidine/ketamine with atipamezole reversal. *Annual Proceedings of the American Association of Zoo Veterinarians* 54–57.

26 Boardman, W.W., Lethbridge, M.R., Hampton, J.O. et al. (2014). Evaluation of medetomidine-ketamine and medeto midine-ketamine-butorphanol for the field anesthesia of free-ranging dromedary camels (*Camelus dromedarius*) Australia. *Journal of Wildlife Diseases* 50 (4): 873–882.

27 Georoff, T.A., James, S.B., Kalk, P. et al. (2010). Evaluation of Medetomidine-ketamine-butorphanol Anesthesia with atipamezole-naltrexone antagonism in captive male guanacos (*Lama guanicoe*). *Journal of Zoo and Wildlife Medicine* 41 (2): 255–262.

28 White, R.J., Bali, S., and Bark, H. (1987). Xylazine and ketamine anaesthesia in the dromedary camel under field conditions. *Veterinary Record* 120 (5): 110–113.

29 Waldbridge, B.M., Lin, H.C., DeGraves, F.J. et al. (1997). Sedative effects of medetomidine and its reversal by atipamezole in llamas. *Journal of the American Veterinary Medical Association* 211 (12): 1562–1565.
30 Aarnes, T.K., Fry, P.R., Hubbell, J.A. et al. (2013). Pharmacokinetics and pharmacodynamics of midazolam after intravenous and intramuscular administration in alpacas. *American Journal of Veterinary Research* 74 (2): 294–299.
31 Seddighi, R., Elliot, S.B., Whitlock, B.K. et al. (2013). Physiologic and antinociceptive effects following intramuscular administration of Xylazine hydrochloride in combination with Tiletamine-Zolazepam in llamas. *American Journal of Veterinary Research* 74 (4): 530–534.
32 Ballweber, L.R. (2009). Ecto- and Endoparasites of New World Camelids. *Veterinary Clinics Food Animal* 25: 295–310.
33 Fowler, M.E. (2010). Parasites. In: *Medicine and Surgery of Camelids*, 231–269. Ames, IA: Wiley Blackwell.
34 Eo, K.Y., Kwan, D., and Kwon, O.D. (2014). Severe whipworm (*Trichuris spp.*) infection in the dromedary (*Camelus dromedarius*). *Journal of Zoo and Wildlife Medicine* 45 (1): 190–192.
35 Burkholder, T.H., Jensen, J., Chen, H. et al. (2004). Plasma evaluation for ivermectin in llamas (*Lama glama*) after standard subcutaneous dosing. *Journal of Zoo and Wildlife Medicine* 35 (3): 395–396.
36 Oukessou, M., Badri, M., Sutra, J.F. et al. (1996). Pharmacokinetics of ivermectin in the camel (*Camelus dromedarius*). *Veterinary Record* 139: 424–425.
37 Opferman, R.R. (1985). Treatment of Sarcoptic mange in a dromedary camel. *Journal of the American Veterinary Medical Association* 187 (11): 1240–1241.

25

Giraffes and Okapis

Drug name	Drug dose	Species	Comments
Antimicrobials and Antifungals			
Amikacin	15–21 mg/kg IV SID × 12d [1, 2]	Giraffes, Okapis	n = 2 animals, 1st: 16 mo, reticulated, captive, mycoplasma-associated polyarthritis. No adverse effects noted. 2nd: 10 yr old female Okapi with chronic fibrinous pleuritis.
	14.7 mg/kg IV [3]	Giraffes	n = 2 animals treated while immobilized, for signs of colic.
	6600 mg IM once [4]	Okapis	n = 1 animal in case series of 3 adult female animals mid-gestation with acute congestive heart failure treated with a variety of antibiotics and cardiac medications.
Ampicillin sodium	22 mg/kg IV BID × 22d [2]	Giraffes	16 mo, reticulated, captive, mycoplasma-associated polyarthritis – initially responsive to ampicillin + Amikacin + flunixin, but kept recurring until cultured mycoplasma and treated with enrofloxacin instead. No adverse effects noted.
Ceftiofur	6–9 mg/kg IM or SC SID or q3–14d [5]	Giraffes	Infection, n = 1 calf.
Ceftiofur sodium (Naxcel)	0.9 mg/kg IM [6]	Giraffes	n = 3 adult male giraffe undergoing surgical castration.
	1.22 mg/kg IM [3]	Giraffes	n = 2 animals treated while immobilized, for signs of colic.

(*Continued*)

Zoo and Wild Mammal Formulary, First Edition. Alicia Hahn.

Drug name	Drug dose	Species	Comments
Ceftiofur short-acting (Naxcel)	3.3 mg/kg IV BID, 1000 mg IM once [1, 4]	Okapis	n = 2, 1st animal, 10 yr old female Okapi with chronic fibrinous pleuritis, 2nd: 1 animal in case series of 3 adult female animals with mid-gestation acute congestive heart failure treated with a variety of antibiotics and cardiac medications.
Ceftiofur long-acting (Excede)	8 mg/kg SQ q72 hrs, 2000 mg SQ q72 hrs × 8 doses [4]	Okapis	n = 3, 1st: 10 yr old female Okapi with chronic fibrinous pleuritis, 2nd: 2 animals in case series of 3 adult female animals with mid-gestation acute congestive heart failure treated with a variety of antibiotics and cardiac medications.
Doxycycline	1500 mg PO SID × 56d [4]	Okapis	n = 1 animals in case series of 3 adult female animals with mid-gestation acute congestive heart failure treated with a variety of antibiotics and cardiac medications.
	4–5 mg/kg PO SID [5]	Giraffes	For infection, sometimes used in combination with rifampin.
Enrofloxacin	2 mg/kg IM [6]	Giraffe	n = 3 adult male giraffe undergoing surgical castration.
	4–8 mg/kg PO SID × 5d [5]	Giraffe	Infection
Enrofloxacin	10 mg/kg PO SID × 14d [2]	Giraffes	16 mo, reticulated, captive, mycoplasma-associated polyarthritis – initially responsive to ampicillin + Amikacin + flunixin, but kept recurring until diagnosed Mycoplasma and treated with enrofloxacin instead. No adverse effects noted.
Neopredef	Powder applied topically to aural canals for suspected ear infection [7]	Okapis	Flushed with dilute chlorhexidine first then applied Neopredef powder.
Oxytetracycline (LA200)	6000 mg SQ q72 hrs × 6 doses [4]	Okapis	n = 2 animals in case series of 3 adult female animals with mid-gestation acute congestive heart failure treated with a variety of antibiotics and cardiac medications.
Penicillin G benzathine and Penicillin G procaine (Penben)	32 432–35 865 IU/kg IM [6]	Giraffes	n = 3 adult male giraffe undergoing surgical castration.
Potassium penicillin G	130 000 IU/kg/day IV [1]	Okapis	n = 1, 10 yr old female Okapi with chronic fibrinous pleuritis.

Drug name	Drug dose	Species	Comments
Panalog ointment	Given topically into aural canal BID × 10d [7]	Okapis	To treat ear infection.
Trimethoprim sulfadiazine (Uniprim)	20 mg/kg PO SID × 6d [6]	Giraffes	n = 3 adult male giraffe post-surgical castration.
	30–45 mg/kg PO SID [5]	Giraffes	For some individuals oral dosing is easier with powder instead of pill formations.
Trimethoprim sulfadimethoxazole	8600 mg PO BID × 10 day [4]	Okapis	n = 2 animals in case series of 3 adult female animals with mid-gestation acute congestive heart failure treated with a variety of antibiotics and cardiac medications.
Tulathromycin	2.5 mg/kg SC q3d [5]	Giraffes	n = 1 animal, for infection.
Rifampin	6–7 mg/kg PO SID [5]	Giraffes	Sometimes used in combination with doxycycline.
Analgesia			
Carprofen	2 mg/kg PO SID to BID [8]	Giraffids	
Etodolac	2.5–5 mg/kg PO SID to BID [8]	Giraffids	
Firocoxib	0.045–0.3 mg/kg PO SID [9]	Giraffes	Retrospective survey of 45 institutions holding giraffe. 9/10 institutions that used fircoxib orally reported fair to excellent perceived efficacy.
	0.1–0.3 mg/kg PO SID [5]	Giraffes	Used for arthritis, phalanx 3 fracture, laminitis and swelling.
Flunixin meglumine	1–2 mg/kg IV, IM, PO SID [2, 8]	Giraffes	
	0.23–1.9 PO SID to BID [9]	Giraffes	Retrospective survey of 45 institutions holding giraffe. 24/28 institutions that used Flunixin reported fair to excellent perceived efficacy (1 reported poor). Adverse events reported: subjective elevation of renal values and taste aversion.
	0.5 mg/kg IM perioperatively and PO × 3d afterward [6]	Giraffes	n = 3 adult males undergoing surgical castration.
Flunixin meglumine	0.6–0.9 mg/kg IM or IV [3]	Giraffes	n = 3 sub adult to adult giraffe treated for signs of colic, ultimately colonic obstruction was diagnosed on histopathology.

(*Continued*)

Drug name	Drug dose	Species	Comments
	0.5–1.1 mg/kg IM SID to BID [9]	Giraffes	Retrospective survey of 45 institutions holding giraffe. 8/13 institutions that used flunixin IM reported fair to excellent perceived efficacy. Adverse events reported: pain at injection site at 2 institutions.
	1.1 mg/kg IV once [9]	Giraffes	Retrospective survey of 45 institutions holding giraffe. 2/2 institutions that used flunixin IV reported good perceived efficacy. No adverse events reported.
	1.1 mg/kg SC SID for 1–3d [5]	Giraffes	Used for arthritis, phalanx 3 fracture, laminitis and swelling.
Gabapentin	1–5 mg/kg PO SID to BID [5]	Giraffes	For suspected spinal injury or chronic lameness. Consider starting at lower dose and tapering up as needed. Has been given with NSAIDS and tramadol.
	2–5 mg/kg PO SID [8]	Giraffids	
	0.2–16 mg/kg PO BID [9]	Giraffes	Retrospective survey of 45 institutions holding giraffe. 5/8 institutions that used gabapentin reported fair to excellent perceived efficacy (3 reported poor response). Adverse events reported: possible lethargy at higher doses.
Glucosamine chondroitin	4–21.6 mg/kg PO SID to BID [9]	Giraffes	Retrospective survey of 45 institutions holding giraffe. 10/15 institutions that used glucosamine chondroitin reported fair to good perceived efficacy. Adverse events reported: taste aversion to some equine apple-flavored products.
Ketoprofen	0.5–2 mg/kg IM, IV SID [8]	Giraffes	
	0.5–3 mg/kg PO SID [9]	Giraffes	Retrospective survey of 45 institutions holding giraffe. 9/9 institutions that used ketoprofen orally reported fair to good perceived efficacy. Adverse events reported were mild hematuria at two institutions.
Lidocaine hydrochloride 2%	20 ml injected into each testicle and around spermatic cord [6]	Giraffes	n = 3 adult male giraffe undergoing surgical castration.

Drug name	Drug dose	Species	Comments
	2000 mg or 2.45 mg/kg SC and intradermal injection once [3]	Giraffes	n = 1 animal undergoing local analgesia for laparotomy in an "inverted L pattern".
Meloxicam	0.1 mg/kg PO SID [8]	Giraffids	
	0.2 mg/kg SC once or 0.3–0.5 mg/kg PO SID [5]	Giraffes	Used for arthritis, phalanx 3 fracture, laminitis and swelling.
	0.05–0.6 mg/kg PO QOD or SID [9]	Giraffes	Retrospective survey of 45 institutions holding giraffe. 6/7 institutions that used meloxicam orally reported good to excellent perceived efficacy.
Meloxicam (Metacam)	0.6 mg/kg SID [10]	Giraffes	n = 1 juvenile with angular limb deformities, used meloxicam for 1 week with bandaging and no improvement, ultimately required periosteal transection and postoperative care.
Methocarbamol	12–25 mg/kg PO SID [5]	Giraffes	Used for a spinal injury or abnormal body posture.
Phenylbutazone	0.75–2 mg/kg PO QOD to BID [9].	Giraffes	Retrospective survey of 45 institutions holding giraffe. 34/39 institutions that used phenylbutazone reported good to excellent perceived efficacy (7 reported no to fair response). Adverse events reported softer stools, possible GI discomfort, and taste aversion.
	1–3 mg/kg PO SID to BID [8]	Giraffes	
	2–6 mg/kg PO SID or 7–8 mg/kg PO EOD [5]	Giraffes	Recommend washout period after 7–14 days of daily dosing. Used for arthritis, phalanx 3 fracture, laminitis and swelling.
Therapy laser	3000 J/digit topical q72 hrs for 1 month then weekly; 8000 J to lateral hock q72 hrs for 1 month [5]	Giraffes	Used for arthritis and cellulitis respectively. Thermography may help identify inflammation and quantify if treatment is helping. If treating digit target from coronary band to proximal to fetlock joint – avoid hoof wall. Consider using noncontact laser on PVC extension.
Tramadol	0.5 mg/kg PO SID [5]	Giraffes	Used for arthritis, phalanx 3 fracture, laminitis and swelling.

(*Continued*)

Drug name	Drug dose	Species	Comments
	0.48–3 mg/kg PO SID to BID [9]	Giraffes	Retrospective survey of 45 institutions holding giraffe. 2/5 institutions that used tramadol orally reported good to excellent perceived efficacy (2 reported no to poor response). Adverse events reported included drowsiness and possible decreased fecal production at higher doses.
Anethesia and Sedation			
Azaperone	0.2–0.5 mg/kg IM [8, 11]	Giraffes, Okapis	Short-acting, calming, and stress-reducing agent.
Detomidine	14–40 μg/kg IM; antagonize with yohimbine 0.1–0.2 mg/kg IV or IM, or atipamezole 0.1–0.2 mg/kg IV or IM [8].	Giraffes	Standing sedation.
Azaperone + detomidine	A: 0.2–0.5 mg/kg + D: 15–30 μg/kg IM; antagonize with yohimbine 0.1–0.2 mg/kg IV/IM, or atipamezole 0.01–0.05 mg/kg IV/IM and naltrexone 2 mg/1 mg butorphanol [11, 12]	Giraffes	Standing sedation: Combination produces good tranquilization and moderate analgesia. Facilitates blood sampling, reproductive exams, tuberculin testing, joint taps, radiographs, suturing, and dystocia corrections. For deeper sedation add 10 mg butorphanol IV in adult animals.
Detomidine + butorphanol	D: 40–100 μg/kg IM + B: 80–200 μg/kg IM; antagonize with yohimbine 0.1–0.2 mg/kg IV/IM, or atipamezole 0.01–0.05 mg/kg IV/IM and naltrexone 1–2 mg/mg butorphanol IM or IV [8, 12].	Okapis	Standing restraint for minor procedures. Animals will move around a bit but otherwise satisfactory sedation.
Detomidine + acepromazine + butorphanol + methadone	D: 30–40 μg/kg + Ace: 15–25 μg/kg + B: 20–30 μg/kg + Meth: 20–30 μg/kg; antagonize with atipamezole 0.05 mg/kg IM/IV + naltrexone 40–60 μg/kg IM/IV [11]	Giraffes	For deeper sedation add xylazine 20–50 μg/kg.

Drug name	Drug dose	Species	Comments
Detomidine + butorphanol+ acepromazine + midazolam	D: 40–60 µg/kg + B: 40–60 µg/kg + A: 30–40 µg/kg + Mid: 30–40 µg/kg; antagonize with atipamezole 0.03–0.06 mg/kg and naltrexone 40–60 µg/kg IM/IV [11].	Okapis	Standing sedation.
Detomidine + azaperone ± butorphanol	D: 15–30 µg/kg IM + A: 0.25–0.3 mg/kg IM. Butorphanol if needed 10–20 mg/kg total IV; antagonize with yohimbine 0.1–0.2 mg/kg IM/IV or atipamezole 0.05–0.1 mg/kg IM/IV. Naltrexone 2 mg/mg of butorphanol IV [8].	Giraffes	Chemically-assisted mechanical restraint.
Detomidine + butorphanol	D: 0.04–0.06 mg/kg + B: 0.03–0.06 mg/kg IM [13]	Giraffes, reticulated	Standing sedation for minor procedures.
	D: 40–100 µg/kg + 80–200 µg/kg IM.; antagonize with yohimbine 0.1–0.2 mg/kg IM/IV or atipamezole 0.05–0.1 mg/kg IM/IV [11].	Okapis	Standing sedation. If indicated, reverse butorphanol with naltrexone 1–2 × dose of butorphanol IM/IV.
Carfentanil + xylazine	X: 0.12 mg/kg wait 10–20 min, then C: 5 µg/kg IM; antagonize with naltrexone 0.5 mg/kg IM [11].	Okapis	Anesthesia, add azaperone 50 mg/adult in stressed animals.
Carfentanil + xylazine	X: 0.1–0.14 mg/kg IM (adult total dose 30–45 mg IM) then wait 15–20 min before darting with 3.9–5.5 µg/kg carfentanil with total dose of 0.9–1.5 mg; antagonize with naltrexone 100 mg/mg carfentanil split into half IV and SQ or all IM. Yohimbine 0.1–0.2 mg/kg IV or IM, or tolazoline 100 mg IV or IM total, or RX82110 5 mg IV or atipamezole 0.125 mg/kg IV or IM. Reversals smoother when all given IM [8, 11].	Okapis	n = 170+ procedures, requires less opioid, smoother induction and excellent muscle relaxation. Azaperone 50 mg/adult can be added to increase sedation and improve induction in stressed animals. When expecting significant stimuli during procedure can add 1–1.5 mg/kg ketamine to carfentanil dart. To improve muscle relaxation or deepen anesthesia can add 2–5 mg IV boluses of xylazine, or 50–200 mg IV boluses of ketamine, or 5% guaifenesin CRI. Renarcotization can be seen for up to 24 hrs so monitor closely and administer supplemental naltrexone as needed.

(*Continued*)

Drug name	Drug dose	Species	Comments
Etorphine ± thiafentanil	Etorphine alone or thiafentanil or 1 : 1 mix. 10–14 mg/subadult. 14–15 mg/adult female. Up to 18 mg/adult male; antagonize with 2 mg of diprenorphine or 100 mg naltrexone per mg etorphine [11]	Giraffes	Immediate reversal required!.
Etorphine	Bull 11 mg, Cow: 9 mg, young: 6 mg, antagonize with diprenorphine 22 mg, 18 mg, 12 mg respectively, or 100 mg of naltrexone per mg etorphine IM [14]	Giraffes	
	8–15 mg/adult [8]	Giraffes	Free-ranging capture, with or without hyaluronidase.
Etorphine + xylazine	1 : 1 ratio, X: 0.1–0.2 mg/kg IM, wait 10–20 min. E: 8–15 µg/kg IM; antagonize with atipamezole 0.05 mg/kg IM/IV and naltrexone 0.2–0.3 mg/kg IM/IV [11]	Okapis	Anesthesia. Do not use Immobilon due to risk of regurgitation from acepromazine.
	X: 40–50 mg/adult given followed by 4–5 mg etorphine 15–20 min later; antagonize with naltrexone 30–50 mg/mg etorphine or diprenorphine 2 mg/mg etorphine and yohimbine or atipamezole for xylazine [8, 11]	Okapis	Increased risk of regurgitation with etorphine versus carfentanil.
Haloperidol	15–20 mg/adult female, 20–30 mg/adult male IM [11, 14]	Giraffes	Tranquilization lasting 12–24 hrs (onset 15 min) is often useful for loading as animals will often start walking in 15–20 min.
	80–100 µg/kg IM or 0.9–1.5 mg/kg PO [11]	Okapis	

Drug name	Drug dose	Species	Comments
Medetomidine + ketamine	M: 0.05 mg/kg + K: 0.55 mg/kg IM, supplemented with M: 0.0036 mg/kg + K: 0.67 mg/kg IV; antagonized with atipamezole 0.085 mg/kg IM [3]	Giraffes	One adult female Giraffe immobilized for anorexia and lack of fecal production.
Thiafentanil + medetomidine + ketamine	T: 0.005–0.006 mg/kg + M: 0.008–0.011 mg/kg + K: 0.55–1.12 mg/kg IM; antagonize with naltrexone 0.15–0.27 mg/kg + atipamezole 0.05–0.06 mg/kg and yohimbine (in an effort to reduce resedation) 0.1 mg/kg IM [6].	Giraffes	n = 3 captive adult males to undergo surgical castration. After reversals 2/3 regurgitated while endotracheal tubes were still in place, then recovered without complication. One animal required an additional dose of atipamezole as 3 hrs after initial dose it resedated.
Thiafentanil + xylazine or detomidine + ketamine	X: 0.9–0.15 mg/kg IM (total adult dose 30–45 mg) or D: 0.04–0.06 mg/kg IM (total dose 12–20 mg/adult). Wait 15–20 min then dart with T: 5–5.6 μg/kg IM + K: 0.5–0.7 mg/kg IM; antagonize with naltrexone 30 mg/1 mg thiafentanil, yohimbine 0.1–0.2 mg/kg IM or atipamezole 0.125 mg/kg IM [8].	Okapis	Inductions are rapid in 2–6 min, and similar responses to carfentanil + xylazine combo except much shorter duration (25–40 min). No renarcotization seen with this protocol.
Etorphine + thiafentanil	E: 4 mg/adult + T: 8–16 mg/adult IM [8]	Giraffes	Free-ranging capture, with or without hyaluronidase.
Medetomidine + butorphanol	M: 60–90 μg/kg + B: 45–55 μg/kg IM. Atipamezole 5 mg/mg medetomidine IM and naltrexone 1–2 mg per mg butorphanol IM or IV [8, 11]	Okapis	Standing restraint for minor procedures.

(*Continued*)

Drug name	Drug dose	Species	Comments
Ketamine + medetomidine (± midazolam)	K: 1–4 mg/kg IM + M: 60–155 µg/kg IM. ± Mid: 0.1 mg/kg IM; antagonize with atipamezole 5 mg/mg Medetomidine IV or IM [8, 11]	Okapis	Minor procedure with deep sedation, need deep IM injection 50–60 mm needles and upper end of medetomidine dosing 100–155 µg/kg produces better anesthesia without need for supplementation. Recumbent in 3–34 min with 15–20 min procedure time. Adding midazolam 0.1 mg/kg IM speeds up and makes for a smoother induction. Okapi can still kick and rouse unlike with opioid procedures. Wait at least 20 min to reverse. Some reports of postanesthesia ileus or fatalities.
Ketamine + medetomidine	Adult male: K: 1200 mg + M: 70 mg; Adult female K: 900 mg + M: 50 mg; Subadult: K: 500 mg + M: 20 mg, antagonize with 5 mg atipamezole for every mg medetomidine given [14, 15]	Giraffes	
Ketamine + medetomidine	M: 40–60 µg/kg + K: 1–1.5 mg/kg IM. Approximately equal to 150 µg medetomidine + 3 mg ketamine per centimeter of shoulder height; antagonize with atipamezole 0.05–0.15 mg/kg IV/IM [8, 11].	Giraffes	Smaller, calm animals had a rapid uneventful induction. Larger animals less desirable. Tachypnea common, high potential for re-sedation from medetomidine. Consider re-dose atipamezole at 4 and possibly 8 hrs if needed.
	M: sub adult 18–20 mg, adult female 40–50 mg and adult male 50–70 mg + K: 300–500 mg subadult, 800–900 mg adult female and 1000–1200 mg adult male. Atipamezole to antagonize at 350 µg/cm shoulder height or 5 × medetomidine dose IM [8].	Giraffes	n = 30 captive. Smooth induction with sitting sternal then rolling lateral. More excitement prior to darting results in less success. Characteristic tachypnea with 50–60 bpm, inadequate analgesia for painful procedures. Resedation possible 3–28 hrs post recovery – most common in Rothschilds and Southern giraffe, less so in Reticulated. Signs of resedation included decreased awareness, dull eyes, inappetence, lowered neck, widened stance, tongue protrusion and salivation, ataxia, leaning for support, and recumbency.

Drug name	Drug dose	Species	Comments
Ketamine + medetomidine + butorphanol	K: 2–3 mg/kg + M: 60–70 μg/kg + B: 50–100 μg/kg IM [8, 11]	Okapis	For minor surgical procedures and hoof trimming. For more invasive procedures animals were intubated and maintained on isoflurane.
Perphenazine enanthate	100–250 mg IM [8]	Giraffes	Tranquilization for 7–10 days with onset of 2–3 days.
	Adult male 100 mg, subadult 150 mg [14]	Giraffes	
Thiafentanil	8–16 mg/adult [8]	Giraffes	Free-ranging capture, with or without hyaluronidase.
Thiafentanil + ketamine + medetomidine	T: 5–6 μg/kg + M: 8–13 μg/kg + K: 0.6–1 mg/kg IM; antagonize with atipamezole 0.05 mg/kg and naltrexone 0.02 mg/kg IM [11]	Giraffes	Anesthesia of calm or captive giraffe. Beware of potential resedation from medetomidine.
	T: 6–10 μg/kg + M: 10–14 μg/kg + K: 0.5 mg/kg; antagonize with atipamezole 0.05 mg/kg and naltrexone 0.2–0.3 mg/kg [11]	Giraffes	Free-ranging capture. Beware of potential resedation from medetomidine.
	Free-ranging helicopter dart: T: 6–14 μg/kg, M: 5.6–23.4 μg/kg + K: 0.19–0.59 μg/kg IM. Captive: T: 4.3–7.3 μg/kg + M: 7.8–18 μg/kg + K: 0.43–0.83 μg/k IM. Free-ranging ground dart: T: 5.1–8.1 μg/kg + M: 12.2–19.6 μg/kg + K: 0.29–0.69 μg/kg IM [8].	Giraffes	In calm animals, rapid onset of 2–5 min with excellent muscle relaxation and safe to work around, good analgesia, and long duration of action, with apneustic respiratory pattern, and moderate to severe hypoxia. Resedation seen in some post recovery so close monitoring is important. Reversal with naltrexone 30 mg/mg thiafentanil IV or IM and atipamezole 3–5 × dose of medetomidine IV or IM.
Xylazine (± atropine) + carfentanil	X: 70–80 mg adult or 30–40 mg yearling. + A: 7–8 mg Adult or 2–3 mg yearling. 15–20 min later: carfentanil 1.2–2.1 mg/adult or 0.3–0.9 mg/yearling IM. Supplement if not recumbent with either 0.5–1 mg etorphine, 5% guaifenesin, or 100–400 mg ketamine IV [8].	Giraffes, yearling, Captive	5–10 min post xylazine (± atropine) sedation with stargazing, ataxia, and tongue protrusion. At 15–20 min adminster etorphine – may see recumbency in another 15–20 min. If not recumbent supplement with additional etorphine, IV guaifenesin 5% to effect or ketamine. Reversal with naltrexone 50–100 mg/mg etorphine 50: 50 IV IM or all IM, and yohimbine 0.1–0.2 mg/kg IV or IM or atipamezole 50–100 mg total IM or 25% IV and 75% IM.

(*Continued*)

Drug name	Drug dose	Species	Comments
Xylazine + etorphine + ketamine	X: 0.05–0.1 mg/kg, then 20 min later E: 5–8 µg/kg + K: 0.5–1 mg/kg; antagonize with atipamezole 0.05 mg/kg IM/IV, naltrexone 0.3 mg/kg IM/IV [11]	Giraffes	Etorphine may be replaced with carfentanil.
Xylazine + etorphine ± atropine	X: 70–80 mg adult or 30–40 mg yearling. + At: 7–8 mg Adult or 2–3 mg yearling. 15–20 min later: etorphine 1.5–2.5 mg/adult or 0.5–1.25 mg/yearling IM. Supplement if not recumbent with either 0.5–1 mg etorphine, 5% guaifenesin, or 100–400 mg ketamine IV [8].	Giraffes, captive	Staged protocol for captive giraffe anesthesia. 5–10 min post xylazine + atropine sedation with stargazing, ataxia, and tongue protrusion. At 15–20 min adminster carfentanil – may see recumbency in another 15–20 min. Reversal with naltrexone 50–100 mg/mg etorphine 50 : 50 IV IM or all IM, and yohimbine 0.1–0.2 mg/kg IV or IM or atipamezole 50–100 mg total IM or 25% IV and 75% IM. Caution should be exercised when using alpha-2 agonists and atropine due to deleterious effects.
Xylazine + azaperone, ± butorphanol	X: 0.1–0.2 mg/kg + Aza: 0.2–0.5 mg/kg IM. If butorphanol needed 10–20 mg total IV; antagonize with yohimbine 0.1–0.2 mg/kg IM or OV, or atipamezole 0.1–0.2 mg/kg IV or IM. Naltrexone 2 mg/mg butorphanol IV [8].	Giraffes	
Xylazine	0.1–0.2 mg/kg IM; antagonize with yohimbine 0.1–0.2 mg/kg IM or IV, or atipamezole 0.1–0.2 mg/kg IV or IM [8, 11].	Giraffes	Standing sedation, mild i.e. to allow calf to nurse.
	125–300 mg/adult IM; or give 0.5–1.2 mg/kg IM. Can add azaperone 0.2–0.4 mg/kg IM [8, 11].	Okapis	Standing sedation for minor procedures. Reverse with yohimbine 0.1–0.2 mg/kg IM or IV or tolazoline 0.5 mg/kg IM or IV, or RX821002 5 mg/kg IV, or yohimbine or tolazoline + atipamezole 30–100 µg/kg IM or IV.

Drug name	Drug dose	Species	Comments
Xylazine + butorphanol	X: 0.4–0.8 mg/kg + B: 80–200 μg/kg IM; antagonize with yohimbine 0.1–0.2 mg/kg IV/IM, or atipamezole 0.05–0.1 mg/kg IV/IM [11].	Okapis	Standing sedation. If indicated, reverse butorphanol with naltrexone 1–2 × dose of butorphanol IM/IV.
Xylazine + ketamine	X: 0.4–0.6 mg/kg + K: 0.4–0.6 mg/kg IM; antagonize with yohimbine 0.1–0.2 mg/kg IV/IM or atipamezole 0.0B-0.6 mg/kg IV/IM [11]	Okapis	Standing sedation. Normally, the animal will stay standing, but may lie down.
Thiafentanil	20 mg, supplemental 5 mg, antagonize with naltrexone 150 mg IM [14]		
Thiafentanil + ketamine + medetomidine	T: 0.007 mg/kg + K: 0.5 mg/kg + M: 0.016 mg/kg, antagonize with 30 mg naltrexone per mg thiafentanil and 5 mg atipamezole for every mg medetomidine given [8, 14]	Giraffes	Free-ranging, ground darted animals only.
Zuclopenthixol	1 mg/kg IM [14]	Giraffes	
Zuclopenthixol acetate	0.5 mg/kg IM, or 100–300 mg IM [8, 11]	Giraffes, Okapis	Tranquilization for 3 days.
	0.4–1 mg/kg IM [8, 11]	Okapis	
Zuclopenthixol decanoate	2 mg/kg IM [11]	Giraffes, Okapis	Tranquilization for 21 days, onset 1–6 hrs.
Antiparasitic			
Copper oxide wire particles	3.2–25 g/animal for assistance in treating *Haemonchus spp.* [16]	Giraffes	Pharmacodynamic study evaluating effect of wire particles on fecal egg count (FEC) per gram of feces on fecal parasite exam. Resulted in FEC reduction of 27–95%. Administered in loose feed or by capsules being incorporated into fruit. Appears to be effective in controlling Haemonchus in giraffe, but potential toxicity should be measured closely.
Ivermectin	0.2 mg/kg SC [6]	Giraffes	n = 3 animals given opportunistically while under anesthesia.

(*Continued*)

Drug name	Drug dose	Species	Comments
Ivermectin (Eqvalan 1%) + fenbendazole (Panacur 10%) + moxidectin (Quest 2% gel)	I: 0.2 mg/kg PO once + F: 5 mg/kg PO SID × 3d [17]	Giraffes	One young male Giraffe dewormed while in quarantine. Resulted in 80% reduction of strongyle type eggs when rechecked 3 weeks later. And at that time treated with moxidectin and was clear on fecal parasite exam 1 and 3 wks later.
Moxidectin (Cydectin 5%) + fenbendazole (Panacur granules 22.2%) + ivermectin (Eqvalan 1%)	M: 0.5 mg/kg Topical dose + F: 6.8 mg/kg PO SID × 3d, followed by I: 0.2 mg/kg PO once, 15d after finishing F. After I, a second dose of M: 0.5 mg/kg topically was also given [17].		One young male giraffe, 7 weeks after entering a new facility with another giraffe, had diarrhea. DrenchRite assay indicated resistance to avermectins. After 2nd dose of moxidectin the diarrhea resolved and a negative simple fecal flotation test was recorded. A few weeks later PCV was decreased and a high Egg per gram of feces (11 900) was noted on fecal exam so M: 1.2 mg/kg topical application in addition to copper oxide wire particles 6 g PO were given. Within 24 days the EPG was 25.
Moxidectin	1 mg/kg PO once (2% equine oral gel) [2, 18]	Giraffes	3 male captive giraffe given oral and topical. The latter did not reach expected efficacious serum levels at 1 mg/kg dose. Pharmacokinetic, not efficacy study. No adverse effects.
Other			
Adequan	0.75 mg/kg IM; loading dose of q5d for 7 doses, then q30d [5]	Giraffes	Arthritis
Clostridial vaccine (Caliber 7)	2 ml SC once [6]	Giraffes	n = 3 adult male giraffe undergoing surgical castration.
Cold water therapy	5–10 min topical water therapy to affected area SID to BID [5]	Giraffes	Some animals prefer a footbath over a hose.
DMSO	Topical SID to affected inflammation [5]	Giraffes	WEAR GLOVES when applying.
Doxapram	0.1 mg/kg IV [11]	Giraffes, Okapis	Used as a respiratory stimulant and to stimulate animals that are reluctant to get up during recovery.
Enalapril	160–200 mg PO BID [4]	Okapis	n = 3 animals in case series of 3 adult female animals with mid-gestation acute congestive heart failure treated with a variety of antibiotics and cardiac medications.
Epsom salts	Foot bath SID [5]	Giraffes	For hoof abscess or foreign body.

Drug name	Drug dose	Species	Comments
Furosemide	0.6 mg/kg IV and IM [3]	Giraffes	One adult giraffe that developed acute ventral cervical and submandibular edema that resolved in 48 hrs with furosemide and prednisolone sodium succinate.
	300–500 IM BID × 5d [4]	Okapis	n = 3 animals in case series of 3 adult female animals with mid-gestation acute congestive heart failure treated with a variety of antibiotics and cardiac medications.
	1000–1600 mg PO BID [4]	Okapis	n = 3 animals in case series of 3 adult female animals with mid-gestation acute congestive heart failure treated with a variety of antibiotics and cardiac medications.
Hyaluronon	Loading dose: 0.3–0.5 mg/kg PO SID × 14d, Maintenance dose: 0.15–0.3 mg/kg PO SID [5]	Giraffes	Arthritis
Pancreatic enzyme therapy	30 tablets PO SID (each containing 24 IU trypsin, 1 IU amylase, 5 IU lipase) for sub-adult [19]	Giraffes	4 giraffe at 4–6 yrs. of age with chronic (>2 mo) gray-green voluminous diarrhea. Fecal evaluation revealed low amylase and lipase values. Within 7–10 days post administration levels improved and stool normalized.
Pentobarbitol sodium + phenytoin sodium (Euthasol)	0.18 ml/kg IV or 150 ml for 815 kg animal [3]	Giraffes	One adult Giraffe under standing sedation in a chute, collapsed after 2 seizures. Sedated with 10 mg detomidine IV then euthanized humanely.
Prednisolone sodium succinate (Solu Delta Cortef)	0.6 mg/kg IV once [3]	Giraffes	One adult giraffe that developed acute ventral cervical and submandibular edema that resolved in 48 hrs with furosemide and prednisolone sodium succinate.
Rabies vaccine (Imrab 3)	2 ml SC once [6]	Giraffes	n = 3 adult male giraffe undergoing surgical castration.
Spironolactone	150–200 mg PO SID To BID to effect [4]	Okapis	n = 3 adult female animals with mid-gestation acute congestive heart failure treated with a variety of antibiotics and cardiac medications.
Tetanus vaccine (tetanus toxoid)	2 ml IM once [6]	Giraffes	n = 3 adult male giraffe undergoing surgical castration.

(*Continued*)

Species	Weight [14]
Giraffe *(Giraffa camelopardalis)*	550–1800 kg
Okapi *(Okapi johnstoni)*	200–350 kg

References

1 Franzen, D., Lamberski, N., Zuba, J. et al. (2015). Diagnosis and medical and surgical management of chronic infectious fibrinous pleuritis in an Okapi (*Okapi johnstoni*). *Journal of Zoo and Wildlife Medicine* 46 (2): 427–430.

2 Hammond, E.E., Miller, C.A., Sneed, L. et al. (2003). Mycoplasma-associated polyarthritis in a reticulated giraffe. *Journal of Wildlife Diseases* 3 (1): 233–237.

3 Davis, M.R., Langan, J.N., Mylniczenko, N.D. et al. (2009). Colonic obstruction in three captive reticulated giraffe (*Giraffa camelopardalis*). *Journal of Zoo and Wildlife Medicine* 40 (1): 181–188.

4 Warren, J.D., Aitken-Palmer, C., Weldon, A.D. et al. (2017). Congestive heart failure associated with pregnancy in okapi (*Okapi johnstoni*). *Journal of Zoo and Wildlife Medicine* 48 (1): 179–188.

5 Dadone, L. (2019). Lameness diagnosis and management in zoo giraffe. In: *Fowler's Zoo and Wild Animal Medicine Current Therapy*, vol. 9 (ed. R.E. Miller, N. Lamberski and P.P. Calle), 623–629. St. Louis, MO: Elsevier Saunders.

6 Borkowski, R., Citino, S., Bush, M. et al. (2009). Surgical castrat399ion of subadult giraffe (*Giraffa camelopardalis*). *Journal of Zoo and Wildlife Medicine* 40 (4): 786–790.

7 Allender, M.C., Langan, J., and Citino, S. (2008). Investigation of aural bacterial and fungal flora following otitis in captive okapi (*Okapia johnstoni*). *Veterinary Dermatology* 19 (2): 95–100.

8 Citino, S.B. and Bush, M. (2007). Giraffidae. In: *Zoo Animal and Wildlife Immobilization and Anesthesia*, 2e (ed. G. West, D. Heard and N. Caulkett), 809–821. Ames, IA: Wiley Blackwell.

9 Boothe, M., Kottwitz, J., Harmon, R. et al. (2016). Results of the megavertebrate analgesia survey: giraffe and hippopotamus. *Journal of Zoo and Wildlife Medicine* 47 (4): 1049–1056.

10 Neilsen, A.M.W., Meneghetti, N., Doles, J. et al. (2018). Correction of Flexor and Angular Front Limb Deformities in a Juvenile giraffe with tendonitis (*Giraffa camelopardalis*). *Annual Proceedings of the American Association of Zoo Veterinarians*. 103.

11 Bertelsen, M.F. (2015). Giraffidae. In: *Fowler's Zoo and Wild Animal Medicine*, vol. 8 (ed. R.E. Miller and M. Fowler), 602–610. St. Louis, MO: Elsevier Saunders.

12 Bush, M., Citino, S.B., and Lance, W.R. (2012). The use of butorphanol in anesthesia protocols for zoo and wild mammals. In: *Fowler's Zoo and Wild Animal Medicine*, vol. 8 (ed. R.E. Miller and M. Fowler), 596–603. St. Louis, MO: Elsevier Saunders.

13 Bouts, T., Dodds, J., Berry, K. et al. (2017). Detomidine and butorphanol for standing sedation in a range of zoo kept ungulate species. *Journal of Zoo and Wildlife Medicine* 48 (3): 616–626.

14 Kreeger, T.J., Arnemo, J.M., and Raath, J.P. (2012). *Handbook of Wildlife Chemical Immobilization*. Fort Collins, Colorado, U.S.A: Wildlife Pharmaceuticals Inc.

15 Lamberski, N., Newell, A., and Radcliffe, R.W.(2004). Thirty immobilizations of captive giraffe (*Giraffa camelopardalis*) using a combination of Medetomidine and Ketamine. *Annual Proceedings of the American Association of Zoo Veterinarians*. 118–120.

16 Kinney, A., Burton, M.S., Miller, J.E. et al. (2007). Effect of Copper oxide wire particles for controlling the parasitic nematode Haemonchus spp. in Giraffe (*Giraffa camelopardalis*). *Annual Proceedings of the American Association of Zoo Veterinarians*. 101.

17 Garretson, P.D., Hammond, E.E., Craig, T.M. et al. (2009). Anthelmintic resistant Haemonchus contortus in a Giraffe (*Giraffa camelopardalis*) in Florida. *Journal of Zoo and Wildlife Medicine* 40 (1): 131–139.
18 West, G., Hammond, E.E., and KuKanich, B. (2017). Pilot study: pharmacokinetics of oral and topical moxidectin in the reticulated Giraffe (*Giraffa camelopardalis*). *Journal of Zoo and Wildlife Medicine* 48 (2): 536–539.
19 Lechowski, R., Pisarski, J., Gosławski, J. et al. (1991). Exocrine pancreatic insufficiency-like syndrome in giraffe. *Journal of Wildlife Diseases* 27 (4): 728–730.

26

Deer

Drug name	Drug dose	Species	Comments
Antimicrobials and Antifungals			
Amikacin	7.5 mg/kg IM q4–6 hrs [1]	Fallow deer	n = 6 adult fallow deer, pharmacokinetic study.
Ceftiofur hydrochloride	3.5–3.8 mg/kg IM BID [2]	Fallow deer	n = six female adult deer/ pharmacokinetic study.
Ceftiofur sodium	250 mg IM BID [3]	Red deer	
Florfenicol (Nuflor)	40 mg/kg SC SID [4]	North American elk	
Penicillin G benzathine with procaine	22 000 IU/kg q48 hrs for 2 treatments [5]	Elk	n = 1 adult male with urinary obstruction, anesthetized for perineal urethrostomy and given postoperative antibiotics and pain control.
Penicillin G benzathine with procaine	44 000 IU/kg (20% IM, 80% SC) [6]	White-tailed deer	n = 19 female, free-ranging deer captured for tubal ligation for population control.
Tulathromycin	2.5 mg/kg SC [7]	White-tailed deer	n = 10 deer, single injection, pharmacokinetic study, effective at this dose, tissue concentrations persisted for 56 days indicating a longer withdrawal time than for cattle.
Analgesia			
Butorphanol	0.1–0.2 mg/kg IM [6]	White-tailed deer	n = 19 female, free-ranging deer captured for tubal ligation for population control.
Methadone	0.5–1 mg/kg IM [8]	Sika deer	n = 9 adult healthy deer, with a terminal elimination half-life of 8.19 hrs. No adverse effects.
Phenylbutazone	4 mg/kg SC EOD for 2 treatments [5]	Elk	n = 1 adult male with urinary obstruction, anesthetized for perineal urethrostomy.
Anesthesia and Sedation			
Acepromazine	DO NOT GIVE [9]	Fallow deer	Contraindicated due to hyperthermia and respiratory depression.

(*Continued*)

Zoo and Wild Mammal Formulary, First Edition. Alicia Hahn.

Drug name	Drug dose	Species	Comments
Azaperone + zuclopenthixol	A: 0.3 mg/kg + Z: 1 mg/kg [9]	White-tailed deer	Effective for translocating deer.
Butorphanol + azaperone + medetomidine	B: 0.51–0.65 mg/kg + A: 0.17–0.22 mg/kg + M: 0.2–0.26 mg/kg IM [10]	Caribou	n = 4 adult captive females, Worked well, smooth induction and recovery.
	B: 0.6 mg/kg + A: 0.4 mg/kg + M: 0.2 mg/kg IM; antagonize with naltrexone 1.2 mg/kg + atipamezole 1 mg/kg [9, 11–13]	Mule and White-tailed deer	In white tailed deer, BAM protocol is appropriate for semen collection.
	B: 0.11 mg/kg A: 0.07 mg/kg + M: 0.05 mg/kg IM [9, 12]	Elk	
Carfentanil	C: 0.006–0.03 mg/kg IM; antagonize with diprenorphine 0.06–0.3 mg/kg or naltrexone 0.06–0.03 mg/kg [12]	All cervids	
	C: 0.01 mg/kg; antagonize with naltrexone 1 mg/kg [9, 14]	Moose, Sika deer	Moose: If animal not down in 15 min repeat full dose. Addition of xylazine increases risk for aspiration pneumonia.
Carfentanil	C: 0.02 mg/kg IM [5]	Elk	n = 1 adult male with urinary obstruction, anesthetized for perineal urethrostomy.
	C: 0.06 mg/kg IM; antagonize with naltrexone 6 mg/kg [9]	Roe deer	
	C: 0.45 mg/kg IM; antagonize with naltrexone 1 mg/kg [9]	Hog deer	If animal not down in 20 min repeat full dose.
	C: 2.1 mg IM; antagonize with naltrexone 1 mg/kg [9]	Barasingha	If animal not down in 20 min repeat full dose. Prone to sudden leg kicks.
Carfentanil + xylazine	C: 0.001 mg/kg + X: 0.055 mg/kg IM; antagonize with tolazoline 1 mg/kg 1/4 IV and 3/4 IM [15]	Moose	n = 10 captive female moose anesthetized for a rumen bolus transmitter administration. Free-ranging animals were later anesthetized with C: 4–6 mg + X: 30–150 mg total per animal (n = 46) or thiafentanil 16 mg + X: 25 mg (n = 27). With tolazoline antagonized with 300–600 mg half IV, half IM.
	C: 0.004 mg/kg + X: 0.125 mg/kg IM; antagonize with naltrexone 0.4 mg/kg + yohimbine 0.125 mg/kg [9]	Axis deer	

Drug name	Drug dose	Species	Comments
	C: 0.004 mg/kg + X: 0.15 mg/kg IM; antagonize with naltrexone 0.4 mg/kg + tolazoline 2 mg/kg [9]	Red deer	
	C: 0.007 mg/kg + X: 0.05 mg/kg IM; antagonize with naltrexone 0.7 mg/kg + yohimbine 0.125 mg/kg [9]	Muntjacs	
	C: 0.01 mg/kg + X: 0.1 mg/kg IM; antagonize with naltrexone 1 mg/kg + tolazoline 2 mg/kg [9, 12, 14]	North American elk	Supplement with carfentanil 0.005 mg/kg as needed. For highly excited elk, dose of carfentanil can be increased to 0.013 mg/kg. Once immobilized, a small amount of naloxone 2 mg/mg carfentanil can improve oxygenation. However, monitor closely for spontaneous recovery.
	C: 0.013 mg/kg + X: 0.125 mg/kg; antagonize with naltrexone 1.3 mg/kg and yohimbine 0.125 mg/kg [9]	Fallow deer	
	C: 0.02 mg/kg + X: 0.24 mg/kg; antagonize with naltrexone 2 mg/kg and yohimbine 0.125 mg/kg [9]	Tule elk	If animal not down in 20 min repeat full dose.
	C: 0.03 mg/kg + X: 0.3 mg/kg; antagonize with naltrexone 3 mg/kg + yohimbine 0.15 mg/kg [9]	White-tailed deer	
Carfentanil + xylazine	C: 0.03 mg/kg + X: 0.7 mg/kg; antagonize with naltrexone 3 mg/kg + yohimbine 0.125 mg/kg [9]	Mule deer	
	C: 0.6 mg + X: 15 mg; antagonize with naltrexone 100 mg + yohimbine 0.125 mg/kg [9]	Sunda sambars	If animal not down in 15 min, repeat full dose.
	C: 2.1 mg + X: 30 mg in males; C: 1.2 mg + X: 15 mg in females [9]	Sambars	If animal not down in 15 min, repeat full dose. Antagonize with naltrexone 1 mg/kg + yohimbine 0.125 mg/kg.
Diazepam	0.5–2 mg/kg IV or PO [12]	All cervids	Sedation. Antagonize with flumazenil 0.04–0.15 mg/kg.
Diazepam + butorphanol + ketamine	D: 0.2 mg/kg IV + B: 0.05 mg/kg + K: 2–3 mg/kg [14]	White-tailed deer	Anesthesia in fawns.

(*Continued*)

Drug name	Drug dose	Species	Comments
Etorphine	E: 7.5 mg total (Adults); antagonize with diprenorphine 12 mg [9, 14]	Moose	For calves use half of etorphine dose. Addition of xylazine increases risk for aspiration pneumonia.
Etorphine + acepromazine	E: 0.02–0.05 mg/kg + A: 0.08–0.2 mg/kg IM [12]	All cervids	Antagonize with diprenorphine 0.027–0.066 mg/kg.
	E: 0.035 mg/kg + A: 0.14 mg/kg; antagonize with diprenorphine 0.7 mg/kg [9]	Red deer	
	E: 0.05 mg/kg + A: 0.2 mg/kg; antagonize with diprenorphine 0.1 mg/kg [9]	Sunda sambars, Sika deer	
	E: 0.06 mg/kg + A: 0.25 mg/kg; antagonize with diprenorphine 0.12 mg/kg [9]	Brow-antlered and Chinese water deer	
	E: 0.06 mg/kg + A: 0.025 mg/kg; antagonize with 2 mg diprenorphine per mg etorphine [9]	Reeve's muntjacs	
	E: 10 mg + A: 20 mg IM; antagonize with diprenorphine 2 mg/mg etorphine [9]	Roosevelt elk	Supplement with etorphine 5 mg as needed.
Etorphine hydrochloride + acepromazine maleate (Large Animal Immobilon solution)	(E: 2.45 mg/ml + A: 10 mg/ml) = LAI: 0.3 ml [9]	Pampas deer	If animal not down in 20 min repeat full dose. Antagonize with diprenorphine 2 mg per mg etorphine given.
	(E: 2.45 mg/ml + A: 10 mg/ml) = LAI: 4 ml [9]	Roosevelt elk	
Etorphine + acepromazine + xylazine	E: 0.01–0.06 mg/kg + A: 0.04–0.024 mg/kg + X: 0.25–0.6 mg/kg IM [12]	All cervids	Antagonize with diprenorphine 0.013–0.08 mg/kg IV + yohimbine or atipamezole.
Etorphine hydrochloride + acepromazine maleate (Large Animal Immobilon solution) + xylazine	(E: 2.45 mg/ml + A: 10 mg/ml) = LAI: 0.1 ml + X: 3 mg; antagonize with diprenorphine 2 mg per mg etorphine given [9].	Muntjacs	
	(E: 2.45 mg/ml + A: 10 mg/ml) = LAI: 0.3 ml + X: 5 mg; antagonize with diprenorphine 2 mg per mg etorphine given + yohimbine 0.125 mg/kg [9]	Roe deer	

Drug name	Drug dose	Species	Comments
	(E: 2.45 mg/ml + A: 10 mg/ml) LAI: 0.7 ml + X: 30 mg; antagonize with diprenorphine 2 mg per mg etorphine and yohimbine 0.125 mg/kg [9]	Sambars	
	(E: 2.45 mg/ml + A: 10 mg/ml) = LAI: 1.7 ml + X: 30 mg; antagonize with diprenorphine 2 mg and yohimbine 0.125 mg/kg [9]	Axis deer	
Etorphine + ketamine + xylazine	E: 1 mg + K: 100 mg + X: 100 mg IM; antagonize with diprenorphine 2 mg + yohimbine 0.125 mg/kg [9]	Barasinghas	
	E: 1 mg + K: 5 mg + X: 5 mg IM; antagonize with diprenorphine 2 mg + yohimbine 0.125 mg/kg [9]	Brocket deer	Supplement with ketamine 15 mg, IV if possible.
Etorphine + xylazine	E: 0.002 mg/kg + X: 0.2 mg/kg; antagonize with diprenorphine 2 mg per mg etorphine + yohimbine 0.125 mg/kg [9]	Roe deer	
	E: 0.015 mg/kg + X: 0.5 mg/kg; antagonize with diprenorphine 0.03 mg/kg + yohimbine 0.125 mg/kg [9]	Barasinghas	
	E: 0.02 mg/kg + X: 0.3 mg/kg; antagonize with diprenorphine 0.04 mg/kg + yohimbine 0.125 mg/kg [9]	Fallow deers	
	E: 0.03 mg/kg + X: 0.2 mg/kg; antagonize with diprenorphine 0.06 mg/kg + yohimbine 0.125 mg/kg [9]	Pere David's deer	
Etorphine + xylazine	E: 0.06 mg/kg + X: 0.3 mg/kg; antagonize with diprenorphine 0.12 mg/kg + yohimbine 0.125 mg/kg [9]	Caribou	
Etorphine + xylazine	E: 3 mg + X: 30 mg IM; antagonize with diprenorphine 6 mg + yohimbine 0.125 mg/kg [9]	Mule deer	

(*Continued*)

Drug name	Drug dose	Species	Comments
	E: 4 mg + X: 20 mg; antagonize with diprenorphine 8 mg [9]	Tule elk	
	E: 6 mg + X: 50 mg IM; antagonize with diprenorphine 12 mg + tolazoline 2 mg [9]	North American elk	Underdosing with etorphine can cause hyperexcitability, use a minimum of 0.02 mg/kg.
Etorphine + xylazine + acepromazine	E: 3.37 mg + X: 75 mg + A: 15 mg IM dart via helicopter [16]	Moose	n = 15 adult free-ranging animals, most to all were markedly hypoxemic, marked acidemia, and mild hypercapnia. Suggest alternate dose or treat with supplemental oxygen.
Fentanyl + azaperone	F: 0.21 mg/kg + A: 1.7 mg/kg [9]	Red deer	
Fentanyl + azaperone + xylazine	F: 3 mg + A: 24 mg + X: 30 mg IM; antagonize with naloxone 10 mg/mg fentanyl, tolazoline 2 mg/kg [9]	Axis Deer	
	F: 10 mg + A: 80 mg + X: 100 mg IM; antagonize with naloxone 0.2 mg/kg, tolazoline 2 mg/kg [9]	Sambars	
Ketamine + dexmedetomidine	K: 3 mg/kg + D: 0.04 mg/kg; antagonize with atipamezole 0.3 mg/kg [9]	Chinese water deer	
Ketamine + medetomidine	K: 0.8–3.2 mg/kg + M: 0.05–0.1 mg/kg IM; antagonize with atipamezole 0.25–0.5 mg/kg half IV half IM [12]	All cervids	
	K: 1 mg/kg + M: 0.03 mg/kg; antagonize with atipamezole 0.15 mg/kg half IV half IM [9]	Pere David's deer	Supplement with ketamine 0.5 mg/kg as needed.
	K: 1 mg/kg + M: 0.2 mg/kg; antagonize with atipamezole 1 mg/kg [9]	Caribou, Rein deer	Supplement with ketamine 0.5 mg/kg as needed. Reindeer: If not down in 20 min, repeat full dose.
	K: 200 mg + M: 10 mg IM dart from ground or helicopter, antagonize with atipamezole at 50 mg total [17].	Svalbard and Norwegian reindeer	n = 7 of each species, 7/7 Norwegian and 5/7 Svalbard were hypoxemic, 1–2 l/min nasal insufflation was required in all to correct.
	K: 1.5 mg/kg + M: 0.05 mg/kg IM; antagonize with atipamezole 0.25 mg/kg [9, 14]	Hog and Roe deer	
Ketamine + medetomidine	K: 1.5 mg/kg + M: 0.06–0.1 mg/kg IM; antagonize with atipamezole 0.3 mg/kg [9, 12]	Moose	

Drug name	Drug dose	Species	Comments
	K: 2 mg/kg + M: 0.07 mg/kg; antagonize with atipamezole 0.35 mg/kg [9]	North American elk	
	K: 2 mg/kg + M: 0.09 mg/kg; antagonize with atipamezole 0.4 mg/kg [9]	Huemals	Supplement with ketamine 1 mg/kg as needed.
	K: 2.2 mg/kg + M: 0.11 mg/kg IM; antagonize with atipamezole 0.5 mg/kg [9, 12, 14]	Red deer	Supplement with ketamine 1.1 mg/kg as needed.
	K: 2.5 mg/kg + M: 0.1 mg/kg IM; antagonize with atipamezole 0.5 mg/kg [9, 12, 14]	Fallow and White-tailed deer, Reindeer/Caribou	
	K: 1–2.5 mg/kg + M: 0.1–0.2 mg/kg IM; antagonize with atipamezole 0.5 mg/kg [14]	Reindeer	
	K: 2.5 mg/kg + M: 0.25 mg/kg IM, antagonized with atipamezole at 3 × the dose of medetomidine in mg [18].	Woodland caribou	n = 13 free-ranging animals.
	K: 3 mg/kg + M: 0.08 mg/kg IM; antagonize with atipamezole 0.4 mg/kg [9]	Chinese water deer	Supplement with ketamine 2 mg/kg as needed.
	K: 3 mg/kg + M: 0.1 mg/kg IM; antagonize with atipamezole 0.4 mg/kg [9]	Brow-antlered deer	Supplement with ketamine 1.5 mg/kg as needed.
	K: 3 mg/kg + M: 0.1 mg/kg IM; antagonize with atipamezole 0.5 mg/kg [9]	Mule deer	Supplement with ketamine 2 mg/kg as needed.
	K: 3.5 mg/kg + M: 0.1 mg/kg IM; antagonize with atipamezole 0.5 mg/kg [9, 14]	Axis deer	Supplement with ketamine 2 mg/kg as needed.
	K: 4 mg/kg + M: 0.06 mg/kg IM; antagonize with atipamezole 0.3 mg/kg [9]	Sika deer	Supplement with ketamine 2 mg/kg as needed.
Ketamine + medetomidine + Telazol	K: 1.5 mg/kg + M: 0.07 mg/kg + T: 1 mg/kg IM; antagonize with atipamezole 0.35 mg/kg [9]	White-tailed deer	
Ketamine + midazolam + xylazine	K: 7 mg/kg + Mid: 0.5 mg/kg + X: 0.3 mg/kg IM [14]	Brocket deer	
	K: 5 mg/kg + Mid: 0.5 mg/kg + X: 0.5 mg/kg IM [14]	Marsh deer	

(*Continued*)

Drug name	Drug dose	Species	Comments
Ketamine + xylazine	K: 1.5 mg/kg + X: 1 mg/kg IM; antagonized with yohimbine 5–10 mg/kg IV [19]	Axis deer	n = 25 females, good induction, no adverse effects,.
Ketamine + xylazine	K: 2.5 mg/kg + X: 0.5 mg/kg IM; antagonized with yohimbine 5–10 mg/kg IV [19]	Axis deer	n = 10 males, rapid induction of anesthesia,.
Ketamine + xylazine	K: 2.7–18.7 mg/kg + X: 0.5–23 mg/kg; antagonize with yohimbine or atipamezole [12]	All cervids	
Ketamine + xylazine	K: 2.5 mg/kg + X: 3 mg/kg; antagonize with yohimbine 0.125 mg/kg [9]	Sika deer	
Ketamine + xylazine	K: 3–4 mg/kg + X: 2 mg/kg IM; antagonize with atipamezole or yohimbine [12]	Mule and White-tailed deer	
Ketamine + xylazine	K: 3.3 mg/kg + X: 3.3 mg/kg; antagonize with yohimbine 0.125 mg/kg [9]	Muntjacs, Reeve's muntjacs	Supplement with ketamine 2 mg/kg as needed.
Ketamine + xylazine	K: 3–4 mg/kg + X: 1 mg/kg IM; antagonize with yohimbine or atipamezole [9, 12]	North American elk	
Ketamine + xylazine	K: 4 mg/kg + X: 2 mg/kg IM; antagonize with tolazoline 2 mg/kg [9]	North American elk	
Ketamine + xylazine	K: 4 mg/kg + X: 4 mg/kg; antagonize with yohimbine 0.125 mg/kg [9]	Axis Deer	Lower doses could be used on captive deer.
Ketamine + xylazine	K: 4 mg/kg + X: 4 mg/kg; antagonize with tolazoline 2 mg/kg [9]	Red deer	
Ketamine + xylazine	K: 4.5 mg/kg + X: 1.5 mg/kg; antagonize with yohimbine 0.125 mg/kg [9]	Himalayan musk deer	Supplement with ketamine 2.5 mg/kg as needed.
Ketamine + xylazine	K: 5 mg/kg + X: 3 mg/kg IM; antagonize with yohimbine 0.15 mg/kg [9]	Roe deer	Supplement with ketamine 2.5 mg/kg as needed.
Ketamine + xylazine	K: 5 mg/kg + X: 5 mg/kg IM; antagonize with yohimbine 0.125 mg/kg [9]	Fallow deer	
Ketamine + xylazine	K: 6 mg/kg + X: 1.2 mg/kg; antagonize with yohimbine 0.125 mg/kg [9]	Caribou	
Ketamine + xylazine	K: 7 mg/kg + X: 7 mg/kg IM; antagonize with yohimbine 0.125 mg/kg or tolazoline 2 mg/kg [9]	Chinese water and Mule deer	

Drug name	Drug dose	Species	Comments
Ketamine + xylazine	K: 7.5 mg/kg + X: 1.5 mg/kg IM; antagonize with yohimbine 0.125 mg/kg or tolazoline 2 mg/kg [9]	White-tailed deer	
Medetomidine	M: 0.08 mg/kg IM; antagonize with atipamezole 0.3 mg/kg [9]	Red deer	Calm or captive animals only.
Medetomidine + azaperone + alfaxalone	M: 0.15 mg/kg + Az: 0.2 mg/kg + Al: 0.5 mg/kg IM [20]	White-tailed deer	n = 8 captive deer, Provided deep sedation for handling and minor procedures.
Medetomidine + azaperone + alfaxalone	M: 0.15 mg/kg + Az: 0.2 mg/kg + Al: 0.5 mg/kg IM; antagonize with atipamezole at 5 × medetomidine dose in mg [21]	Mule deer	n = 28 deer, calm and rapid induction, supplemental drugs required in 5, 4 of which had dart failure, one debilitated nonurban animal died after antagonism.
Propofol	1 mg/kg IV q15 min [22]	Fallow deer	n = 6 cases used as adjunct for anesthetic procedure, with a relatively short period of respiratory depression seen after given.
Sufentanil + xylazine	S: 0.1 mg/kg + X: 0.5 mg/kg IM; antagonize with naltrexone 1 mg/kg + tolazoline 2 mg/kg [9]	North American elk	
Telazol	T: 2.6 mg/kg IM [9]	Axis deer	
Telazol	T: 2.9–20 mg/kg IM (33 mg/kg Fallow deer) [12]	All cervids	Antagonize with flumazenil 0.11–0.77 mg/kg.
Telazol	T: 5 mg/kg [9]	Caribou, Pere David's and Sika deer	
Telazol	T: 6 mg/kg IM [9]	Brow-antlered deer	
Telazol	T: 6.6 mg/kg IM [9]	Sambars, Philippine sambars	Philippine sambar: supplement with ketamine 3.3 mg/kg as needed.
Telazol	T: 8 mg/kg [9]	Reeve's muntjacs	
Telazol + medetomidine	T: 0.7–1.3 mg/kg + M: 0.08–0.12 mg/kg IM [12]	All cervids	
Telazol + medetomidine	T: 1 mg/kg + M: 0.1 mg/kg; antagonize with atipamezole 0.5 mg/kg half IV and half IM [9, 12, 14]	Fallow deer	

(*Continued*)

Drug name	Drug dose	Species	Comments
Telazol + xylazine (CRI Xylazine + ketamine + midazolam)	T: 1.5–2 mg/kg + X: 1.5–2 mg/kg IM, Then IV CRI of X: 0.45–0.55 mg/kg/hr + K: 1.8–2.2 mg/kg/hr + Mid: 0.027–0.033 mg/kg/hr [23]	Red deer	n = 16 captive female red deer. Antagonize with atipamezole 0.08–0.1 mg/kg + sarmazenil 7.5–9.8 µg/kg. Smooth induction, stable anesthesia, rapid recovery but supplemental oxygen is needed.
Telazol + xylazine	T: 2 mg/kg + X: 1 mg/kg IM [14]	White-tailed deer	
Telazol + xylazine	T: 2 mg/kg + X: 0.8 mg/kg IM [14]	Marsh deer	Free-ranging.
Telazol + xylazine	T: 2.5 mg/kg + X: 2.5 mg/kg IM; antagonize with tolazoline 2 mg/kg [9, 14]	Red deer	
Telazol + xylazine	T: 3 mg/kg + X: 0.2 mg/kg IM; antagonize with yohimbine 0.125 mg/kg [9]	Pere David's deer	
Telazol + xylazine	T: 3 mg/kg + X: 0.3 mg/kg IM; antagonize with yohimbine 0.125 mg/kg [9]	Brow-antlered deer	
	T: 3 mg/kg + X: 0.4 mg/kg IM; antagonize with tolazoline 2 mg/kg [9, 14]	North American elk	
	T: 3 mg/kg + X: 1.5 mg/kg IM [9, 12, 14]	Moose, White-tailed and Mule deer	
	T: 4.4 mg/kg + X: 2.2 mg/kg IM; antagonize with yohimbine 0.125 mg/kg or tolazoline 2 mg/kg [9, 12, 14]	Mule and White-tailed deer	Supplement with ketamine 2.2 mg/kg as needed.
	T: 5 mg/kg + X: 1 mg/kg [9]	Fallow deer	
Thiafentanil	T: 3 mg total IM; antagonize with 10 mg/kg naltrexone IM [12]	White-tailed deer	
	T: 10 mg total IM; antagonize with naltrexone 10 mg/kg IM [12]	Moose	OR: T: 0.03 mg/kg IM; antagonize with naltrexone 0.6 mg/kg.
	T: 0.04 mg/kg; antagonize with naltrexone 1 mg/kg [9, 14]	North American elk	T: 0.05–0.1 mg/kg range.

Drug name	Drug dose	Species	Comments
Thiafentanil + azaperone + xylazine	T: 1.5 mg + A: 25 mg + X: 20 mg IM, antagonized with tolazoline 2 mg/kg and 33 mg of naltrexone per 1 mg thiafentanil [24]	Caribou	n = 15 free-ranging female calves, anesthetized. medetomidine in place of xylazine resulted in 3 respiratory arrests and one death.
Thiafentanil + xylazine	T: 0.15 mg/kg + X: 1 mg/kg; antagonize with naltrexone 2 mg/kg + tolazoline 2 mg/kg [9, 14]	Mule deer	
	T: 0.1 mg/kg + X: 1 mg/kg; antagonize with naltrexone 2 mg/kg + tolazoline 2 mg/kg (or yohimbine 0.125 mg/kg) [9, 14]	Mule deer	
	T: 12–15 mg + X: 50 mg IM; antagonize with naltrexone [12]	North American elk	
	T: 10–12 mg + X: 100 mg (Or: T: 0.15–0.2 mg/kg + X: 100 mg total) [12]	Mule deer	Antagonize with naltrexone.
Thiafentanil + ketamine + xylazine	T: 0.02 mg/kg + K: 2 mg/kg + X; 1 mg/kg; antagonize with naltrexone 1 mg/kg + atipamezole 0.1 mg/kg [9]	Fallow deer	Supplement with 1/2 the original dose as needed.
Xylazine	X: 0.4–8 mg/kg IM (1/2 dose can be given IV) [12]	All cervids	Antagonize with yohimbine 0.1–0.2 mg/kg half IV and half IM.
	X: 0.5–1 mg/kg IM [12]	Red deer	
	X: 1 mg/kg IM; antagonize with atipamezole 0.04–0.8 mg/kg IV [9, 12, 14]	North American elk	
	X: 1 mg/kg IM; antagonize with yohimbine 0.125 mg/kg [9]	Pere David's deer	Only captive, calm animals.
	X: 2 mg/kg IM; antagonize with tolazoline 2 mg/kg [9]	North American Elk	Only captive, calm elk.
	X: 2–3 mg/kg IM [9, 12, 14]	White-tailed deer	Sedation
	X: 3 mg/kg IM; antagonize with tolazoline 2 mg/kg [9]	Red deer	Calm animals only.
	X: 3–4 mg/kg IM; antagonize with yohimbine 0.2 mg/kg or atipamezole 1 mg/8 mg xylazine [9]	Axis, Mule, and Roe deer	Calm animals only, sedation.

(Continued)

Drug name	Drug dose	Species	Comments
	X: 4 mg/kg; antagonize with yohimbine 0.2 mg/kg [9]	Hog and Sika deer	Calm animals only.
	X: 5 mg/kg IM; antagonize with idazoxan 0.06 mg/kg or yohimbine 0.125 mg/kg [9]	Caribou	Calm animals only.
Yohimbine	Y: 0.125 mg/kg [9]		Can be used instead of tolazoline.
Zuclopenthixol	1 mg/kg IM [25]	North American elk	n = not defined, but animals divided into treated and control groups and treated animals spent more time lying down and eating, while control animals had higher rectal temperatures, serum cortisol levels, blood lactate, acidosis, and CK levels. Drug appeared effective for 2–3 days.
Zuclopenthixol	1 mg/kg [26]	Waipiti	n = 32 males given 24 hrs prior to antler removal, suggest lidocaine ring block.
Antiparasitic			
Abamectin	0.2 mg/kg SC once [27]	Fallow deer	Pharmacokinetic study in adult deer, suggested effective parasite control at this dose.
Imidocarb dipropionate (Imizol)	3 mg/kg SC or IM on days 1, 2, 6, 9, and 21 [28]	Reindeer	n = 1 clinical animal and 2 non clinical animals with Babesia odocoilei successfully treated after a herd mate died.
Ivermectin	0.2–0.4 mg/kg SC [29]	White-tailed deer	n = 7 animals with Paralephostrongylus andersoni infestations – overall drug suppressed larval production by adult females for several weeks or destroyed first stage larvae in the lungs. Did not clear infestations.
	0.2 mg/kg in medicated corn/day/deer for several days or 0.4 mg/kg IM [30]	White-tailed deer	n = 11 animals with Psoroptes cuniculi (rabbit ear mites) infestation of the ears and body hair. Treated successfully.
Ivermectin	0.2 mg/kg SC [31]	Red deer	n = 5 calves given ivermectin then later euthanized and was 100% efficient in removing immature and mature Dictyocaulus viviparous. Plasma levels persist for over a week.
Ivermectin (Ivomec ovine liquid drench, Equine paste, or SC injection)	Do not use equine past as negatively affected plasma concentrations [32]	Reindeer	n = 26, 8 mo old calves administered 1 of 3 treatment solutions and equine oral paste was not as effective as ovine oral drench or SC administration.

Drug name	Drug dose	Species	Comments
Ivermectin sustained release varnish (Eudragit)	Varnish applied topically to wounds after larvae removed [33]	Persian fallow deer	n = 3 animals receiving injectable ivermectin 0.2 mg/kg SC, versus 5 animals with varnish painted on lesions. The former usually required 2 immobilizations with treatment and the latter, 1 anesthetic event.
Triclabendazole	10–14 mg/kg in medicated corn at bait stations combined with environmental control [34]	Fallow deer	Semi-free-ranging deer with management of environment and feeding medicated corn led to removal of parasite in population over 7 years.
	50–60 mg/kg PO rubmen drench [35]	Rocky Mountain elk	n = 12 animals (free-ranging, captured) given medication then culled at 4, 6, or 8 wks post treatment. Efficacy was 90% for immature flukes Fascioloides magna at 4 wks and 98% for adult flukes at all 3 time points.
Other			
Clostridium bacterin (Ultrabac 7)	4 ml SC [5]	Elk	n = 1 adult male with urinary obstruction, anesthetized for perineal urethrostomy and vaccinated.
Levetiracetam	40 mg/kg PO BID [36]	Reeve's muntjacs	n = 1 animal with seizures refractory to phenobarbitol that had only 1 breakthrough seizure in 10 months on levetiracetam.

Species	Weight [9, 12]
Barasingha *(Cervus duvauceli)*	172–181 kg
Caribou *(Rangifer tarandus)*	80–318 kg
Chevrotain *(Moshiola spp)*	2.4–3 kg
Chevrotain, Water *(Hyemoschus spp.)*	7–16 kg
Deer, Axis *(Axis axis)*	40–110 kg
Deer, Brocket *(Mazama rufina)*	8–25 kg
Deer, Brow-antlered *(Cervus eldi)*	75–150 kg
Deer, Chinese water *(Hydroptes inermis)*	11–30 kg
Deer, Fallow *(Dama dama)*	40–100 kg
Deer, Himalayan musk *(Moschus chrysogasters)*	7–17 kg
Deer, Hog *(Axis procinus)*	27–110 kg
Deer, Marsh *(Blastocerus spp.)*	70–130 kg
Deer, Mouse *(Tragulus spp.)*	1.5–4.5 kg
Deer, Mule *(Odocoileus hemionus)*	75–135 kg
Deer, Pampas *(Ozotoceros bezoarticus)*	25–40 kg
Deer, Pere David's *(Elaphurus davidianus)*	159–214 kg

(Continued)

Species	Weight [9, 12]
Deer, Red *(Cervus elaphus hippelaphus)*	60–180 kg
Deer, Roe *(Capreolus capreolus)*	15–50 kg
Deer, Sika *(Cervus nippon)*	40–80 kg
Deer, White-tailed *(Odocoileus virginianus)*	60–150 kg
Elk, North American *(Cervus canadensis)*	230–318 kg
Elk, Roosevelt *(Cervus canadensis roosevelti)*	Female 265–284 kg, Male 318–499 kg
Elk, Tule *(Cervus canadensis nannodes)*	150–182 kg
Huemal *(Hippocamelus bisculus)*	45–85 kg
Moose *(Alces alces)*	300–500 kg
Muntjac *(Muntiacus muntjak)*	14–28 kg
Muntjac, Reeves *(Muntiacus reevesi)*	14–28 kg
Pudu *(Pudu spp.)*	5–14 kg
Reindeer *(Rangifer tarandus tarandus)*	50–90 kg
Sambar *(Cervus unicolor)*	109–260 kg
Sambar, Phillipine *(Cervus mariannus)*	40–60 kg
Sambar, Sunda *(Cervus timorensis)*	53–73 kg

References

1 Heatley, J. (1997). Disposition of Amikacin in fallow deer (*Dama dama*). *Journal of Veterinary Pharmacology and Therapy* 20 (3): 243–245.

2 Kottwitz, J., Blue-McLendon, A., Monarski, C. et al. (2015). Disposition of ceftiofur and its active metabolites in fallow deer (*Dama dama*) following single-dose intravenous and intramuscular administration. *Journal of Zoo and Wildlife Medicine* 46 (2): 255–261.

3 Drew, M.L., Waldrup, K., Kreeger, T. et al. (2004). Pharmacokinetics of ceftiofur in red deer (*Cervus elephaus*). *Journal of Veterinary Pharmacology and Therapy* 27 (1): 7–11.

4 Alcorn, J., Dowling, P., Woodbury, M. et al. (2004). Pharmacokinetics of florfenicol in North American elk (*Cervus elaphus*). *Journal of Veterinary Pharmacology and Therapeutics* 27 (5): 289–292.

5 Larsen, R.S., Cebra, C.K., and Wild, M.A. (1997). Surgical correction of urethral obstruction in an elk (*Cervuselaphus*) by perinealurethrostomy. *Proceedings of the American Association of Zoo Veterinarians*. 51–53.

6 MacLean, R.A., Mathers, N.E., Frank, E.S. et al. (2002). Tubal ligation as a means of controlling a population of urban White-tailed deer: Preliminary results. *Proceedings of the American Association of Zoo Veterinarians*. 226–231.

7 Bachtold, K.A., Alcorn, J.M., Boison, J.O. et al. (2016). Pharmacokinetics and lung and muscle concentrations of tulathromycin following subcutaneous administration in white-tailed deer (*Odocoileus virginianus*). *Journal of Veterinary Pharmacology and Therapeutics* 39 (3): 292–298.

8 Scala, C., Marsot, A., Limoges, M.J. et al. (2015). Population pharmacokinetics of methadone hydrochloride after a single intramuscular administration in adult Japanese sika deer (*Cervus nippon nippon*). *Veterinary Anaesthesia and Analgesia* 42 (2): 165–172.

9 Kreeger, T.J. and Arnemo, J.M. (2012). *Handbook of Wildlife Chemical Immobilization*. China: Kreeger.

10 Hansen, C.M. and Beckmen, K.B. (2018). Butorphanol-azaperone-medetomidine for the immobilization of captive caribou (*Rangifer tarandus granti*). *Journal of Wildlife Diseases* 54 (3): 650–652.

11 Kirschner, S.M. (2017). Assessment of butorphanol-azaperone-medetomidine combination as anesthesia for semen collection and evaluation of semen quality in white-tailed deer (*Odocoileus virginianus*). *Animal Reproduction Science* 184: 196–203.

12 Masters, N.J. and Flach, E. (2015). Tragulidae, Moschidae, and Cervidae. In: *Fowler's Zoo and Wild Animal Medicine*, vol. 8 (ed. R.E. Miller and M. Fowler), 611–625. St. Louis, MO: Elsevier Saunders.

13 Siegal-Willott, J. (2009). Butorphanol, azaperone and medetomidine anesthesia in free-ranging white-tailed deer (*Odocoileus virginianus*) using radiotransmitter darts. *Journal of Wildlife Diseases* 45 (2): 468–480.

14 Caulkett, N. and Arnemo, J.M. (2014). Cervids. In: *Zoo Animal and Wildlife Immobilization and Anesthesia*, 2e (ed. G. West, D. Heard and N. Caulkett), 823–830. Ames, IA: Wiley Blackwell.

15 Minicucci, L., Carstensen, M., Crouse, J. et al. (2018). A technique for deployment of rumen bolus transmitters in free-ranging moose (*Alces alces*). *Journal of Zoo and Wildlife Medicine* 49 (1): 227–230.

16 Evans, A.L. (2012). Physiological evaluation of free-ranging moose (*Alces alces*) immobilized with etorphine-xylazine-acepromazine in Northern Sweden. *Acta Veterinaria Scandinavica* 31: 540.

17 Evans, A.L. (2013). Physiologic evaluation of medetomidine-ketamine anesthesia in free-ranging Svalbard (*Rangifer tarandus platyrhynchus*) and wild Norwegian reindeer (*Rangifer tarandus tarandus*). *Journal of Wildlife Diseases* 49 (4): 1037–1041.

18 Caulkett, N., Rettie, W.J., and Haigh, J.C. (1996). Immobilization of free-ranging woodland caribou (*Rangifer tarandus caribou*) with Medetomidine-Ketamine and reversal with atipamezole. *Proceedings of the American Association of Zoo Veterinarians*. 389–393.

19 Sontakke, S.D. (2007). Anesthesia induced by administration of xylazine hydrochloride alone or in combination with ketamine hydrochloride and reversal by administration of yohimbine hydrochloride in captive Axis deer (*Axis axis*). *American Journal of Veterinary Research* 68 (1): 20–24.

20 Pon, K., Caulkett, N., and Woodbury, M. (2015). Efficacy and safety of Medetomidine-Azaperone-Alfaxalone combination in captive white-tailed deer (*Odocoileus virginianus*). *Proceedings of the American Association of Zoo Veterinarians*. 76–77.

21 Mathieu, A. (2017). Capture of free-ranging mule deer (*Odocoileus hemionus*) with a combination of medetomidine, azaperone and alfaxalone. *Journal of Wildlife Diseases* 53 (2): 296–303.

22 Jalanka, H.H. and Teravained, E. (1992). Propofol: A potentially useful intravenous anesthetic agent in Nondomestic ruminants and camelids. *Proceedings of the American Association of Zoo Veterinarians*. 264–270.

23 Auer, U., Wenger, S., Begelbock, C. et al. (2010). Total intravenous anesthesia with midazolam, ketamine, and xylazine or detomidine following induction with tiletamine, zolazepam, and xylazine in red deer (*Cervus elaphus hippelaphus*) undergoing surgery. *Journal of Wildlife Diseases* 46 (4): 1196–1203.

24 Lian, M., Bechmen, K.B., Bentzen, T.W. et al. (2016). Thiafentanil-azaperone-xylazine and carfentanil-xylazine immobilizations of free-ranging caribou (*Rangifer tarandus granti*) in Alaska, USA. *Journal of Wildlife Diseases* 52 (2): 327–334.

25 Read, M.R., Caulkett, N.A., and McCallister, M. (2000).Use of Zuclopenthixol acetate to decrease handling stress in waipiti (*Cervus elaphus*). *Proceedings of the International Association of Aquatic Animal Medicine.*

26 Woodbury, M.R. (2001). Comparison of analgesic techniques for antler removal in wapiti. *Canadian Veterinary Journal* 42 (12): 929–935.

27 Zele, D., Tavcar-Kalcher, G., and Kobal, S. (2011). Plasma pharmacokinetics of abamectin in fallow deer (*Cervus dama dama*) following subcutaneous administration. *Journal of Veterinary Pharmacology and Therapy* 34 (5): 455–459.

28 Bartlett, S.L., Abou-madi, N., Messick, J.B. et al. (2009). Diagnosis and treatment of Babesia odocoilei in captive reindeer (*Rangifer tarandus tarandus*) and recognition of three novel host species. *Journal of Zoo and Wildlife Medicine* 40 (1): 152–159.

29 Samuel, W.M. and Gray, J.B. (1988). Efficacy of ivermectin against Paralephostrongylus andersoni (*Nematoda metastrongyloidea*) in white-tailed deer (*Odocoileus virginianus*). *Journal of Wildlife Diseases* 24 (3): 491–495.

30 Garris, G.I., Prullage, J.B., Prullage, J.L. et al. (1991). Control of Psoroptes cuniculi in captive white tailed deer with ivermectin treated corn. *Journal of Wildlife Diseases* 27 (2): 254–257.

31 Mackintosh, C.G., Mason, P.C., Manley, T. et al. (1985). Efficacy and pharmacokinetics of febantel and ivermectin in red deer (*Cervus elaphus*). *New Zealand Veterinary Journal* 33 (8): 127–131.

32 Oksanen, A., Asbakk, K., Raekallio, M. et al. (2014). The relative plasma availabilities of ivermectin in reindeer (*Rangifer tarandus tarandus*) following subcutaneous and two different oral formulation applications. *Acta Veterinaria Scandinavica* 25: 56–63.

33 Avni-Magen, N., Eshar, D., Friedman, M. et al. (2018). Retrospective evaluation of a novel sustained release ivermectin varnish for treatment of wound myiasis in zoo house animals. *Journal of Zoo and Wildlife Medicine* 49 (1): 201–205.

34 Trailovic, S.M., Marinikovic, D., and Kulisic, Z. (2016). Diagnosis and therapy of liver fluke (*Fascioloides magna*) infection in fallow deer (*Dama dama*). *Journal of Wildlife Diseases* 52 (2): 319–326.

35 Pybus, M.J., Onderka, D.K., and Cool, N. (1991). Efficacy of triclabendazole against natural infections of Fascioloides magna in wapiti. *Journal of Wildlife Diseases* 27 (4): 599–605.

36 Blatt, E.R., Seeley, K.E., Lovett, M.C. et al. (2017). Management of a reeve's muntjac (*Muntiacus reevesi*) with seizures using levetiracetam. *Journal of Zoo and Wildlife Medicine* 48 (4): 1197–1199.

27

Nondomestic Cattle and Antelope

Drug name	Drug dose	Species	Comments
Antimicrobials and Antifungals			
Amikacin	2.5% solution instilled into ear canal, and 6.5 mg/kg IM on day 1, 3, 17, and 31 [1]	Bongo	n = 1 animal with severe otitis media interna. Tried treating with enrofloxacin and trimethoprim sulfa orally to no avail, then started Amikacin and gave topical and IM treatments when immobilized. Resolved 24 days after starting Amikacin.
Amikacin or cefazolin mixed with polymethyl methacrylate (PMMA)	A: 1.25 g mixed with 20 g PMMA powder and solution [1]	Bongo	n = 1 captive animal with severe otitis media-interna that eventually underwent a total ear canal ablation and bulla osteotomy. Antibiotic impregnated PMMA beads placed in surgical site. Unfortunately incision dehisced postop and beads fell out. Managed as open wound and healed.
Ampicillin sodium + enrofloxacin	A: 20 mg/kg IV + E: 10 mg/kg IV [2]	Gerenuk	n = 1 captive female with ectopic pregnancy that during removal was treated with IV antibiotics.
Amoxicillin trihydrate + enrofloxacin	A: 15 mg/kg SC BID and E: 5 mg/kg SC BID × 14d [2]	Gerenuk	n = 1 captive female with ectopic pregnancy that during removal was treated SC postoperatively.
Cefovecin	10 mg/kg SID to BID [3]	Soemmering's, Arabian, and Speke's gazelles	Not long-acting in these species.
Ceftiofur (Naxcel)	4.5 mg/kg IM [4]	Lesser kudu	n = 1 animal with vasculitis and edema of hind limbs secondary to leptospirosis infection. Initially improved with supportive care, then required long-term steroids for full resolution.

(Continued)

Zoo and Wild Mammal Formulary, First Edition. Alicia Hahn.

Drug name	Drug dose	Species	Comments
	2 mg/kg IM SID × 10d [5]	Eastern Bongo	n = 1 animal with chronic vaginal prolapse, treated with ovariohysterectomy and postoperative antibiotics.
Ceftiofur hydrochloride 5%	2.2 mg/kg IM q48 h–72 hrs [6]	Asian water buffalo	5% solution, Guangxi Beidouxing Animal Drugs company.
Ceftiofur hydrochloride 5% (Excenel)	2.2 mg/kg IM SID [6]	Asian water buffalo	Excenel 5% Pfizer Inc.
Ceftiofur sodium	1–2 mg/kg nebulized SID [7]	Tibetan yaks	n = 2 animals post castration (recumbent). Severe pneumonia. 1 died and 1 survived.
	1.1 mg/kg IM SID × 36d [8]	Roan antelope	n = 1 animal with fractured femur. Given 2 days prior and for 34 days post repair.
Difloxacin (Dicurel)	6.7 mg/kg PO BID or 12.2 mg/kg PO SID [1]	Bongo	May have improved palatability and oral acceptance by ruminants over enrofloxacin orally. Given in 1 bongo with severe otitis interna-media along with topical treatment.
Enrofloxacin	1.6 mg/kg IV q6–8 hrs [9]	Scimitar-horned oryx	n = 5 animals for pharmacokinetic study.
	2.7 mg/kg IM SID [4]	Lesser kudu	n = 1 animal with vasculitis and edema of hind limbs secondary to leptospirosis infection. Initially improved with supportive care, then required long-term steroids and antibiotics for full resolution.
Enrofloxacin	100 mg PO SID [10]	Dorcas gazelles	n = 1 animal postoperative surgical repair of stifle. 2 wks later 50% reduction in joint motion. Later euthanized for severe pedal osteoarthritis.
Florfenicol	20 mg/kg SC SID × 7d [2]	Gerenuk	n = 1 female with pneumonia that appeared to improve/resolve.
Fluconazole	10 mg/kg PO SID (lower doses did not result in sufficient serum levels) [11]	Kirk's dik-diks	n = 1 animal diagnosed with coccidioidomycosis and treated for 23 mo with resolution of clinical signs and improvement in blood work and titer values.
Gentamicin + trimethoprim sulfamethoxazole (TMS)	G: 2 mg/kg IM SID × 10d and TMS: 30 mg/kg PO SID × 40d [12]	Bongo	n = 1 male with urethral rupture and ultimately surgical removal of penis and scrotal urethrostomy. Treated postoperatively with antibiotics and allowed to heal with 2nd intention, Resolved.

Drug name	Drug dose	Species	Comments
Oxytetracycline (LA 200)	20 mg/kg IM q48 hrs × 30d [1]	Bongo	n = 1 captive animal with severe otitis media-interna that eventually underwent a total ear canal ablation and bulla osteotomy. Treated postoperatively with antibiotics and resolved.
Procaine penicillin G	40 000 IU/kg BID SQ [4]	Lesser kudu	n = 1 animal with vasculitis and edema of hind limbs secondary to leptospirosis infection. Initially improved with supportive care, then required long-term steroids for full resolution.
Penicillin G with benzathine and procaine (Pen BP 48)	300 000 IU q48 hrs for 3 treatments [10]	Dorcas gazelles	n = 1 animal post necrotic mass excision.
Trimethoprim sulfadimethoxine	35.5 mg/kg PO BID × 20d [1]	Bongo	n = 1 animal with severe otitis media-interna. Treated with oral antibiotics and topical solution of gentamicin 100 mg + dimethylsulfoxide 5 ml + 10 ml silver sulfadiazine ointment instilled into canal daily for 4 days, Resolved.
Trimethoprim sulfadimethoxazole	24 mg/kg PO SID [5]	Eastern bongo	n = 1 animal with chronic vaginal prolapse post dystocia.
Tulathromycin	2.5 mg/kg SC q120 hrs [7]	Tibetan yaks	n = 2 animals post castration (recumbent). Severe pneumonia. 1 died and 1 survived.
Analgesia			
Aspirin	650 mg PO SID × 3d [10]	Dorcas gazelles	n = 1 animal postoperative repair of medial patellar luxation and torn cruciate ligament.
Detomidine	0.04 mg/kg IM epidural administration [13]	Domestic cattle	
Etodolac	75 mg PO SID [10]	Dorcas gazelles	n = 1 animal postoperative surgical repair of stifle injury.
Flunixin meglumine	0.5 mg/kg SID IM [8]	Roan antelope	n = 1 animal with fractured femur. Given 2 days prior and for 2 days post repair.
	1.1–2.2 mg/kg IM, IV, or PO [4, 5, 13]	Dairy and beef cattle, Lesser kudu (n = 1), Eastern bongo (n = 1)	1 mg/kg PO SID in an Eastern bongo with chronic vaginal prolapse.
Flunixin meglumine	1.1 mg/kg IV q12 hr [7]	Tibetan yaks	n = 2 animals post castration (recumbent). Severe pneumonia. One died and 1 survived.

(Continued)

Drug name	Drug dose	Species	Comments
Gabapentin + meloxicam (JS1)	G: 10 mg/kg PO (capsules or powder) + M: 0.5 mg/kg [13, 14]	Domestic cattle	For neuropathic pain.
Ketoprofen	30 mg IV once [10]	Dorcas gazelles	n = 1 animal pre-operative surgical repair of stifle injury.
	2 mg/kg PO SID × 5d [5]	Eastern bongo	n = 1 animal postoperative analgesia after ovariohysterectomy.
	3 mg/kg IV [13]	Domestic calves and bulls	Calves undergoing horn debudding and bulls for castration.
	0.13 mg/kg IM [12]	Bongo	n = 1 male with urethral rupture and ultimately surgical removal of penis and scrotal urethrostomy that was treated intraoperatively with ketoprofen.
Meloxicam	0.5 mg/kg PO SID [13]	Domestic cattle	
	1 mg/kg PO SID × 4d [7]	Tibetan yaks	n = 1 animal post castration (recumbent). Postoperative analgesia.
	52.5 mg PO SID × 10d [15]	Greater kudu	n = 1, 5 yr old male with front-foot phalanx 3 fractures bilaterally. Treated intermittently with phenylbutazone. Spent 5 mo mostly lying down, but treatment with meloxicam resulted in more standing. Ultimately healed.
Phenylbutazone	2.8 mg/kg PO BID for 7–14d [15]	Lesser kudu	n = 1 animal with phalanx 3 avulsion fracture. Healed ultimately with wooden blocks on contralateral toes over 3 mo.
	10–20 mg/kg PO then 2.5–5 mg/kg SID or 10 mg/kg q48 hrs. Another option: 9 mg/kg PO then 4.5 mg/kg q48 hrs [13]	Domestic cattle	
	750 mg PO SID × 5d [15]	Greater kudu	n = 1 female with lameness associated with fracture of phalanx 3 and avulsion of tendon. Mild lameness persisted for 2 mo despite treatment. Corrective hoof trimming assisted every 2–3 mo. 9 mo later radiographs confirmed resolution.

Drug name	Drug dose	Species	Comments
	1000 mg po SID × 10d [15]	Greater kudu	n = 1, 5 yr. old male with front foot phalanx 3 fractures bilaterally. Spent 5 mo mostly lying down, but treatment with meloxicam at 52.5 mg PO SID for 14 days resulted in more standing. Ultimately healed.
Anethesia and Sedation			Additional doses for neuroleptics in African antelope species can be found in West 2: CH 60, Ball and Hofmeyr.
Acepromazine	0.05–0.1 mg/kg IM [13]	Domestic cattle	Sedation, onset in 10–20 min. Duration: 4–12 hrs.
Atipamezole	Antagonist for: medetomidine 5 mg/mg IM, for detomidine: 0.1 mg/kg IM, for xylazine: 0.1 mg/kg IM [16]	Bovidae	
Azaperone	IV or IM [16]	Bovidae	IV onset: <10 min, duration: ≤6 hrs. IM onset: 30 min, IM duration ≤6 hrs.
	0.5 mg/kg [16]	Aepycerotinae	
	0.3–1 mg/kg [16]	Alcelaphinae	
	0.25–0.5 mg/kg [16]	Antilopinae	
	0.1–0.5 mg/kg [16]	Bovinae	
	0.5–1 mg/kg [16]	Cephalophinae	
	0.5 mg/kg [16]	Hippotraginae	
	0.5–1 mg/kg [16]	Reduncinae	
	0.1 mg/kg [13]	African buffalo	Sedation
Butorphanol + azaperone + medetomidine	B: 0.3 mg/kg + A: 0.14 mg/kg + M: 0.07 mg/kg; antagonize with tolazoline 4 mg/kg + naltrexone 0.2 mg/kg [17]	American bison	
	B: 0.75 mg/kg + A: 0.7 mg/kg + M: 0.3 mg/kg [17]	Pronghorn	
Butorphanol + detomidine + midazolam	B: 0.15–0.25 mg/kg + D: 0.15–0.25 mg/kg and Mid: 0.23–0.38 mg/kg IM; antagonized with atipamezole 0.25 mg/kg IM [18]	Nile lechwes	n = 9 captive animals, hyperthermia in 3 with insufficient immobilization post darting. Recovery was smooth.

(*Continued*)

Drug name	Drug dose	Species	Comments
Butorphanol + ketamine + medetomidine	B: 0.36–0.44 mg/kg + K: 4.3–5.5 mg/kg + M: 0.036–0.043 mg/kg IM via hand injection; antagonize with naloxone 0.02 mg/kg + atipamezole 0.17–0.23 mg/kg IM [19]	Thompson's gazelles	n = 9 captive juveniles, 7 undergoing castration. Bradycardia <60 bpm and hypoventilation seen. Recommend to add supplemental oxygen. Local lidocaine (see other drug section) administered for castrations.
Carfentanil	0.006–0.008 mg/kg; antagonize with naltrexone 0.6–0.8 mg/kg IM [13]	African buffalo	
	0.016–0.02 mg/kg IM; antagonized with naltrexone 1.5–2.1 mg/kg half IV half SC [20]	Dama gazelles	n = 16 captive born animals, weighing 38–58 kg. Supplemental oxygen recommended.
	0.018–0.2 mg/kg; antagonize with naltrexone 2 mg/kg [16, 17]	Lechwes	If animal is not down in 20 min, repeat full dose.
	0.018–0.2 mg/kg [21]	Gazelles and small antelope	
	0.02 mg/kg [16]	Gaur	
	0.025 mg/kg; antagonize with naltrexone 2.5 mg/kg [16, 17]	Addax, Black, Jentink's, Maxwell's, Red-flanked, Yellow-backed and Zebra duikers	If animal is not down in 20 min, repeat full dose. Duiker: 0.026 mg/kg carfentanil.
	0.03 mg/kg; antagonize with naltrexone 3 mg/kg [16, 17]	Springbok	
Carfentanil	0.035 mg/kg; antagonize with naltrexone 3.5 mg/kg [16, 17]	Dama, Dorcas, Grant's, Mountain, Persian, Slender-horned, and Soemmering's gazelles	If animal is not down in 20 min, repeat full dose. Captive animals 0.018 mg/kg carfentanil may be suitable. Species prone to excessive running during induction with carfentanil.
	0.05 mg/kg [16]	Blackbuck	
	0.05–0.1 mg/kg [16]	Saigas	
	1 mg; antagonize with naltrexone 100 mg [17]	Sitatunga	
	Males: 1.2 mg, Females: 1 mg; antagonize with naltrexone 120 mg [17]	Thompson's gazelles	Or consider: 0.02–0.03 mg/kg. If animal is not down in 20 min, repeat full dose.
	1.5 mg; antagonize with naltrexone 1 mg/kg [17]	Blackbuck, Bongo	Bongo: 2 mg males, 1.5 mg females.

Drug name	Drug dose	Species	Comments
	Males: 2.1 mg (Females: 1.5 mg); antagonize with naltrexone 1 mg/kg [17]	Nile lechwes	If animal is not down in 20 min, repeat full dose.
	Males: 4 mg, Females: 3 mg; antagonize with naltrexone 100 mg/mg carfentanil [17]	Nilgais	Or consider: 0.02 mg/kg IM. If animal is not down in 20 min, repeat full dose.
Carfentanil + acepromazine + detomidine + ketamine	C: 0.012 mg/kg + A: 0.04 mg/kg + D: 0.12 mg/kg + K: 0.4 mg/kg IM; antagonize with naltrexone 1.2 mg/kg and yohimbine 0.33 mg/kg [13]	Watusi/Ankole	
Carfentanil + azaperone	Females: C: 1.8–2.2 mg + A: 40 mg IM; Males: C: 2.2–2.3 mg + A: 40 mg IM; antagonize with naltrexone at 100 × the dose of carfentanil in mg [22]	Addax	n = 65 routine exams from 2008 through 2018, no significant complications reported.
Carfentanil + detomidine	C: 0.008 + D: 0.03 mg/kg [16]	Giant eland	
Carfentanil + detomidine + ketamine	C: 0.006–0.01 mg/kg + D: 0.019–0.029 mg/kg + K: 0.3 mg/kg IM; antagonize with atipamezole 0.1 mg/kg + naltrexone 0.6–1 mg/kg IM [13]	Watusi/Ankole	
	C: 0.01–0.017 mg/kg + D: 0.009–0.014 mg/kg + K: 0.33–2.78 mg/kg IM; antagonize with atipamezole 0.05 mg/kg + naltrexone 1–1.7 mg/kg IM [13]	Bantengs	Immobilization.
Carfentanil + ketamine + xylazine	C: 0.005 mg/kg + K: 0.06–0.09 mg/kg + X: 0.125 mg/kg; antagonize with naltrexone 0.5 mg/kg [13]	Gaur	
Carfentanil + ketamine + xylazine	C: 0.007 mg/kg + K: 0.15 mg/kg + X: 0.11 mg/kg; antagonize with naltrexone 0.7 mg/kg [13, 17]	Bantengs	
	C: 0.011–0.012 mg/kg + K: 1.55–2.5 mg/kg + X: 0.06–0.13 mg/kg; antagonize with naltrexone 1.1–1.2 mg/kg, yohimbine 0.11–0.12 mg/kg [13]	Forest buffalo	

(*Continued*)

Drug name	Drug dose	Species	Comments
	C: 0.015–0.025 mg/kg + K: 1.5–2.5 mg/kg + X: 0.2–0.35 mg/kg [16]	Bontebok/Blesbok	
	C: 0.02 mg/kg + K: 1–2 mg/kg + X: 0.25 mg/kg [16]	Nile lechwes	
	C: 1.4 mg + K: 80 mg + X: 20 mg; antagonize with naltrexone 140 mg + yohimbine 1.5 mg/kg [16, 17]	Bongo	Or consider: C: 0.01 mg/kg + K: 0.5 mg/kg + X: 0.15–0.2 mg/kg. For adults. If animal is not down in 20 min, repeat full dose.
	C: 2.5 mg + K: 40 mg + X: 40 mg; antagonize with naltrexone 1 mg/kg + yohimbine 0.125 mg/kg [17]	Greater kudu	
	C: 3 mg + K: 50 mg + X: 50 mg; antagonize with naltrexone 1 mg/kg + yohimbine 0.125 mg/kg [17]	Sable antelope	
Carfentanil + xylazine	C: 0.0075 mg/kg + X: 0.1 mg/kg; antagonize with naltrexone 0.75 mg/kg [13]	Yaks	
	C: 0.001–0.008 mg/kg + X: 0.05–0.25 mg/kg; antagonize with naltrexone 0.1–0.8 mg/kg [13]	Bantengs	
Carfentanil ± xylazine	C: 0.015–0.029 mg/kg ± X: 0.1–0.25 mg/kg [16, 23]	Nyala	
	C: 0.015–0.02 mg/kg ± X: 0.2 mg/kg [16]	Addra gazelles	
Carfentanil + xylazine	C: 0.004 mg/kg + X: 0.07 mg/kg; antagonize with naltrexone 0.4 mg/kg + yohimbine 0.125 mg/kg [17]	Feral cattle	Supplement with carfentanil 0.004 mg/kg as needed.
	C: 0.002–0.005 mg/kg + X: 0.028–0.05 mg/kg; antagonize with naltrexone 02–0.5 mg/kg + yohimbine 0.05 mg/kg [13, 16, 17]	African buffalo	If animal is not down in 20 min, repeat full dose.
Carfentanil + xylazine	C: 0.005–0.007 mg/kg + X: 0.05–0.1 mg/kg [16, 24]	Giant eland	n = 6 adult females for pharmacokinetic study. Also consider for adult females: C: 0.016–0.017 mg/kg IM + X: 0.2–0.26 mg/kg IM; antagonize with naltrexone 1.6–1.74 mg/kg IM.

Drug name	Drug dose	Species	Comments
	C: 0.004–0.008 mg/kg + X: 0.05–0.1 mg/kg; antagonize with naltrexone 0.5 mg/kg + yohimbine 0.125 mg/kg [16, 17, 25]	American bison	Supplement with X: 0.05–0.1 mg/kg IV to improve relaxation.
	C: 0.006 mg/kg + X: 0.15 mg/kg; antagonize with naltrexone 0.6 mg/kg + yohimbine 0.125 mg/kg [17]	Impala	
	C: 0.006–0.03 mg/kg + X: 0.05–0.25 mg/kg; antagonize with naltrexone 0.75–3 mg/kg + yohimbine 0.1 mg/kg [13, 16, 17]	Gaur	Supplement with carfentanil 0.0075 mg/kg as needed.
	C: 0.008–0.03 mg/kg + X: 0.05–0.25 mg/kg; antagonize with naltrexone 1–3 mg/kg [13,]	Anoa	
	C: 0.008 mg/kg + X: 0.08 mg/kg [16]	Wildebeests	
	C: 0.008–0.016 mg/kg + X: 0.15–0.2 mg/kg; antagonize with naltrexone 0.8 mg/kg + yohimbine 0.1 mg/kg [16, 17, 23]	Eland	If animal is not down in 20 min, repeat full dose.
	C: 0.01 mg/kg + X: 0.1 mg/kg; antagonize with naltrexone 1 mg/kg + yohimbine 0.125 mg/kg [17]	Roan antelope, Bontebok/Blesbok, Hartebeests, Greater kudu, Steenbok, Topi/Tsessebe's Waterbuck, Lechwes	Hartebeest: Difficult to immobilize, may substitute azaperone 70 mg for xylazine. Topi/Tsessebe: hyaluronidase 1500–3000 IU may be added to decrease induction time.
	C: 0.01 mg/kg + X: 0.15 mg/kg [16]	Hartebeests, Bongo	
	C: 0.01 mg/kg + X: 0.1–0.25 mg/kg [16]	Waterbuck	
	C: 0.015–0.02 mg/kg + X: 0.15–0.2 mg/kg [16, 23]	Roan antelope	
	C: 0.01 mg/kg + X: 0.25 mg/kg; antagonize with naltrexone 1 mg/kg + atipamezole 0.0025 mg/kg [17]	Yaks	Supplement with carfentanil 0.005 mg/kg as needed.
	C: 0.01 mg/kg + X: 0.4 mg/kg; antagonize with naltrexone 1 mg/kg + yohimbine 0.25 mg/kg [16, 17, 26]	Gray rhebok	A study of 12 adults showed that etorphine 0.01 mg/kg instead of carfentanil, resulted in better anesthetic episodes and shorter recovery times.

(*Continued*)

Drug name	Drug dose	Species	Comments
Carfentanil + xylazine	C: 0.015–0.02 mg/kg + X: 0.15–0.2 mg/kg [16, 23]	Sable antelope	
	C: 0.01–0.02 mg/kg + X: 0.1–0.2 mg/kg; antagonize with naltrexone 2 mg/kg + yohimbine 0.125 mg/kg [16, 17]	Gemsbok	If animal is not down in 20 min, repeat full dose.
	C: 0.02 mg/kg ± X: 0.2–0.5 mg/kg IM [21]	Gazelles and small antelope	
	C: 0.02–0.03 mg/kg ± X: 0.1–0.2 mg/kg [16]	Impala, Yellow-backed duikers	
	C: 0.021 mg/kg ± X: 0.21 mg/kg IM [23]	Blue wildebeests	
	C: 0.022 mg/kg ± X: 0.22 mg/kg IM [23]	Defassa Water-buck	
	C: 0.024 mg/kg + X: 0.24 mg/kg [23]	Bongo	
	C: 0.025 mg/kg + X: 0.15–0.25 mg/kg [16, 23]	Addax, Bontebok/Blesbok	
	C: 0.026 mg/kg + X: 0.26 mg/kg [23]	Greater kudu	Higher dose of narcotic reduces pacing but is still common.
	C: 0.035 mg/kg + X: 0.35 mg/kg [23]	Uganda kobs	
	C: 0.03–0.05 mg/kg + X: 0.1–0.25 mg/kg [16]	Slender-horned gazelles	
	C: 0.03 mg/kg + X: 0.2 mg/kg [23]	Impala	
	C: 0.035 mg/kg + X: 0.35 mg/kg [16]	Uganda kobs	
	C: 0.04 mg/kg + X: 0.3 mg/kg [16, 23]	Sitatungas	
	C: 0.05 mg/kg + X: 1 mg/kg; antagonize with naltrexone 5 mg/kg + yohimbine 0.125 mg/kg [16, 17]	Pronghorn	If animal is not down in 20 min, repeat full dose.
	C: 1.5 mg + X: 35 mg; antagonize with naltrexone 100 mg/mg carfentanil and yohimbine 0.125 mg/kg [17]	European bison	If animal is not down in 20 min, repeat full dose.
	Males: C: 2.1 mg (Females: C: 1.5 mg) + X: 5 mg; antagonize with naltrexone 1 mg/kg + yohimbine 0.125 mg/kg [17]	Uganda kobs	

Drug name	Drug dose	Species	Comments
	C: 3 mg + X: 5 mg; antagonize with naltrexone 3 mg/kg + yohimbine 0.125 mg/kg [16, 17, 23]	Arabian oryx	Or consider: C: 0.03–0.04 mg/kg + X: 0.25 mg/kg IM. If animal is not down in 15 min, repeat full dose.
Carfentanil + xylazine	C: Males: 3 mg (Females: 2.5 mg) + X: 10 mg; antagonize with naltrexone 3 mg/kg + yohimbine 0.125 mg/kg [17, 23]	Scimitar-horned oryx	Or consider: C: 0.015–0.3 mg/kg + X: 0.15–0.3 mg/kg IM. If animal is not down in 15 min, repeat full dose.
Detomidine	0.01 mg/kg IV [13]	Non domestic cattle	Standing sedation. To prolong effect add butorphanol 0.05 mg/kg. In domestic cattle, 0.04 mg/kg detomidine used for standing sedation. For domestic calves 0.01 mg/kg for light sedation and 0.02–0.04 mg/kg for deeper sedation.
Detomidine + butorphanol	D: 0.04–0.06 mg/kg + B: 0.03–0.06 mg/kg IM [27]	Wisents, Yaks, Asian water buffalo	Standing sedation.
	D: 0.06–0.08 mg/kg + B: 0.05–0.09 mg/kg; antagonize with yohimbine 0.2–0.22 mg/kg and naltrexone 0.84–0.88 mg/kg [13]	Bantengs	Sedation
	D: 0.05–0.08 mg/kg + B: 0.08–0.2 mg/kg; antagonize with atipamezole 0.03–0.15 mg/kg and naltrexone 0.05–1 mg/kg [13]	Watusi/Ankole	Sedation
	D: 0.15–0.2 mg/kg + B: 0.13–0.15 mg/kg IM [27]	Bongo	Standing sedation.
Detomidine + butorphanol + ketamine	D: 0.07–0.104 mg/kg + B: 0.07–0.083 mg/kg + K: 0.7–2.13 mg/kg IM; antagonize with yohimbine 0.2 mg/kg + naltrexone 0.7–0.9 mg/kg [13]	Bantengs	Immobilization.
Detomidine + diazepam + ketamine	Det: 0.01 mg/kg + Dia: 0.01 mg/kg + K: 3 mg/kg [13]	Asian water buffalo calves	
Detomidine + xylazine	D: 0.0025–0.01 mg/kg + X: 0.05–0.2 mg/kg IV or IM [13]	Non domestic cattle	Sedation
Diazepam	0.5–1 mg/kg IM or IV [21]	Gazelles and small antelope	Sedation for several hours.

(*Continued*)

Drug name	Drug dose	Species	Comments
Etorphine	0.01–0.02 mg/kg [16]	Gaur	
	0.023 mg/kg; antagonize with diprenorphine 0.05 mg/kg [17]	Bongo	
	0.03–0.06 mg/kg IM [16]	Addra gazelles	
	0.03 mg/kg IM [16]	Gaur	
	0.05 mg/kg [16]	Klipspringers	
	2.4 mg; antagonize with diprenorphine 5.8 mg [17]	Dama gazelles	
	2.5 mg/kg; antagonize with diprenorphine 5 mg/kg [17]	Mountain gazelles	
	3 mg; antagonize with diprenorphine 6 mg [16, 17]	Blackbuck	Or consider: 0.1 mg/kg.
Etorphine	5 mg; antagonize with diprenorphine 2 mg/mg etorphine given [17]	Sitatungas	
	6 mg; antagonize with diprenorphine 2 mg/mg etorphine given [17]	Nilgais	Or consider: 0.03 mg/kg IM.
	8 mg; antagonize with diprenorphine 16 mg [17]	Zebus	
Etorphine + acepromazine	E: 0.015 mg/kg + A: 0.15 mg/kg; diprenorphine 0.03 mg/kg [13, 28]	African buffalo, Impala	n = 9 female Impala. Resulted in good induction, muscle relaxation and recovery when compared to Ket + Med.
	E: 0.018–0.024 mg/kg + A: 0.07–0.1 mg/kg; diprenorphine 0.036–0.048 mg/kg [13]	Forest buffalo	
	E: 0.02 mg/kg + A: 0.1 mg/kg; antagonize with diprenorphine 2 mg/mg etorphine [17]	Tamaraws	Supplement with etorphine 0.01 mg/kg as needed.
	E: 0.024–0.034 mg/kg + A: 0.1–0.14 mg/kg; antagonize with diprenorphine 0.048–0.068 mg/kg [13]	Watusi/Ankole	
Etorphine + acepromazine maleate (Large Animal Immobilon solution = E: 2.45 mg/ml + A: 10 mg/ml)	LAI: 1 ml; antagonize with diprenorphine 2 mg/mg etorphine [17]	Uganda kobs	

Drug name	Drug dose	Species	Comments
Etorphine + acepromazine + detomidine + ketamine	E: 0.016 + 0.019 mg/kg + A: 0.04–0.05 mg/kg + D: 0.005 mg/kg + K: 0.48–0.5 mg/kg IM; antagonize with naltrexone 1.8 mg/kg [13]	Watusi/Ankole	
Etorphine + acepromazine + xylazine (Large Animal Immobil on solution = E: 2.45 mg/ml + A: 10 mg/ml)	LAI: 0.1 ml + X: 2.5 mg; antagonize with diprenorphine 2 mg/mg etorphine and yohimbine 0.125 mg/kg [17]	Dorcas gazelles	
	LAI: 0.4 ml + X: 2 mg; antagonize with diprenorphine 2 mg/mg etorphine and yohimbine 0.125 mg/kg [17]	Dama gazelles	
	LAI: 0.7 ml + X: 5 mg; antagonize with diprenorphine 2 mg/mg etorphine and yohimbine 0.15 mg/kg [17]	Nyala	
Etorphine + acepromazine + xylazine	1.4 ml + X: 5 mg; antagonize with diprenorphine 2 mg/mg etorphine and yohimbine 0.125 mg/kg [17]	Greater kudu	
(Large Animal Immobilon solution = E: 2.45 mg/ml + A: 10 mg/ml)			
Etorphine + acepromazine + xylazine (Large Animal Immobilon solution = E: 2.45 mg/ml + A: 10 mg/ml)	LAI: 1.6 ml + X: 25 mg; antagonize with diprenorphine 2 mg/mg etorphine [17]	Waterbuck	
	LAI: 1.8 ml + X: 50 mg; antagonize with diprenorphine 2 mg/mg etorphine and yohimbine 0.125 mg/kg [17]	Nilgais	
	LAI: 1.8 ml + X: 50 mg; antagonize with diprenorphine 2 mg/mg etorphine and yohimbine 0.125 mg/kg [17]	European bison	
	LAI: 2 ml + X: 50 mg; antagonize with diprenorphine 2 mg/mg etorphine and yohimbine 0.125 mg/kg [17]	Bantengs	Supplement as needed with 1 ml LAI.

(Continued)

Drug name	Drug dose	Species	Comments
	LAI: 2.3 ml + X: 10 mg; antagonize with diprenorphine 2 mg/mg etorphine and yohimbine 0.125 mg/kg [17]	Blackbuck	
	LAI: 2.5 ml + X: 50 mg; antagonize with diprenorphine 2 mg/mg etorphine and yohimbine 0.125 mg/kg [13, 17]	Yak	Or consider: E: 0.006–0.024 mg/kg + A: 0.025–0.1 mg/kg + X: 0.05–0.2 mg/kg; antagonize with diprenorphine 0.012–0.05 mg/kg IM.
	LAI: 2.5 ml + X: 100 mg; antagonize with diprenorphine 2 mg/mg etorphine and yohimbine 0.125 mg/kg [13, 17]	Gaur	Or consider: E: 0.01–0.022 mg/kg + A: 0.04–0.09 mg/kg + X: 0.12–0.22 mg/kg; antagonize with diprenorphine 0.02–0.044 mg/kg.
Etorphine + acepromazine + xylazine	E: 0.005–0.007 mg/kg + A: 0.02–0.03 mg/kg + X: 0.08–0.18 mg/kg; antagonize with diprenorphine 0.01–0.014 mg/kg [13]	African buffalo	
	E: 0.005–0.012 mg/kg + A: 0.02–0.05 mg/kg + X: 0.056–0.125 mg/kg; antagonize with diprenorphine 0.01–0.024 mg/kg [13]	Bantengs	
	E: 0.027–0.033 mg/kg + A: 0.11–0.12 mg/kg + X: 0.27–0.33 mg/kg; antagonize with diprenorphine 0.054–0.066 mg/kg [13]	Anoa	
	E: 0.031–0.036 mg/kg + A: 0.13–0.14 mg/kg + X: 0.14–0.18 mg/kg; antagonize with diprenorphine 0.062–0.072 mg/kg [13]	Forest buffalo	
Etorphine Xylazine ++ acepromazine + butorphanol	E: 0.028 mg/kg + A: 0.114 mg/kg + X: 0.16 mg/kg + B: 0.05 mg/kg IM [21]	Gazelles and small antelope, preferred for Dama gazelles	
Etorphine + acepromazine + xylazine + ketamine	E: 0.01–0.012 mg/kg + A: 0.04–0.05 mg/kg + X: 0.4–1.67 mg/kg + K: 0.04–1.67 mg/kg; antagonize with diprenorphine 0.02–0.024 mg/kg [13]	Yaks	

Drug name	Drug dose	Species	Comments
Etorphine + azaperone	Females: E: 3.0 mg + A: 40 mg IM; Males: E: 3.3 mg + A: 40 mg IM; antagonize with naltrexone at 50 × the dose of etorphine in mg [22]	Addax	n = 9 routine exams from 2008 to 2018, no significant complications reported.
	E: 0.015 mg/kg + A: 0.15 mg/kg; antagonize with diprenorphine 0.03 mg/kg [16, 17]	African buffalo	
	E: 0.025 mg/kg + A: 0.3 mg/kg; antagonize with diprenorphine 0.05 mg/kg [17]	Roan antelope	If confined in bomas can decrease dose. hyaluronidase 1500–3000 IU can be added to reduce induction time.
	E: 0.1 mg/kg + A: 2 mg/kg; antagonize with diprenorphine 2 mg/mg etorphine [17]	Oribis	Supplement with etorphine 0.05 mg/kg as needed.
	E: 1.5 mg + A: 20 mg total IM; antagonize with diprenorphine 3 mg [16, 17]	Impala	Or consider: E: 0.08–0.1 mg/kg + X: 0.1–0.3 mg/kg IM.
	E: 1.5 mg + A: 50 mg total IM; antagonize with diprenorphine 2 mg/mg etorphine [17]	Bushbucks	Supplement with etorphine 1 mg as needed.
	E: 2 mg + A: 40 mg; antagonize with diprenorphine 2 mg/mg etorphine given [17]	Mountain reed-buck	Supplement with etorphine 1 mg as needed.
	Male: E: 3–4 mg, (Female E: 3 mg) + A: 80 mg; antagonize with diprenorphine 2.5 mg/mg etorphine, or Naltrexone at 15 × etorphine dose in mg [23]	Black wildebeests, Topi/Tsessebe	Immobilization. hyaluronidase is frequently added to decrease induction time.
Etorphine + azaperone	E: 4 mg + A: 80 mg; antagonize with diprenorphine 8 mg/kg [17]	Topi/Tsessebe	
	Male: E: 4–5 mg, (Female E: 3–4 mg) + A: 80 mg; antagonize with diprenorphine 2.5 mg/mg etorphine, or naltrexone at 15 × etorphine dose in mg [23]	Red hartebeests, Gemsbok	Immobilization. hyaluronidase is frequently added to decrease induction time.

(Continued)

Drug name	Drug dose	Species	Comments
Etorphine + azaperone	Male: E: 4–5 mg, (Female E: 3–4 mg) + A: 100 mg; antagonize with diprenorphine 2.5 mg/mg etorphine, or naltrexone at 15 × etorphine dose in mg [23]	Sable and Roan antelope, Blue wildebeests	Immobilization. hyaluronidase is frequently added to decrease induction time.
	E: 5 mg + A: 80 mg; antagonize with naltrexone 1 mg/kg [17]	Lichtenstein's hartebeests	
	Male: E: 5–6 mg, (Female E: 4–5 mg) + A: 150 mg; antagonize with diprenorphine 2.5 mg/mg etorphine, or naltrexone at 15 × etorphine dose in mg [23]	Greater kudu, Waterbuck	Immobilization. hyaluronidase is frequently added to decrease induction time.
	Male: E: 10–12 mg, (Female E: 6–8 mg) + A: 180–200 mg; antagonize with diprenorphine 2.5 mg/mg etorphine, or naltrexone at 15 × etorphine dose in mg [23]	Eland	Immobilization. hyaluronidase is frequently added to decrease induction time.
Etorphine + detomidine	E: 0.04 mg/kg + D: 0.025 mg/kg; antagonize with diprenorphine 0.08 mg/kg + atipamezole 0.15 mg/kg [16, 17, 29]	Addax	n = 15 adults in 35 anesthetic events with either E + D or Ket: 1–1.5 mg/kg + Med: 0.048–0.066 mg/kg; antagonized with atipamezole 0.18–0.3 mg/kg. Both protocols were satisfactory but had bradycardia.
	E: 0.045–0.05 mg/kg + D: 0.045–0.05 mg/kg [16, 23]	Arabian oryx	
Etorphine + ketamine + xylazine	E: 1 mg + K: 60 mg + X: 60 mg; antagonize with diprenorphine 2 mg/mg etorphine + yohimbine 0.15 mg/kg [17]	Nyala	
	E: 1.25 mg + K: 15 mg + X: 15 mg; antagonize with diprenorphine 2.5 mg + yohimbine 0.125 mg/kg [16, 17]	Bontebok/Blesbok	Or consider: E: 0.02–0.025 mg/kg + K: 0.2–0.3 mg/kg + X: 0.2–0.3 mg/kg IM.
	E: 1.5 mg + K: 10 mg + X: 10 mg; antagonize with diprenorphine 3 mg + yohimbine 0.125 mg/kg [17]	Thompson's gazelles	Or consider: E: 0.05–0.07 mg/kg + K: 0.2–0.45 mg/kg + X: 0.2–0.45 mg/kg IM.

Drug name	Drug dose	Species	Comments
	E: 1.5 mg + K: 30 mg + X: 30 mg; antagonize with diprenorphine 3 mg + yohimbine 0.15 mg/kg [17]	Lechwes	
Etorphine + ketamine + xylazine	E: 3 mg + K: 150 mg + X: 150 mg; antagonize with diprenorphine 6 mg + yohimbine 0.125 mg/kg [17]	Greater kudu	
	E: 5.5 mg + K: 50 mg + X: 50 mg; antagonize with diprenorphine 7 mg + yohimbine 0.125 mg/kg [17]	Gemsbok	
Etorphine + medetomidine	E: 0.05 mg/kg + M: 0.005 mg/kg [16, 23]	Scimitar-horned oryx	
	E: 0.05 mg/kg + M: 0.05 mg/kg; antagonize with diprenorphine 0.1 mg/kg + 0.025 mg/kg atipamezole [17]	Arabian oryx	
	E: 0.05 mg/kg + M: 0.05–0.055 mg/kg; then IV continuous infusion of E: 0.04 mg/kg/hr + ketamine: 1.5 mg/kg/hr + M: 0.005 mg/kg/hr IV; antagonized with 13 mg atipamezole and 42 mg naltrexone [30]	Impala	n = 10 wild-caught adults. Resulted in severe hypoxemia/hypercapnia and acidosis. Thus supplemental oxygen is mandatory with this protocol.
Etorphine + xylazine	E: 0.006 mg/kg + X: 0.04 mg/kg; antagonize with diprenorphine 0.012 mg/kg + yohimbine 0.125 mg/kg [13, 17]	Yaks	
	E: 0.01 mg/kg + X: 0.05 mg/kg; antagonize with diprenorphine 0.02 mg/kg + yohimbine 0.125 mg/kg [16, 17]	American bison	
	E: 0.01 mg/kg + X: 0.4 mg/kg; antagonize with diprenorphine 0.02 mg/kg + yohimbine 0.125 mg/kg [16, 17]	Kirk's dik-diks, Sunis, Klipspringers, Blue duikers	
	E: 0.01 mg/kg + X: 0.4 mg/kg; antagonize with naltrexone 1 mg/kg + yohimbine 0.25 mg/kg [16, 17]	Gray rhebok	

(*Continued*)

Drug name	Drug dose	Species	Comments
	E: 0.01 mg/kg + X: 0.5 mg/kg antagonize with diprenorphine 0.02 mg/kg + yohimbine 0.125 mg/kg [17]	European bison	
	E: 0.012–0.05 mg/kg + X: 0.09–0.33 mg/kg; antagonize with diprenorphine 0.024–0.1 mg/kg + atipamezole 0.027–0.033 mg/kg [13]	Forest buffalo	
	E: 0.0125 mg/kg + X: 0.1 mg/kg; antagonize with diprenorphine 0.025 mg/kg + yohimbine 0.05 mg/kg [13, 17]	African buffalo	
	E: 0.014–0.038 mg/kg + X:0.14–0.7 mg/kg [13]	Watusi/Ankole	
	E: 0.015 mg/kg + X: 0.15–0.25 mg/kg [16]	Gemsbok	
Etorphine + xylazine	E: 0.02 mg/kg + X: 0.4 mg/kg; antagonize with diprenorphine 0.04 mg/kg + 0.125 mg/kg yohimbine [16, 17].	Eland	Can substitute azaperone 200 mg for xylazine. Hyaluronidase 1500–3000 IU is recommended.
	E: 0.02 mg/kg + X: 0.5–0.15 mg/kg [16]	Bongo	
	E: 0.02 mg/kg + X: 1 mg/kg; antagonize with diprenorphine 0.5 mg/kg + 0.05 mg/kg yohimbine [16, 17].	Black, Maxwell's, Red-flanked, Yellow-backed, and Zebra duikers	Monitor for respiratory depression.
	E: 0.025 mg/kg + X: 0.15–0.25 mg/kg [16]	Roan antelope	
	E: 0.03 mg/kg + X: 0.1–0.25 mg/kg; antagonize with diprenorphine 0.06 mg/kg + 0.125 mg/kg yohimbine [16, 17].	Waterbuck	
	E: 0.03 mg/kg + X: 0.2 mg/kg; antagonize with diprenorphine 0.5 mg/kg + 0.05 mg/kg yohimbine [17].	Asian water buffalo	If animal is not down in 20 min, repeat full dose. Induction may be >20 min.
	E: 0.03 mg/kg + X: 0.25 mg/kg; antagonize with diprenorphine 0.06 mg/kg + 0.125 mg/kg yohimbine [16, 17].	Gemsbok	Species is very sensitive to xylazine and it must be antagonized. Could substitute with azaperone 100 mg or detomidine 10 mg. Hyaluronidase 1500–3000 may be added to increase drug absorption. Once down 100 mg ketamine IV may improve anesthesia.

Drug name	Drug dose	Species	Comments
	E: 0.03 mg/kg + X: 0.3 mg/kg; antagonize with diprenorphine 0.06 mg/kg + 0.125 mg/kg yohimbine [16, 17].	Arabian oryx	
	E: 0.04 mg/kg + X: 0.005 mg/kg [16]	Arabian oryx	
	E: 0.04 mg/kg + X: 0.4 mg/kg; antagonize with diprenorphine 0.04 mg/kg + 0.15 mg/kg yohimbine [17].	Steenbok	
	E: 0.04 mg/kg + X: 0.3 mg/kg [16]	Nyala	
	E: 0.025–0.04 mg/kg + X: 0.15–0.5 mg/kg; antagonize with diprenorphine 0.08 mg/kg + 0.125 mg/kg yohimbine [16, 17].	Scimitar-horned oryx	
	E: 0.05 mg/kg + X: 0.15 mg/kg; antagonize with diprenorphine 2 mg/mg of etorphine given [17].	Bontebok/Blesbok	If animal is not down in 20 min, repeat full dose.
Etorphine + xylazine	E: 0.08 mg/kg + X: 0.2 mg/kg; antagonize with diprenorphine 2 mg/mg etorphine + yohimbine 0.125 mg/kg [17]	Nyala	
	E: 0.1 mg/kg + X: 1 mg/kg; antagonize with diprenorphine 0.2 mg/kg + yohimbine 0.125 mg/kg [16, 17]	Pronghorn	
	E: 0.1 mg/kg + X: 0.4 mg/kg; antagonize with diprenorphine 0.02 mg/kg + yohimbine 0.15 mg/kg [17]	Klipspringers, Sunis	Klipspringer: Fentanyl is superior to etorphine in this species-see below F + A.
	E: 1 mg + X: 80 mg; antagonize with diprenorphine 2 mg + yohimbine 0.125 mg/kg [17]	Uganda kobs	
	E: 1.2 mg + X: 10 mg; antagonize with diprenorphine 2.4 mg + yohimbine 0.125 mg/kg [16, 17]	Springbok	Or consider E: 0.05–0.1 mg/kg + X: 0.15–0.25 mg/kg.

(*Continued*)

Drug name	Drug dose	Species	Comments
	E: 3 mg + X: 5 mg; antagonize with diprenorphine 6 mg + yohimbine 0.15 mg/kg [17]	Reedbuck	
	E: 4 mg + X: 10 mg; antagonize with diprenorphine 8 mg + yohimbine 0.15 mg/kg [16, 17]	Lechwes	Red lechwe: E: 0.02–0.05 mg/kg + X: 0.1–0.4 mg/kg IM.
	E: 6 mg + X: 20 mg; antagonize with diprenorphine 12 mg + yohimbine 0.125 mg/kg [16, 17]	Sable antelope	Or consider E: 0.015–0.025 mg/kg + X: 0.1–0.2 mg/kg ± Ket: 0.1–0.2 mg/kg.
	Bull: E: 6 mg + X: 10 mg; Cow: E: 5 mg + X: 10 mg; antagonize with diprenorphine 2 mg/mg etorphine + yohimbine 0.15 mg/kg [17]	Hartebeests	Supplement with etorphine 2 mg as needed.
	E: 10 mg + X: 70 mg total, antagonize with diprenorphine 20 mg + yohimbine 0.125 mg/kg [16, 17]	Greater kudu	Or consider for greater kudu: E: 0.02–0.03 + X: 0.2–0.3 mg/kg IM.
Fentanyl + azaperone	F: 0.4 mg/kg + A: 1 mg/kg; antagonize with 0.2 mg/kg naloxone [17]	Steenbok	Supplement with fentanyl 0.3 mg/kg as needed.
	F: 0.5 mg + A: 1.56 mg [17]	Dorcas, Mountain, Persian, Soemmering's, and Thompson's gazelles	
	F: 0.6 mg + A: 2.5 mg; antagonize with naltrexone 0.2 mg/kg [17]	Klipspringers	
Fentanyl + azaperone	F: 0.8 mg + A: 2 mg [17]	Oribis	
	F: 3 mg + A: 5 mg; antagonize with naloxone 0.2 mg/kg [17]	Dik-diks, Blue and Red duikers, Sunis	Supplement with fentanyl 1.5–2.5 mg as needed. Red duiker: 5 mg fentanyl initially.
	F: 10 mg + A: 20 mg IM [17]	Gray rhebok	
	F: 12 mg + A: 75 mg IM [17]	Reedbuck	
	F: 15 mg + A: 50 mg IM [17]	Bontebok/Blesbok, Bushbucks	Bushbuck: 80 mg azaperone.
	F: 25 mg + A: 150 mg; antagonize with naltrexone or naloxone 0.2 mg/kg [17]	Pukus	If animal is not down in 20 min, repeat full dose.

Drug name	Drug dose	Species	Comments
	F: 50 mg + A: 300 mg [17]	Waterbuck	
	F: 60 mg + A: 200 mg; antagonize with naloxone 0.2 mg/kg [17]	Roan antelope, African buffalo	African Buffalo: 300 mg azaperone.
Fentanyl + xylazine	F: 0.2 mg/kg + X: 0.4 mg/kg IM [17]	Kirk's dik-diks, Blue duikers, Gray rhebok, Sunis	
Flumazenil	Antagonist for zolazepam: 0.01 mg/kg IV [16]	Bovidae	
Fluphenazine decanoate	IM [16]	Bovidae	Neuroleptic. Onset: 3 days, duration: 21–28 days.
	0.5–1 mg/kg [16]	Aepycerotinae	
	0.25–0.5 mg/kg [16]	Alcelaphinae	
	0.5–1 mg/kg [16]	Antilopinae	
	0.25–0.5 mg/kg [16]	Bovinae	
	0.25–0.5 mg/kg [16]	Hippotraginae	
	0.25–0.5 mg/kg [16]	Reduncinae	
Haloperidol decanoate	IM [16]	Bovidae	Neuroleptic, onset: 2–3 days, duration: 21–30 days.
Haloperidol lactate	IV or IM [16]	Bovidae	Neuroleptic. IV onset: <5 min, IV duration: ≤8 hrs; IM onset: <15 min, IM duration: 8–18 hrs.
	0.2–0.5 mg/kg	Aepycerotinae	
	0.05–0.1 mg/kg	Alcelaphinae	
	0.1–1 mg/kg	Antilopinae	
	0.025–0.2 mg/kg	Bovinae	
	0.25–0.5 mg/kg	Cephalophinae	
Haloperidol lactate	0.1–0.2 mg/kg	Hippotraginae	Neuroleptic. IV onset: <5 min, IV duration: ≤8 hrs; IM onset: <15 min, IM duration: 8–18 hrs.
	0.1–0.2 mg/kg	Reduncinae	
Haloperidol	0.3 mg/kg [21]	Arabian gazelles	
Haloperidol	5 mg Adults [17]	Sunis	Animals transport well in dark individual crates.
	Adult male: 15 mg, Adult female: 10 mg, Subadult: 7.5 mg, neonate: 5 mg [17]	Bontebok/Blesbok, Gray duikers, Eland, Nyala	Eland: Adult 20 mg, Subadult 10 mg.
	Adult male: 20 mg, Adult female: 15 mg, Subadult: 8 mg [17]	Waterbuck	
	Adult male: 20 mg, Adult female: 15 mg, Subadult: 7.5 mg, neonate: 5 mg [17]	Springbok	

(*Continued*)

Drug name	Drug dose	Species	Comments
	Adult male: 20 mg, Adult female: 15 mg, Subadult: 10 mg, neonate: 5 mg [17]	Impala, Mountain reedbuck, Gray rhebok, Sable antelope	Sable: Adult 15 mg, Subadult 10 mg.
	Adult male: 30 mg, Adult female: 20 mg, Subadult: 10 mg [17]	Hartebeests, Greater kudu, Topi/Tsessebe	Kudu 20 mg adult, 10 mg subadult.
	Adults, not to exceed 20 mg [17]	Gemsbok	
Ketamine	10 mg/kg IV after manual restraint [17]	Sunis	
	15 mg/kg [17]	Four-horned antelope	Supplement with ketamine 8 mg/kg as needed.
Ketamine + diazepam	K: 2–4 mg/kg + D: 0.2 mg/kg IV [25]	Bison calves	To give 5–10 min of light anesthesia. If depressed calves, use D: 0.2 mg/kg + butorphanol 0.1 mg/kg IV instead. If a calf is difficult to work with can use xylazine 0.1–0.2 mg/kg + butorphanol 0.1 mg/kg IM prior to K + D IV.
Ketamine + medetomidine	K: 0.05–2 mg/kg + M: 0.025–0.1 mg/kg; antagonize with atipamezole 0.12–0.5 mg/kg [13]	Anoa	
	K: 1 mg/kg + M: 0.1 mg/kg; antagonize with atipamezole 0.25 mg/kg [17]	Reedbuck	
	K: 1–1.3 mg/kg + M: 0.0.5–0.09 mg/kg [16]	Bontebok/Blesbok	
	K: 1–1.5 mg/kg + M: 0.05–0.07 mg/kg; antagonize with atipamezole 0.25 mg/kg [16, 17, 29]	Addax	See etorphine + xylazine for same species for alternate protocol.
	K: 1.5–2 mg/kg + M: 0.06–0.07 mg/kg [16]	Gerenuk	
	K: 1.8–4 mg/kg + M: 0.06–0.1 mg/kg [16]	Addra gazelles	
	K: 2 mg/kg + M: 0.25 mg/kg; antagonize with atipamezole 1 mg/kg [16, 17]	Blackbuck	
Ketamine + medetomidine	K: 2.1 mg/kg + M: 0.16 mg/kg; antagonize with atipamezole 0.8 mg/kg [16, 17]	Klipspringers	

Drug name	Drug dose	Species	Comments
	K: 2.2 mg/kg + M: 0.2 mg/kg; antagonize with atipamezole 1 mg/kg [16, 17]	Blue and Gray duikers	Supplement with ketamine 1.1–2 mg/kg as needed.
	K: 1.5–2.5 mg/kg + M: 0.05–0.08 mg/kg; antagonize with atipamezole 0.4 mg/kg [16, 17]	American and European bison	Higher end of dose ranges used for European bison.
	K: 2.4 mg/kg + M: 0.07 mg/kg IM [21]	Beiras	Long induction time. Requires quiet surroundings during induction.
	K: 3 mg/kg + M: 0.07 mg/kg IM [21]	Gerenuk	Long induction time. Requires quiet surroundings during induction.
	K: 3 mg/kg + M: 0.1 mg/kg; antagonize with atipamezole 0.5 mg/kg [13, 17]	Yaks	
	K: 3–5 mg/kg + M: 0.2–0.25 mg/kg [16]	Impala	
	K: 4 mg/kg + M: 0.05–0.07 mg/kg IV [21]	Gazelles and small antelope	Long induction time. Requires quiet surroundings during induction.
	K: 5 mg/kg + M: 0.3 mg/kg; antagonize with atipamezole 1.5 mg/kg [16, 17, 31]	Pronghorn	Another option: A study of 10 hand-raised pronghorn given M: 0.1 mg/kg IM then placed a jugular IV catheter and given either ketamine or propofol: 1–2 mg/kg IV every 10–20 sec until laterally recumbent. Total dose: ketamine 3.3–5.5 mg/kg IV or propofol 5–11.5 mg/kg IV. Then antagonized 15 min later with atipamezole 0.2 mg/kg IM. Oxygen supplementation is required. Protocol worked well.
	K: 8 mg/kg + M: 0.04 mg/kg; antagonize with atipamezole 0.12 mg/kg [17]	Impala	
Ketamine + medetomidine + butorphanol	K: 2–4 mg/kg + M: 0.04–0.07 mg/kg + B: 0.2–0.4 mg/kg IM [21]	Gazelles and small antelope	
	K: 4 mg/kg + M: 0.2 mg/kg + B: 0.15 mg/kg IM then maintained with Continuous infusion IV of K: 2.4 mg/kg/hr + M: 0.0012 mg/kg/hr + midazolam: 0.036 mg/kg/hr [32]	Impala	n = 10 female impala, worked well with surgical anesthesia in 9/9 animals.

(*Continued*)

Drug name	Drug dose	Species	Comments
Ketamine + midazolam	K: 4 mg/kg + Mid: 0.2 mg/kg IV [21]	Gazelles and small antelope	
Ketamine + xylazine	K: 1.5–2 mg/kg + X: 0.75–1 mg/kg; antagonize with atipamezole 0.06–0.08 mg/kg [13, 17]	Bantengs	
Ketamine + xylazine	K: 3.3–7.1 mg/kg + X: 4.1–8.9 mg/kg IV, or: K: 5.4–5.9 mg/kg + X: 6.8–7.4 mg/kg IM [21]	Arabian gazelles	
	K: 3.6 mg/kg + X: 4.5 mg/kg [21]	Dorcas gazelles	
	K: 4 mg/kg + X: 0.25 mg/kg; antagonize with tolazoline 2 mg/kg [17]	Blackbuck	Captive animals.
	K: 4 mg/kg + X: 0.8 mg/kg; antagonize with yohimbine 0.125 mg/kg [16, 17]	Eland	
	K: 4 mg/kg + X: 0.5–1 mg/kg; antagonize with yohimbine 0.125 mg/kg [17]	Bison	
	K: 4.4 mg/kg + X: 5.5 mg/kg [21]	Red-fronted gazelles	
	K: 5 mg/kg + X: 1 mg/kg [17]	Sitatungas	
	K: 5.6 mg/kg + X: 7 mg/kg [21]	Soemmering's, Mountain, and Speke's gazelles	
	K: 6 mg/kg + X: 1 mg/kg [13]	Anoa	
	K: 6 mg/kg + X: 6 mg/kg [17]	Persian gazelles	
	K: 6.6 mg/kg + X: 1.1 mg/kg; antagonize with yohimbine 0.125 mg/kg [17]	Sitatungas	Supplement with ketamine 3.3 mg/kg as needed.
	K: 6.8 mg/kg + X: 8.5 mg/kg [21]	Chinkara gazelles	
	K: 9 mg/kg + X: 0.5 mg/kg; antagonize with yohimbine 0.125 mg/kg [16, 17]	Springbok	Supplement with ketamine 5 mg/kg as needed.

Drug name	Drug dose	Species	Comments
	Mountain Gazelle/Idmi: K: 9.3–12.2 mg/kg + X: 11.7–15.2 mg/kg IM; Goitred Gazelle: K: 5.4–5.9 mg/kg + X: 6.8–7.4 mg/kg IM. Captive of both sp.: K: 1.4–4 mg/kg + X: 0.4–1 mg/kg IV [21, 33].	Mountain and Persian gazelles	n = 58 animals. 131 immobilizations. Captive required much lower doses IV than wild animals.
	K: 10 mg/kg + X: 0.2 mg/kg [17]	Steenbok	
	K: 10 mg/kg + X: 12 mg/kg [17]	Mountain gazelles	
	K: 13 mg/kg + X: 16 mg/kg IM [17]	Gray duikers	
	K: 15 mg/kg + X: 0.2–0.4 mg/kg IM [16]	Sunis	
	K: 15–25 mg/kg + X: 0.2–0.3 mg/kg IM [16]	Maxwell's duikers	
Medetomidine	0.029–0.049 mg/kg [13]	Free-ranging Norwegian cattle	Sedation
Medetomidine	0.06 mg/kg; antagonize with atipamezole 0.25 mg/kg [17]	Arabian oryx	Calm animals only.
	0.07 mg/kg [13]	Yaks	Deep sedation. Lighter sedation with detomidine 0.025 mg/kg.
Naltrexone	Antagonist for: carfentanil: 100 mg/mg IM, for etorphine: 50 mg/mg, for butorphanol 5 mg/mg [16]	Bovidae	May be given partially IV.
Perphenazine enanthate	IM [16]	Bovidae	Neuroleptic. Onset in hours, duration: 7–10 days. Doses suggested by subfamily.
	1 mg/kg [16]	Aepycerotinae	
	0.25–1 mg/kg [16]	Alcelaphinae	
	1–5 mg/kg [16]	Antilopinae	
	0.1–1 mg/kg [16]	Bovinae	
	2–5 mg/kg [16]	Cephalophinae	
	0.5–1 mg/kg [16]	Hippotraginae	
	1 mg/kg [16]	Reduncinae	
Perphenazine	2–5 mg/kg [17]	Impala	
	3.5 mg/kg IM [21]	Mhorr gazelles	
	Adults 20–40 mg [17]	Gray duikers, Mountain reed-buck	Reedbuck: 30 mg.
	Adult: 50–80 mg [17]	Bontebok/Blesbok	

(*Continued*)

Drug name	Drug dose	Species	Comments
	Adult: 50–100 mg [21]	Gazelles 20–40 kg in size	Duration: about 10 d.
	Adult: 100 mg, Subadult: 50 mg [17]	Eland, Sable antelope	
	Adults 100–200 mg [17]	Gemsbok, Hartebeests, Nyala	Hartebeest: 100 mg; Nyala 100–150 mg.
	Adults: 100–150 mg, Subadult: 40 mg [17]	Topi/Tsessebe	
	Adults: 100–200 mg, Subadult: 50 mg [17]	Waterbuck	
	Adult male: 100 mg, Adult female: 70 mg, Subadult: 50 mg, Neonate: 20 mg [17]	Springbok	
	Adult male: 200 mg, Adult female: 100 mg, Subadult: 50 mg [17]	Greater kudu	
	Adult male: 400 mg, Adult female: 200 mg, Subadult: 100 mg, Calf: 50 mg [17]	African buffalo	
Pipothiazine palmitate	IM [16]	Bovidae	Neuroleptic. Onset 2–3 days, duration: 21–28 days. Doses suggested by subfamily.
	4–4.5 mg/kg	Aepycerotinae	
Pipothiazine palmitate	2–4 mg/kg [16]	Alcelaphinae	Neuroleptic. Onset 2–3 days, duration: 21–28 days. Doses suggested by subfamily.
	1–2.5 mg/kg [16]	Antilopinae	
	0.1–1 mg/kg [16]	Bovinae	
	0.25–0.5 mg/kg [16]	Hippotraginae	
	0.3–2 mg/kg [16]	Reduncinae	
Pipothiazine	2 mg/kg [17]	Impala	
Propofol	2–4 mg/kg IV [13]	Domestic cattle	For induction of anesthesia.
	4–6 mg/kg IV [21]	Gazelles and small antelope	
Telazol	2–4 mg/kg IV [21]	Gazelles and small antelope	
	3.6 mg/kg IM [17]	Zebus	Supplement with ketamine 1 mg/kg as needed.
	5 mg/kg IM [17]	African buffalo, Impala, Uganda kobs	
	6 mg/kg [17]	Blackbuck, Kirk's dik-diks, Blue and Red duikers, Greater kudu, Oribis	Supplement with ketamine 3 mg/kg as needed.

Drug name	Drug dose	Species	Comments
	8 mg/kg IM [17]	Bontebok/Blesbok, Steenbok	
	8.8 mg/kg IM [17]	Thompson's gazelles	
	10 mg/kg [17]	Gray and Maxwell's duikers, Dorcas, Grant's, and Slender-horned gazelles, Nyala, Scimitar-horned oryx, Sitatungas, Springbok, Sunis	Nyala: 11 mg/kg IM; Scimitar-horned oryx: 9.4 mg/kg; Springbok: 10.6 mg/kg.
	12 mg/kg IM [17]	Bushbucks	
	15 mg/kg [17]	Steenbok	
Telazol + detomidine	T: 4 mg/kg + D: 0.2 mg/kg; antagonize with atipamezole 0.2 mg/kg [17]	Bantengs	Expect prolonged recoveries.
Telazol + medetomidine	T: 1.2 mg/kg + M: 0.06 mg/kg; antagonize with atipamezole 0.18 mg/kg [17, 25, 34]	American bison	n = 7 male bison, 3–5 yrs. of age. Hypoxemia resulted. Use supplemental oxygen, attempt to keep sternal, and only give half IV instead of both portions IM if can get to safety quickly as recovery is rapid.
	T: 4 mg/kg + M: 0.4 mg/kg; antagonize with atipamezole 0.18 mg/kg [21]	Arabian gazelles	
Telazol + Hy Telazol + medetomidine hydromorphone + xylazine	T: 1.98 mg/kg + H: 0.26 mg/kg + X: 1.32 mg/kg; antagonize with naltrexone 0.09 mg/kg + tolazoline 4 mg/kg [25]	Bison	
Telazol + xylazine	T: 3 mg/kg + X: 1.5 mg/kg IM; antagonize with tolazoline 1.5 mg/kg IV and 1.5 mg/kg IM [34]	Wood bison	n = 7 male bison, 3–5 yrs. of age. Hypoxemia resulted. Use supplemental oxygen, attempt to keep sternal, and only give half IV instead of both portions IM if can get to safety quickly as recovery is rapid.
	T: 2 mg/kg + X: 0.2 mg/kg; antagonize with yohimbine 0.125 mg/kg [17]	Gemsbok, Arabian oryx	
	T: 3 mg/kg + X: 0.2 mg/kg; antagonize with yohimbine 0.15 mg/kg [17]	Sable antelope	

(*Continued*)

Drug name	Drug dose	Species	Comments
	T: 1.5–3 mg/kg + X: 0.75–1.5 mg/kg; antagonize tolazoline 2–3 mg/kg-half IV and half IM [17, 25].	American bison	Use the lower end of dose range for calm animals and higher end for fractious or wild animals. Approximately 1 hour of anesthesia and analgesia for minor procedures.
Thiafentanil	0.017 mg/kg; antagonize with naltrexone 0.5 mg/kg [17]	American bison	Supplement with thiafentanil 0.008 mg/kg as needed.
	0.04 mg/kg; antagonize with naltrexone 0.8 mg/kg [17]	Impala	Supplement with carfentanil 0.02 mg/kg as needed.
	0.08 mg/kg; antagonize with naltrexone 0.4 mg/kg [16, 17]	Lechwes, Impala	
	2 mg; antagonize with naltrexone 150 mg [17]	Bushbucks	
	5 mg IM; antagonize with naltrexone 150 mg [17]	Hartebeests	
Thiafentanil + azaperone	Females: T: 2.0–2.5 mg + A: 40 mg IM; Males: T: 3.8–4.2 mg + A: 40 mg IM; antagonize with naltrexone at 10 × the dose of thiafentanil in mg [22]	Addax	n = 9 routine exams from 2008 to 2018, no significant complications reported.
	T: 0.01 mg/kg + A: 1 mg/kg; antagonize with naltrexone 0.3 mg/kg [17]	Gray rhebok	Supplement with thiafentanil 0.05 mg/kg as needed.
	T: 0.007–0.02 mg/kg + A: 0.06–0.1 mg/kg; antagonize with naltrexone 0.07–0.2 mg/kg [13, 17]	African buffalo	
	T: 0.03 mg/kg + A: 0.3 mg/kg; antagonize with naltrexone 0.6 mg/kg [17]	Roan antelope	Supplement with thiafentanil 0.015 mg/kg as needed.
	T: 0.03 mg/kg + A: 0.4 mg/kg; antagonize with naltrexone 0.6 mg/kg [17]	Sable antelope	If animal is not down in 15 min, repeat full dose.
Thiafentanil + azaperone	T: 0.03 mg/kg + A: 0.5 mg/kg [16]	Bontebok/Blesbok	
	T: 0.03 mg/kg + A: 0.6 mg/kg; antagonize with naltrexone 0.6 mg/kg [17]	Topi/Tsessebe, Waterbuck	Supplement with thiafentanil 0.015 mg/kg as needed. Waterbuck: If animal is not down in 15 min, repeat full dose.

Drug name	Drug dose	Species	Comments
	T: 0.04 mg/kg + A: 1 mg/kg; antagonize with naltrexone 1 0.8–1 mg/kg [17]	Reedbuck, Mountain reedbuck, Steenbok	If animal is not down in 15 min, repeat full dose.
	T: 0.06 mg/kg + A: 0.5 mg/kg antagonize with naltrexone 1 mg/kg [17]	Uganda kobs	If animal is not down in 15 min, repeat full dose.
	T: 0.1 mg/kg + A: 1 mg/kg; antagonize with naltrexone 2 mg/kg [17]	Klipspringers	Supplement with thiafentanil 0.05 mg/kg as needed.
Thiafentanil + detomidine	T: 0.04 mg/kg + D: 0.05 mg/kg; antagonize with naltrexone 0.8 mg/kg + atipamezole 0.2 mg/kg [17]	Greater kudu	
Thiafentanil + ketamine	T: 0.02 mg/kg + K: 1.5–3 mg/kg IM [16]	Nile lechwes	
	T: 0.04 mg/kg + K: 3.5 mg/kg IM [16]	Gerenuk	
Thiafentanil + medetomidine	T: 0.01–0.025 mg ± M: 0.05–0.1 mg [16]	African buffalo	
	T: 0.012 mg/kg + M: 0.02 mg/kg; antagonize with atipamezole 0.1 mg/kg and naltrexone 0.12 mg/kg [13]	Gaur	
	T: 0.045 mg ± M: 0.05 mg [16]	Nyala	
	T: 1.2 mg + M: 2 mg; antagonize with naltrexone 12 mg + atipamezole 10 mg [17]	Impala	
Thiafentanil + medetomidine + ketamine	T: 0.01–0.02 mg/kg + M: 0.005–0.006 mg/kg + K: 0.3–0.6 mg/kg; antagonize with naltrexone 0.6 mg/kg + atipamezole 0.04 mg/kg [16, 17]	Roan antelope	
	T: 0.02 mg/kg + M: 0.008 mg/kg + K: 1 mg/kg; antagonize with naltrexone 0.6 mg/kg IV + atipamezole 0.035 mg/kg IV [17, 35]	Lichtenstein's hartebeests	n = 13 wild animals. If animal is not down in 15 min, repeat full dose.
	T: 0.02–0.04 mg/kg + M: 0.02–0.04 mg/kg + K: 1 mg/kg; antagonize with naltrexone 1.2 mg/kg + atipamezole 0.16 mg/kg [16, 17]	Gemsbok	

(*Continued*)

Drug name	Drug dose	Species	Comments
Thiafentanil + medetomidine + ketamine	T: 0.045 mg/kg + M: 0.07 mg/kg + K: 200 mg; antagonize with naltrexone 1 mg/kg + atipamezole 0.5 mg/kg [17]	Nyala	
Thiafentanil + xylazine	T: 0.015 mg/kg + X: 0.2 mg/kg; antagonize with naltrexone 0.15 mg/kg + tolazoline 2 mg/kg [17]	Gaur	
	T: 0.01–0.02 mg/kg + X: 0.5 mg/kg [16]	Gray duikers	
	T: 0.011–0.018 mg/kg + X: 0.05–0.25 mg/kg [13]	Gaur	
	T: 0.025 mg/kg + X: 0.15 mg/kg; antagonize with naltrexone 1 mg/kg + atipamezole 0.0025 mg/kg [16, 17]	Yaks, Tibetan yaks	
	T: 0.03 mg/kg + X: 0.1 mg/kg [16]	Wildebeests	
	T: 0.03 mg/kg + X: 0.1–0.2 mg/kg [16]	Sable antelope, Waterbuck	
	T: 0.03–0.07 mg/kg + X: 0.1–0.15 mg/kg; antagonize with naltrexone 0.3 mg/kg + yohimbine 0.1 mg/kg [16, 17]	Eland	
Thiafentanil + xylazine (or medetomidine)	T: 0.04 + X: 0.5–1 mg/kg (or Med: 0.025–0.05 mg/kg IM) [16]	Impala	
Thiafentanil + xylazine	T: 0.05 + X: 0.25 mg/kg [16]	Greater kudu	
	T: 0.08–0.1 mg/kg + X: 0.2–0.3 mg/kg; antagonize with 2 mg/kg naltrexone and 0.125 mg/kg yohimbine [16, 17]	Nyala	Supplement with thiafentanil 0.05 mg/kg as needed.
Thiafentanil + xylazine	T: 0.1 mg/kg + X: 0.5 mg/kg [16]	Pronghorn	
Thiafentanil + xylazine + azaperone	T: 0.03 mg/kg + X: 0.1 mg/kg + A: 0.3 mg/kg IM [16]	Topi/Tsessebe	
	T: 0.05–0.07 mg/kg + X: 0.2 mg/kg ± A: 0.1 mg/kg IM [16]	Reedbuck	

Drug name	Drug dose	Species	Comments
Tolazoline	Antagonist for: medetomidine: 1 mg/kg IM, for detomidine: 1 mg/kg IM, for xylazine: 1 mg/kg IM [16]	Bovidae	
Xylazine	0.02 mg/kg IV [13]	Non domestic cattle	Standing sedation. To prolong effect, add butorphanol 0.05 mg/kg. For domestic calves X: 0.025–0.05 IV or 0.1–0.2 mg/kg IM have been used. Free ranging Norwegian cattle X: 0.37–0.73 mg/kg.
Xylazine	0.1–0.2 mg/kg IV [25]	Bison	Standing sedation, If add acepromazine 0.05 mg/kg and butorphanol 0.05 mg/kg. All three may produce deep sedation and possibly recumbency.
	Sedation: 0.05–0.1 mg/kg; Immobilization 0.2–0.4 mg/kg [13]	African buffalo	
	0.5 mg/kg; antagonize with 0.125 mg/kg yohimbine or 0.09 mg/kg atipamezole [17]	Arabian oryx	
	Sedation: 0.3 mg/kg, Immobilization 0.6–1 mg/kg [13]	Yaks	
	1 mg/kg; antagonize with 0.125 mg/kg yohimbine [17]	Uganda kobs, Yaks	
	Sedation: 0.03–0.22 mg/kg; antagonize with yohimbine 0.07–0.18 mg/kg. Immobilization: 1.5 mg/kg IM, antagonize with atipamezole 0.04–0.08 mg/kg [13]	Bantengs	For female animals.
	3 mg/kg; antagonize with yohimbine 0.125–0.2 mg/kg [17]	Roan antelope, Nilgais, Scimitar-horned oryx, Sable antelope, Sitatungas	Calm animals only.
	4 mg/kg; antagonize with yohimbine 0.125 mg/kg [17]	Dama gazelles	Calm animals only.
Xylazine + acepromazine	X: 0.05–0.09 mg/kg + A: 0.06–0.1 mg/kg IM [13].	Bantengs	Sedation of females.

(*Continued*)

Drug name	Drug dose	Species	Comments
Xylazine + ketamine	X: 0.2–0.5 mg/kg IV via tail vein, then 2 mg/kg ketamine IV via jugular vein. To prolong anesthesia 5% guaifenesin and K: 1 mg/kg boluses can be used; antagonize X at procedure end [25].	Bison	For short-term anesthesia.
Zuclopenthixol acetate	IM [16]	Bovidae	Neuroleptic. Onset: 1 hr, duration: 3–4 days.
	IM [36]	Bovidae	Neuroleptic doses suggested by subfamily.
	1 mg/kg [36]	Aepycerotinae	
	1 mg/kg [36]	Alcelaphinae	
	2–5 mg/kg [36]	Antilopinae	
	0.3–2 mg/kg [36]	Bovinae	
	0.5–1 mg/kg [36]	Hippotraginae	
	1–2 mg/kg [36]	Reduncinae	
	1.5 mg/kg [16]	Blue wildebeests	n = 17 animals monitored via visual and telemetry belts and compared to controls. No adverse effects noted.
Zuclopenthixol decanoate	IM [16]	Bovidae	Neuroleptic. Onset: 1 wk, duration 10–21 days.
Zuclopenthixol	1 mg/kg [13, 17]	Bontebok/Blesbok, African buffalo, Gray duikers, Eland, Gemsbok, Impala, Greater kudu, Nyala, Mountain reed-buck, Springbok, Topi/Tsessebe, Waterbuck	African Buffalo: Not to exceed 600 mg. Adequate tranquilization for 3 days.
	10–20 mg Adults [17]	Sunis	
	100 mg Adults [17]	Hartebeests	
	Adult male 300 mg; Adult female 225 mg; Subadult 125 mg [17]	Roan and Sable antelope	Excellent tranquilization for 3 days.
Antiparasitic			
Albendazole	20 mg/kg PO then repeat in 14d [2]	Gerenuk	n = 1 female to treat parasites.
Doramectin	0.4 mg/kg SC, repeat in 14d [2]	Gerenuk	n = 1 female to treat parasites.
Fenbendazole	25 mg/kg PO once [2]	Gerenuk	n = 1 female to treat parasites.

Drug name	Drug dose	Species	Comments
Ivermectin sustained release varnish (Eudragit)	Varnish applied topically to wounds after larvae removed [37]	Addax, Arabian and Scimitar-horned oryx	n = 3 animals receiving injectable ivermectin 0.2 mg/kg sc, versus 5 animals with varnish painted on lesions. The former usually required multiple immobilizations with treatment and the latter only one anesthetic event.
Ivermectin or fenbendazole trial	Ivermectin 0.2 mg/kg PO SID × 3d q5 wks × 3 treatments or fenbendazole 7.5 mg/kg PO × 3d q3 wks × 3 treatments [38]	Arabian and Scimitar-horned oryx, Slender-horned gazelles	Both treatments given in separate years starting in spring to seven herds of captive wild ruminants. Both in their respective year resulted in very low to zero fecal egg counts during summer but by fall egg counts rose again.
Other			
Bovine colostrum (Land o' Lakes)	Calves required ≥4.68 g of IgG/kg divided into 5 feedings over 24 hrs to prevent failure of passive transfer (FPT) [39]	Springbok	n = 10 calves fed bovine colostrum product to correct FPT.
Dexamethasone sodium phosphate	0.75 mg/kg IM SID for 8 wks (last 7–10d decreased by 10% each day) [4]	Lesser kudu	n = 1 animal with vasculitis of hind limbs with edema secondary to leptospirosis infection. Initially improved with supportive care, then required long-term steroids and antibiotics for full resolution.
Dextrose	500 mg/kg or 10 ml/kg 5% solution IV over several minutes. Once hypoglycemia corrected maintain glucose with 250 mg/kg/day [16]	Neonatal ruminants	Maintenance dose, give until accepting food or parenteral nutrition begins.
Ear topical medications	1) Gentamicin 100 mg + DMSO 5 ml + 10 ml Silver sulfadiazine (SSD) ointment into affected canal SID. 2) 100 mg enrofloxacin + 5 ml DMSO + 10 ml SSD ointment into affected ear canal every 2–4 days. 3) Amikacin 2.5% solution instilled into canal weekly along with parenteral Amikacin at each treatment [1].	Bongo	n = 3 captive animals with severe otitis media-interna treated with 3 different topical ear medications. Five animals total have been reported with the condition and 2 ultimately received single or bilateral total ear canal ablation and bulla osteotomy to resolve issue.

(Continued)

Drug name	Drug dose	Species	Comments
Lidocaine 2%	60 mg given as Epidural [5]	Eastern Bongo	n = 1 animal during procedure for vulvoplasty after vaginal prolapse.
	0.75 ml divided into 3 portions of 0.25 ml injected into scrotal skin and each testicle [19]	Thompson's gazelles	n = 7 captive juvenile animals anesthetized for castration.
	Epidural: 0.17–0.38 mg/kg [22]	Addax	n = 3 animals used 22 times. Sedated with acepromazine 0.14–0.34 mg/kg once in a drop chute, then gave lidocaine via 20ga needle at sacrococcygeal intervertebral space or 1st intercoccygeal intervertebral space-for transvaginal ultrasound guided oocyte collection.
Melengesterol acetate (MGA) implant	7–10 g implant given q2 yr 5 times [5]	Eastern Bongo	n = 1 animal for chronic vaginal prolapse, ultimately required ovariohysterectomy. When >2 yr between implant replacement, bull followed female and attempted breeding.
Pantoprazole	1 mg/kg IV SID [7]	Tibetan yaks	n = 2 animal post castration (recumbent). Severe pneumonia with bruxism and suspected abomasal ulceration.
PMMA material	Impregnated with 2 g cefazolin [8]	Roan antelope	n = 1 animal with fractured femur. Placed under metal plate intraop and left in place.
Vitamin B complex	3.4 mg/kg IM once [4]	Lesser kudu	n = 1 animal for supportive care.
Vitamin E (vit E 300)	8.2 IU/kg IM [4]	Lesser kudu	n = 1 animal for supportive care.

Species	Weight
Addax *(Addax nasomaculatus)*	60–125 kg
Anoa *(Bubalus depressicornis)*	150–300 kg
Antelope, Four-horned *(Tetracerus quadricornis)*	17–21 kg
Antelope, Roan *(Hippotragus equinus)*	100–325 kg
Banteng *(Bos javanicus)*	400–900 kg
Beira *(Dorcatragus megalotis)*	9–11.5 kg
Bison, American *(Bison bison)*	350–1000 kg
Bison, European *(Bison bonasus)*	350–1000 kg
Blackbuck *(Antilope cervicapra)*	32–43 kg
Bongo *(Tragelaphus eurycerus)*	150–200 kg

Species	Weight
Bontebok/Blesbok *(Damaliscus pygargus)*	60–75 kg
Buffalo, African *(Syncerus caffer)*	600–900 kg
Buffalo, Asian water *(Bubalus bubalis)*	700–1200 kg
Buffalo, Forest *(Syncerus nanus)*	Female: 260 kg; Male: 320 kg
Bushbuck *(Tragelaphus scriptus)*	Female: 24–42 kg; Male: 30–77 kg
Cattle, feral *(Bos taurus)*	500–1000 kg
Kirk's dik-dik *(Madoqua kirki)*	3–7 kg
Duiker, Black *(Cephalophorus niger)*	20–40 kg
Duiker, Blue *(Cephalophorus monticola)*	3.5–9 kg
Duiker, Gray *(Silivicapra grimmia)*	12–25 kg
Duiker, Jentink's *(Cephalophorus jentinki)*	20–40 kg
Duiker, Maxwell's *(Cephalophorus maxwelli)*	10–15 kg
Duiker, Red *(Cephalophorus natalensis)*	20–40 kg
Duiker, Red-flanked *(Cephalophorus rufilatus)*	20–40 kg
Duiker, Yellow-backed *(Cephalophorus sylvicultor)*	45–80 kg
Duiker, Zebra *(Cephalophus zebra)*	20–40 kg
Eland *(Taurotragus oryx)*	400–700 kg
Eland, Giant *(Taurotragus derbianus)*	440–900 kg
Gaur *(Bos gaurus)*	650–1000 kg
Gazelle, Arabian *(Gazella arabica)*	10–20 kg
Gazelle, Dama *(Nanger dama)*	20–60 kg
Gazelle, Dorcas *(Gazella dorcas)*	20–60 kg
Gazelle, Grant's *(Gazella granti)*	20–60 kg
Gazelle, Mountain *(Gazella gazella)*	20 kg
Gazelle, Persian *(Gazella subgutturosa)*	20–60 kg
Gazelle, Red-fronted *(Eudorcas rufifrons)*	25–30 kg
Gazelle, Slender-horned *(Gazella leptoceros)*	20–30 kg
Gazelle, Speke's *(Gazella spekei)*	15–25 kg
Gemsbok *(Oryx gazella)*	150–240 kg
Gerenuk *(Litocranius walleri)*	Female: 25–45 kg; Male: 30–50 kg
Harebeest, Hunter's/Hirola *(Beatragus)*	80–118 kg
Hartebeest *(Alcelaphus buselaphus)*	140–170 kg
Hartebeest, Lichtenstein's *(Alcelaphus lichtensteinii)*	135–245 kg
Hartebeest, Red *(Alcelaphus caama)*	105–165 kg
Impala *(Aepyceros melampus)*	40–60 kg
Klipspringer *(Oreotragus oreotragus)*	8–14 kg
Kob, Uganda *(Kobus kob)*	100–300 kg
Kudu, Greater (*Tragelaphus strepsiceros*)	160–250 kg
Kudu, Lesser *(Ammelaphus imberbis)*	55–105 kg

(*Continued*)

Species	Weight
Lechwe *(Kobus leche)*	80–125 kg
Lechwe, Nile *(Kobus megaceros)*	50–125 kg
Nilgai *(Boselaphus tragocamelus)*	170–240 kg
Nyala *(Tragelaphus angasi)*	60–110 kg
Oribi (*Ourebia ourebi)*	8–15 kg
Oryx, Arabian *(Oryx leucoryx)*	80–120 kg
Oryx, Scimitar-horned *(Oryx dammah)*	100–210 kg
Pronghorn *(Antilocapra americana)*	40–50 kg
Puku *(Kobus vardoni)*	50–90 kg
Reedbuck *(Redunca arundinum)*	50–75 kg
Reedbuck, Mountain *(Redunca fulvorufula)*	25–35 kg
Rhebok, Gray *(Pelea capreolus)*	20–35 kg
Sable *(Hippotragus niger)*	150–260 kg
Saiga *(Saiga tatarica)*	20–50 kg
Sitatunga *(Tragelaphus spekei)*	50–125 kg
Springbok *(Antidorcas marsupialis)*	30–45 kg
Steenbok *(Raphicerus campestris)*	7–16 kg
Suni *(Neotragus moschatus)*	4–9 kg
Tamaraw *(Bubalus mindorensis)*	700–1200 kg
Topi/Tsessebe *(Damaliscus lunatus)*	120–140 kg
Waterbuck *(Kobus ellipsiprymnus)*	225–260 kg
Watusi/Ankole cattle *(Bos taurus/indicus)*	400–725 kg
Wildebeest, black, White-tailed *(Connochaetes gnou)*	120–180 kg
Yak *(Bos grunniens)*	Female: 250–400 kg; Male: 800–1000 kg
Zebu *(Bos taurus)*	800–1000 kg

References

1 Adkesson, M., Citino, S., Dennis, P. et al. (2009). Medical and surgical management of otitis in captive bongo (*Tragelaphus eurycerus*). *Journal of Zoo and Wildlife Medicine* 40 (2): 332–343.

2 Helmick, K.E. and Citino, S.B. (2001). Surgical resolution of an ectopic pregnancy in a captive gerenuk (*Litocranius walleri walleri*). *Journal of Zoo and Wildlife Medicine* 32 (4): 503–508.

3 Gull, J.M., Muntener, C.R., and Hatt, J.M. (2012). Long-acting antibiotics in zoo animals: What do we know? *Proceedings of the American Association of Zoo Veterinarians.*

4 Fogelberg, K. and Ferrell, S.T. (2010). Vasculitis secondary to presumptive leptospirosis treated with long-term corticosteroids in a captive lesser kudu (*Tragelaphus imberbis australis*). *Journal of Zoo and Wildlife Medicine* 41 (3): 542–544.

5 Gyimesi, Z.S., Linhart, R.D., Burns, R.B. et al. (2008). Management of chronic vaginal prolapse in an eastern bongo (*Tragelaphus eurycerus isaaci*). *Journal of Zoo and Wildlife Medicine* 39 (4): 614–621.

6 Nie, H., Feng, X., Peng, J. et al. (2016). Comparative pharmacokinetics of ceftiofur hydrochloride and ceftiofur sodium after administration to water buffalo (*Bubalus bubalis*). *American Journal of Veterinary Research* 77 (6): 646–652.

7 Smith, J.S., Sheley, M., and Chigerwe, M. (2018). Aspiration pneumonia in two Tibetan yak bulls (*Bos grunniens*) as a complication of ketamine-xylazine-butorphanol anesthesia for recumbent castration. *Journal of Zoo and Wildlife Medicine* 49 (1): 242–246.

8 Heatley, J.J., Hubert, J., Burba, D. et al. (2000). Distal femoral fracture repair with a modified cobra head plate in a roan antelope (*Hippotragus equinus*). *Proceedings of the International Association of Aquatic Animal Medicine.*

9 Gamble, K.C., Boothe, D.M., Jensen, J.M. et al. (1997). Pharmacokinetics of a single intravenous enrofloxacin dose in scimitar-horned oryx (*Oryx dammah*). *Journal of Zoo and Wildlife Medicine* 28 (1): 36–42.

10 Ball, R.L. and Martel, C. (2006). Surgical repair of stifle injuries in small gazelle species. *Proceedings of the American Association of Zoo Veterinarians.*

11 Musgrave, K.E., Phair, K., and West, G. (2017). Long-term management of fungal pneumonia (*Coccidioides immitis*) in a Kirk's Dik-Dik (*Madoqua kirkii*) in a highly endemic area. *Proceedings of the American Association of Zoo Veterinarians.*

12 Fresno, L., Fernández-Morán, J., Fernández-Bellon, H. et al. (2008). Complicated urethral rupture and scrotal urethrostomy in a bongo antelope (*Tragelaphus eurycerus isaaci*). *Journal of Zoo and Wildlife Medicine* 39 (3): 464–467.

13 Napier, J. and Armstrong, D.L. (2014). Nondomestic cattle. In: *Zoo Animal and Wildlife Immobilization and Anesthesia*, 2e (ed. G. West, D. Heard and N. Caulkett), 863–872. Ames, IA: Wiley Blackwell.

14 Coetzee, J.F., Mosher, R.A., Kohake, L.E. et al. (2011). Pharmacokinetics of oral gabapentin alone or co-administered with meloxicam in ruminant beef calves. *Veterinary Journal* 190: 98–102. https://doi.org/10.1016/j.tvjl.2010.08.008.

15 Rivas, A.E., Hausmann, J.C., Gieche, J. et al. (2017). Clinical management of third phalanx fractures in lesser (*Tragelaphus imberbis*) and greater kudu (*Tragelaphus strepsiceros*). *Journal of Zoo and Wildlife Medicine* 48 (1): 171–178.

16 Wolfe, B.A. (2015). Bovidae (except sheep and goats) and Antilocapridae. In: *Fowler's Zoo and Wild Animal Medicine*, vol. 8 (ed. R.E. Miller and M. Fowler), 626–645. St. Louis, MO: Elsevier Saunders.

17 Kreeger, T., Arnemo, J.M., and Raath, J.P. (2002). *Handbook of Wildlife Chemical Immobilization.* Fort Collins, Colorado: Wildlife Pharmaceuticals Inc.

18 Laricchiuta, P., De Monte, V., Campolo, M. et al. (2012). Evaluation of a butorphanol, detomidine, and midazolam combination for immobilization of captive Nile lechwe antelope (*Kobus magaceros*). *Journal of Wildlife Diseases* 48 (3): 739–746.

19 Chittick, E., Horne, W., Wolfe, B. et al. (2001). Cardiopulmonary assessment of medetomidine, ketamine, and butorphanol anesthesia in captive Thomson's gazelles (*Gazella thomsoni*). *Journal of Zoo and Wildlife Medicine* 32 (2): 168–175.

20 Schumacher, J., Heard, D.J., Young, L. et al. (1997). Cardiopulmonary effects of carfentanil in dama gazelles (*Gazella dama*). *Journal of Zoo and Wildlife Medicine* 28 (2): 166–170.

21 Pas, A. (2014). Gazelle and Small Antelope. In: *Zoo Animal and Wildlife Immobilization and Anesthesia*, 2e (ed. G. West, D. Heard and N. Caulkett), 843–856. Ames, IA: Wiley Blackwell.

22 Junge, R.E. (1998). Epidural analgesia in addax (*Addax nasomaculatus*). *Journal of Zoo and Wildlife Medicine* 29 (3): 285–287.

22 Swenson, J. (2018). Personal communication.

23 Ball, R. and Hofmeyr, M. (2014). Antelope. In: *Zoo Animal and Wildlife Immobilization and Anesthesia*, 2e (ed. G. West, D. Heard and N. Caulkett), 831–841. Ames, IA: Wiley Blackwell.

24 Cole, A., Mutlow, A., Isaza, R. et al. (2006). Pharmacokinetics and pharmacodynamics of carfentanil and naltrex one in female common eland (*Taurotragus oryx*). *Journal of Zoo And Wildlife Medicine* 37 (3): 318–326.

25 Caulkett, N. (2014). Bison. In: *Zoo Animal and Wildlife Immobilization and Anesthesia*, 2e (ed. G. West, D. Heard and N. Caulkett), 873–877. Ames, IA: Wiley Blackwell.

26 Howard, L.L., Kearns, K.S., Clippinger, T.L. et al. (2004). Chemical immobilization of rhebok (*Pelea capreolus*) with carfentanil-xylazine or etorphine-xylazine. *Journal of Zoo and Wildlife Medicine* 35 (3): 312–319.

27 Bouts, T., Dodds, K., Berry, A. et al. (2017). Detomidine and butorphanol for standing sedation in a range of zoo-kept ungulate species. *Journal of Zoo and Wildlife Medicine* 48 (3): 616–626.

28 Perrin, K.L., Denwood, M.J., Grøndahl, C. et al. (2015). Comparison of etorphine-acepromazine and medetomidine-ketamine anesthesia in captive impala (*Aepyceros melampus*). *Journal of Zoo and Wildlife Medicine* 46 (4): 870–879.

29 Portas, T.J., Lynch, M.J., and Vogelnest, L. (2003). Comparison of etorphine-detomidine and medetomidine-ketamine anesthesia in captive addax (*Addax nasomaculatus*). *Journal of Zoo and Wildlife Medicine* 34 (3): 269–273.

30 Zeiler, G.E., Stegmann, G.F., Fosgate, G. et al. (2015). Etorphine-ketamine-medetomidine total intravenous anesthesia in wild impala (*Aepyceros melapmus*) of 120-minute duration. *Journal of Zoo and Wildlife Medicine* 46 (4): 755–766.

31 Mama, K.R., Uhrig, S., Miller, D.S. et al. (2009). Evaluation of two short-term anesthetic protocols in captive juvenile pronghorn (*Antilocapra americana*). *Journal of Zoo and Wildlife Medicine* 40 (4): 803–805.

32 Gerlach, C.A., Kummrow, M.S., Meyer, L.C. et al. (2017). Continuous intravenous infusion anesthesia with medetomidine, ketamine, and midazolam after induction with a combination of etorphine, medetomidine, and midazolam or with medetomidine, ketamine, and butorphanol in impala (*Aepyceros melampus*). *Journal of Zoo and Wildlife Medicine* 48 (1): 62–71.

33 Foster, C.A. (1999). Immobilization of goitred gazelles (*Gazella subgutterosa*) and Arabian mountain gazelles (*Gazella gazella*) with xylazine-ketamine. *Journal of Zoo and Wildlife Medicine* 30 (3): 448–450.

34 Caulkett, N.A., Cattet, M.R.I., Cantwell, S. et al. (1998). Anesthesia of wood bison (*Bison bison athabascae*) with medetomidine-Telazol and xylazine-Telazol combinations. *Proceedings of the American Association of Zoo Veterinarians.*

35 Citino, S.B., Bush, M., Grobler, D. et al. (2002). Anesthesia of boma-captured Lichtenstein's hartebeest (*Sigmoceros lichtensteinii*) with a combination of thiafentanil, medetomidine, and ketamine. *Journal of Wildlife Diseases* 38 (2): 457–462.

36 Laubscher, L.L., Hoffman, L.C., Pitts, N.I. et al. (2016). The effect of a slow-release formulation of zuclopenthixol acetate (AcunilÆ) on captive blue wildebeest (*Connochaetes taurinus*) behavior and physiological response. *Journal of Zoo and Wildlife Medicine* 47 (2): 514–522.

37 Avni-Magen, N., Eshar, D., Friedman, M. et al. (2018). Retrospective evaluation of a novel sustained-release ivermectin varnish for treatment of wound myiasis in zoo-housed animals. *Journal of Zoo and Wildlife Medicine* 49 (1): 201–205.

38 Goossens, E., Vercruysse, J., Vercammen, F. et al. (2006). Evaluation of three strategic parasite control programs in captive wild ruminants. *Journal of Zoo and Wildlife Medicine* 37 (1): 20–26.

39 Thompson, K.A., Lamberski, N., Kass, P.H. et al. (2013). Evaluation of a commercial bovine colostrum replacer for achieving passive transfer of immunity in springbok calves (*Antidorcas marsupialis*). *Journal of Zoo and Wildlife Medicine* 44 (3): 541–548.

28

Nondomestic Goats and Sheep

Drug namet	Drug dose	Species	Comments
Antimicrobials and Antifungals			
Amoxicillin/ clavulanic acid	20 mg/kg IM or IV TID [1]	Domestic sheep and goats	
Amoxicillin trihydrate	10 mg/kg IM TID [1]	Domestic sheep and goats	
Ampicillin sodium	10–20 mg/kg IV or IM BID [1]	Domestic sheep and goats	
Cefovecin (Convenia)	10 mg/kg [2]	Domestic goat	Duration <24 hr, not long-acting.
Ceftiofur crystalline free acid (Excede)	6.6 mg/kg SC [2]	Domestic goat	Half-life 36.9, suspect effective for 6–7 days.
Ceftiofur crystalline free acid (Excede)	6.6 mg/kg SC [3]	Domestic Sheep	Maintained serum concentrations >1 μg/ml for treatment of *Pasteurella multocida* and *Mannheimia haemolytica* for 2.6–4.9 days.
Ceftiofur sodium	1–2.2 mg/kg IM SID [1]	Domestic sheep and goats	
Erythromycin	3–5 mg/kg IM q8–12 hrs [1]	Domestic sheep and goats	
Enrofloxacin	10 mg/kg PO SID [1, 4]	Domestic sheep	Prolonged half-life and high oral bioavailability when tablets are crushed and mixed with grain or enrofloxacin solution mixed with grain, and achieve plasma concentration 8–10 × MIC for most microorganisms. Some sources recommend 5 mg/kg IV or IM SID.
Florfenicol	20 mg/kg IM or 40 mg/kg SC [5]	Domestic sheep	n = 16 adults, given either dose with washout period, half-life 13.4 hrs, and 12.5 hrs respectively.
Griseofulvin	7.5–60 mg/kg PO for 7–20 days [1]	Domestic Sheep	For dermatophytosis.

(*Continued*)

Zoo and Wild Mammal Formulary, First Edition. Alicia Hahn.

Drug namet	Drug dose	Species	Comments
Oxytetracycline	Traditional formulation 10 mg/kg once IM, then 8.5 mg/kg IM SID or long-acting at 20 mg/kg IM once, then 14 mg/kg IM every 48 hrs [6]	Domestic goat	IM cleared much slower than IV and is preferred.
Oxytetracycline hydrochloride	10 mg/kg IV or IM BID (sheep), SID to BID (goats) [1]	Domestic sheep and goats	Treat for at least 7 days for listeriosis.
Oxytetracycline, long-acting (LA 200)	20 mg/kg IM q48–72 hrs [1]	Domestic sheep and goats	
Penicillin G, potassium or sodium	20–40 000 IU/kg IV q6rs [1]	Domestic sheep and goats	
Penicillin G procaine	20–45 000 IU IM SID [1]	Domestic sheep and goats	50 000 IU/kg IM for clostridial infections. 70 000 IU/kg For virulent foot rot due to *Dicheloobacter nodosus*.
Rifampin	20 mg/kg PO SID [7]	Domestic sheep	
Sodium iodide	1 g/14 kg IV repeat at 3–7d intervals or 70 mg/kg IV every 7–10d [1]	Domestic sheep	Dermatophytosis.
Trimethoprim sulfonamide	24–30 mg/kg IM SID to BID [1]	Domestic sheep and goats	
Tulathromycin	2.5 mg/kg [2, 8]	Domestic goat	Half-life 91–129 hrs with single dose, with 2 doses 7 days apart, half-life was 47.3–75.5 hours.
Tylosin	20 mg/kg IM BID [1]	Domestic sheep and goats	
Analgesia			
Aspirin	100 mg/kg PO BID [1]	Domestic goats	
Buprenorphine	0.006 mg/kg IV for 4–8 hrs of pain relief [1]	Domestic sheep	
Butorphanol	B: 0.05–0.5 mg/kg IM [1]	Domestic sheep and goats	For sedation and analgesia.
Carprofen	4 mg/kg SC [1]	Domestic sheep	For postoperative analgesia.
Flunixin meglumine	1.1–2 mg/kg IV or IM SID [1]	Domestic sheep and goats	For analgesia.
Ketoprofen	1–3 mg/kg IM, IV [9]	Musk oxen	For potent analgesia, have used in late-term pregnant animals.
Ketoprofen	3 mg/kg IV or IM SID [1]	Domestic sheep and goats	
Meloxicam	0.4 mg/kg PO SID [9]	Musk oxen	Used for up to a week with no side effects observed, well tolerated orally.
Meloxicam	0.5 mg/kg IV or 1 mg/kg PO [10]	Domestic sheep	n = 6 adult domestic sheep, high oral bioavailability.
Phenylbutazone	10 mg/kg PO SID [1]	Domestic goats	For pain relief.

Drug namet	Drug dose	Species	Comments
Anethesia and Sedation			
Acepromazine	A: 0.1 mg/kg IM [11]	Iberian ibex	n = 7 animals, decreased rectal temperature, provided sedation.
Atipamezole	1–3 mg total for adult [9]	Musk oxen	For reversal.
Atipamezole + doxapram	200 kg cow: A: 1–2 mg + D: 10–15 mg IM [9]	Musk oxen	For animals that are too deep with respiratory depression and low blood pressure can partially reverse alpha-2 agonist and stimulate respiration.
Buprenorphine	B: 0.01–0.02 mg/kg IV or IM [9]	Musk oxen	Used as a reversal agent if animal expected to have pain, but need to partially reverse after potent opiod use. Residual analgesia for 6–8 hrs.
Carfentanil	C: 0.022 mg/kg; antagonize with naltrexone 2 mg/kg [12]	Markhor	
Carfentanil	C: 0.035 mg/kg; antagonize with naltrexone 3.5 mg/kg [12, 13]	Mountain goats	If not down in 20 min, repeat full dose.
Carfentanil	C: 0.04 mg/kg; antagonize with naltrexone 4 mg/kg [12]	Feral goats	
Carfentanil + xylazine	C: 0.013 mg/kg + X: 0.08 mg/kg; antagonize with 1.3 mg/kg naltrexone and yohimbine 0.125 mg/kg [12]	Chamois	
Carfentanil + xylazine	C: 0.04 mg/kg + X: 0.15 mg/kg; antagonize naltrexone 4 mg/kg + yohimbine 0.125 mg/kg [12]	Ibex	If animal not down in 20 min, repeat full dose.
Carfentanil + xylazine	C: 0.044 mg/kg + X: 0.2 mg/kg [13]	Bighorn sheep	
Carfentanil + xylazine + ketamine	C: 4 mg + X: 50 mg + K: 100 mg; antagonize with naltrexone 500 mg + yohimbine 15 mg [13]	Argali sheep	Assumed 90 kg.
Detomidine	0.005–0.02 mg/kg IV [1]	Domestic sheep and goats	For standing sedation.
Detomidine + butorphanol + midazolam	Calf 0–3 mo: D: 0.5–1 mg + B: 1–2 mg + Mid: 0.5–1 mg [9]	Musk oxen	Sedation: to supplement manual restraint.

(*Continued*)

Drug namet	Drug dose	Species	Comments
	Calf 4–6 mo: D: 1.5–3 mg + B: 3–6 mg + Mid: 1.5–4 mg [9]	Musk oxen	Sedation
	Calf 7–9 mo: D: 2.5–3.5 mg + B: 4–6 mg + Mid: 2–4 mg [9]	Musk oxen	Sedation
	Calf 10–12 mo: D: 3–5 mg + B: 5–8 mg + Mid: 3–5 mg [9]	Musk oxen	Sedation
Detomidine + butorphanol + methadone	Adult: D: 17 mg + B: 10 mg + M: 10 mg [9]	Musk oxen	Sedation only for very tame or debilitated animals. Used successfully in a 200 kg adult cow with pneumothorax.
Detomidine + ketamine + Telazol	D: 0.19–0.27 mg/kg + K: 1.4–2 mg/kg + T: 6.8 mg/kg [13]	Alpine ibex	Captive animals.
Diazepam	0.05–0.1 mg/kg IM [13]	Musk oxen	To induce muscle relaxation, could instead use 5% guaifenesin.
Etorphine	E: 4–5 mg/animal [13]	Mountain goats	
Etorphine	E: 0.028 mg/kg; antagonize with 0.056 mg/kg diprenorphine [12]	Feral goats	
Etorphine + acepromazine (Large Animal Immobilon = E: 2.45 mg/ml + A: 10 mg/ml)	LAI: Give 0.8 ml IM; antagonize with 2 mg diprenorphine per mg of etorphine given [12]	Chamois	
Etorphine + acepromazine + xylazine (Large Animal Immobilon = E: 2.45 mg/ml + A: 10 mg/ml)	LAI: 0.7 ml + X: 10 mg IM [12]	Markhor	Antagonize with 2 mg diprenorphine per mg of etorphine given plus yohimbine 0.125 mg/kg.
	LAI: 0.8 ml + X: 10 mg IM [12]	Ibex	Antagonize with 2 mg diprenorphine per mg of etorphine given plus yohimbine 0.125 mg/kg.
Etorphine + xylazine	E: 0.05 mg/kg + X: 0.15 mg/kg IM [13]	Musk oxen	n = 133 wild musk oxen.
	E: 3.5 mg + X: 50 mg [13]	Bighorn sheep	
	E: 4 mg + X: 30 mg; antagonize with diprenorphine 8 mg and yohimbine 0.15 mg/kg [12]	Mountain goats	
Etorphine + xylazine + hyaluronidase	E: 2 mg + X: 30 mg + H: 200 IU [13]	Musk oxen	Free-ranging animals.

Drug namet	Drug dose	Species	Comments
Etorphine + ketamine + xylazine	E: 2 mg + K: 20 mg + X: 20 mg; antagonize with diprenorphine 4 mg and yohimbine 0.15 mg/kg [12]	Ibex, Markhor	
Etorphine + ketamine + xylazine + midazolam	Yearling: E: 0.6–0.8 mg + K: 8–10 mg + X: 6–8 mg + Mid: 1 mg [9]	Musk oxen	Anesthesia.
	Subadult 14–18 mo: E: 0.8–1 mg + K: 8–10 mg + X: 8–10 mg + Mid: 1–2 mg [9]	Musk oxen	Anesthesia.
	2 yr. old: E: 1–1.2 mg + K: 10–12 mg + X: 10–12 mg + Mid: 1–2 mg [9]	Musk oxen	Anesthesia.
	Adult cow: per 100 kg weight: E: 0.8–1 mg/kg + K: 10 mg + X: 8–10 mg + Mid: 1 mg [9]	Musk oxen	Anesthesia.
	Adult bull, per 100 kg weight: E: 0.6–1 mg/kg + K: 10 mg + X: 6–10 mg + Mid: 1 mg [9]	Musk oxen	Anesthesia. Bulls usually need less per kg of weight than cows, several times 300 kg docile Bulls have been anesthetized with dose for 200 kg cows.
Fentanyl + xylazine	F: 0.05 mg/kg + 0.5 mg/kg; antagonize with 0.2 mg/kg naloxone + yohimbine 0.125 mg/kg [12]	Chamois, Ibex	Monitor for hyperthermia and respiratory depression.
Haloperidol	H: 0.33 mg/kg IM [11]	Iberian ibex	n = 7 animals, decreased rectal temperature, provided sedation.
Ketamine	K: 20 mg/kg [12]	Feral goats	
Ketamine + medetomidine	K: 1.5 mg/kg + M: 0.05–0.06 mg/kg IM [13]	Musk oxen	Short-term anesthesia.
	K: 1.5 mg/kg + M: 0.08–0.14 mg/kg; antagonize with 0.5 mg/kg atipamezole [12, 13]	Ibex, Barbary sheep, Himalayan tahr	Tahr, captive M: 0.08–0.1 mg/kg; Barbary, captive, M:0.1–0.14 mg/kg.
	K: 1.5 mg/kg + M: 0.06–0.1 mg/kg; antagonize with 0.4 mg/kg atipamezole [13]	Chamois	For captive animals; in free-ranging animals used K: 1.5–2 mg/kg + M: 0.08–0.1 mg/kg to reduce time to recumbency.
	K: 1.6 mg/kg + M: 0.063 mg/kg	Markhor	Moderate hypoxemia but more complete immobilization than etorphine 0.056 mg/kg + acepromazine 0.25 mg/kg.

(Continued)

Drug namet	Drug dose	Species	Comments
	K: 2 mg/kg + M: 0.05 mg/kg; antagonize with 0.25 mg/kg atipamezole [12]	Feral goats	If not down in 15 min, repeat full dose.
	K: 2 mg/kg + M: 0.07 mg/kg; antagonize with atipamezole 0.35 mg/kg half IV and half IM [12]	Mountain goats	For captive animals.
Ketamine + medetomidine	K: 2 mg/kg + M: 0.06–0.08 mg/kg; antagonize with atipamezole 3 × dose in mg of medetomidine [13]	Bighorn Sheep, Dall or Stone's Sheep, Mountain IM, goats	Captive animals; for free-ranging animals use K: 2.6–5.8 mg/kg + M: 0.12–0.2 mg/kg stalked on foot.
	K: 2 mg/kg + M: 0.08 mg/kg; antagonize with atipamezole 0.4 mg/kg half IV and half IM [12]	Markhor	Supplement with ketamine 1 mg/kg as needed; rapid, smooth induction <5 min, and antagonism <10 min.
	K: 2 mg/kg + M: 0.1 mg/kg; antagonize with atipamezole 0.5 mg/kg half IV and half IM [12]	Chamois	Supplement with ketamine 1 mg/kg as needed.
	K: 2.5 mg/kg + M: 0.125 mg/kg IM [13]	Mouflon	Captive animals.
	K: 3 mg/kg + M: 0.1–0.12 mg/kg [13]	Ibex	Free-ranging animals.
Ketamine + xylazine	K: 1.5–2.9 mg/kg + X: 1.4–2.4 mg/kg [13]	Ibex	Free-ranging animals.
	K: 2.5 mg/kg + X: 3 mg/kg IM; antagonize with atipamezole 0.3 mg/kg [12]	Chamois	
Medetomidine + butorphanol	M: 0.03 mg/kg + B: 0.2–0.25 mg/kg OM; antagonize with naltrexone 0.35 mg/kg atipamezole at 5 × medetomidine dose in mg [14]	Takin (Sichuan and Mishmi subspecies)	Immobilizations: Smooth induction and good relaxation, with bradycardia and low SpO2 values, remedied by oxygen at 4–6 l/min. Smooth recovery in 7–8 min.
Midazolam	Mid: 0.5 mg/kg IV or IM [15]	Domestic sheep	n = 8 healthy rams, with drug half-life of 0.35–1.23 hrs and 0.2–0.72 hrs respectively, both are suitable short-term sedative methods.
Naltrexone	100 × the carfentanil dose in mg [16, 17]	Domestic goats	n = 8 adult goats, immobilized with carfentanil, then reversed with IM, IV, or SC naltrexone, with smoothest recoveries with IM administration. Less renarcotization than with naloxone or nalmefene (n = 9).

Drug namet	Drug dose	Species	Comments
Perphenazine (Trilafon Dekanoate)	P: 0.51 mg/kg [9]	Musk oxen	
Propofol	4–6 mg/kg IV [1]	Domestic sheep and goats	For induction of anesthesia.
Telazol	T: 15 mg/kg [12]	Feral goats	
Telazol + xylazine	T: 4.2 mg/kg + X: 0.5 mg/kg IM [13]	Bighorn sheep	Human-habituated sheep.
	T: 2 mg/kg + X: 1 mg/kg [13]	Stone's sheep	Captive animals.
Telazol + xylazine + Hydromorphone	T: 1.64 mg/kg + X: 1.1 mg/kg + H: 0.22 mg/kg IM [13]	Bighorn sheep	Superior to T + X alone in human-habituated sheep; antagonize with atipamezole 0.11 mg/kg and naltrexone 0.18 mg/kg, recovery rapid in ~10 min.
Xylazine	X: 0.5–1 mg/kg ± ketamine at 1–2 mg/kg [13]	Musk oxen	Tame, human-habituated animals.
Xylazine	X: 5 mg/kg [12]	Mountain goats	Only for trapped animals.
Zuclopenthixol-acetate (Cisordinol-Acutard 50 mg/ml) and zuclopenthixol-decanoate (Cisordinol depot 200 mg/ml)	1 ml/80–100 kg [9]	Musk Oxen	Introduction of new herd members, to new enclosure, or transport. Both the short-acting 72 hrs and depot form (21 days), are very effective.
Antiparasitic			
Albendazole	5 mg/kg PO [1]	Domestic sheep	For nematodes and tapeworms. 7.5 mg/kg PO in goats.
Amprolium	25–40 mg/kg PO SID × 5d for treatment, 5 mg/kg PO SID × 21d for prevention [1]	Domestic sheep and goats	
Clorsulon	7 mg/kg PO [1]	Domestic sheep and goats	To treat fluke infestation.
Decoquinate	2 mg/kg PO SID [1]	Domestic sheep	To prevent abortion from *Toxoplasma gondii* throughout gestation.
	0.5 mg/kg in feed for at least 28d [1]	Domestic goats	For coccidiosis.
Doramectin	0.2 mg/kg SC [1]	Domestic sheep and goats	For lungworms, cooperia, and GI parasites.
Eprinomectin	0.5 mg/kg PO [1]	Domestic sheep and goats	
Fenbendazole	5 mg/kg PO [1]	Domestic sheep and goats	Anecdotal reports indicate 10–20 mg/kg PO may be needed for efficacy.

(Continued)

Drug namet	Drug dose	Species	Comments
Ivermectin	0.2 mg/kg PO or SC, two doses 7 days apart [1]	Domestic sheep and goats	Two doses for Psoroptic mites. Anecdotal reports suggest 0.3 mg/kg may be needed for nematode parasite control.
Levamisole	8 mg/kg PO [1]	Domestic sheep and goats	Anecdotal reports indicate 12 mg/kg PO may be needed for efficacy.
Moxidectin	0.2–0.5 mg/kg PO or SC [1]	Domestic sheep and goats	For nematodes.
Praziquantel	10–15 mg/kg PO [1]	Domestic sheep and goats	For tapeworms.
Pyrantel pamoate	25 mg/kg PO [1]	Domestic sheep and goats	
Sulfamethazine	110 mg/kg PO SID × 5d [1]	Domestic sheep and goats	Coccidiosis.
Triclabendazole	40 mg/kg [18]	Bighorn Sheep	n = 9 Sheep were experimentally infected with liver flukes, then 5 sheep treated, 4 untreated; for treated group: at 6 weeks post treatment no eggs detected in feces. Appeared safe and effective.
Other			
Ammonium chloride	450 mg/kg PO SID [19]	Domestic goats	n = 15 male, yearling, castrated goats, this dose required to achieve urinary pH of <6.5 in goats.
Ammonium chloride	0.5% of diet or 100–200 mg/kg PO BID [1]	Domestic sheep	For prevention of urinary calculi.
Calcium borogluconate	50 ml of 20 mg/ml calcium solution IV or SC [1]	Domestic sheep	To treat hypocalcemia.
Calcium borogluconate	60–100 ml of 20–25% solution [1]	Domestic goats	To treat hypocalcemia.
Dexamethasone	0.44 mg/kg IM once [1]	Domestic goats	Anti-inflammatory.
	0.1–1 mg/kg IV or IM [1]	Domestic sheep	For inflammation.
Dexamethasone sodium phosphate	1–2 mg/kg IV [1]	Domestic sheep and goats	For circulatory shock.
Dextrose	60–100 ml of 50% solution IV [1]	Domestic sheep	To treat pregnancy toxemia.
	1 g q4 hrs IV until recovery [1]	Domestic goats	For ketosis.
Diazepam	0.4 mg/kg IV [1]	Domestic goats	To stimulate appetite.
	0.5–1 mg/kg [1]	Domestic goats	For tetany.
Epinephrine	0.02–0.03 mg/kg SC, IM, IV [1]	Ruminants	

Drug namet	Drug dose	Species	Comments
Furosemide	2–5 mg/kg PO or 1–2 mg/kg IV, IM SID to BID [1]	Domestic sheep and goats	For heart failure and fluid retention.
	5–10 mg/kg IV [1]	Domestic sheep and goats	For anuria or lack of urine production.
Insulin	20–40 units IV over 5–10 min [1]	Domestic sheep	For pregnancy toxemia.
Iron (ferrous sulfate)	0.5–2 g/day PO for up to 2 weeks [1]	Domestic sheep and goats	
Lidocaine	1–2 mg/kg IV over 60 sec [1]	Domestic sheep	For ventricular arrhythmias.
	2–4 ml [1]	Domestic goats	For caudal epidural anesthesia. Be careful not to approach toxic dose.
Mannitol	0.25–1.5 g/kg IV over 5 min [1]	Domestic sheep and goats	For diuresis.
Melengesterol acetate	0.125 mg BID for 8–14d [1]	Domestic sheep	For estrus synchronization.
Metoclopramide	0.1 mg/kg IM or IV BID [1]	Domestic sheep	
Mineral oil	0.5–1 l total PO [1]	Domestic sheep	For treatment of bloat.
Oxytocin	30–50 IU IV, IM, SC or 10–20 IU IM q2 hrs [1]	Domestic sheep and goats	Latter dose used for retained placenta in goats.
Propylene glycol	60 ml of 600 mg/ml solution orally [1]	Domestic sheep	PO for mild signs of pregnancy toxemia – i.e. non-comatose.
Propylene glycol	1–2 oz PO [1]	Domestic goats	For treatment of ketosis.
Vitamin B12 (Cyanocobalamin)	1000 µg/head IM [1]	Domestic sheep and goats	For deficiency.
Vitamin K1 (Phylloquinone)	0.5–2.5 mg/kg IM [1]	Domestic sheep and goats	For poisoning by warfarin and related compounds.

Species	Weight [20]
Aoudad/Barbary Sheep *(Ammotragus lervia)*	40–145 kg
Bharal/Blue sheep *(Pseudois nayaur)*	35–75 kg
Bighorn sheep *(Ovis canadensis)*	Female 55–90 kg, Male 55–135 kg
Chamois *(Rupicapra rupicapra or Rupicapra pyrenica)*	Female 30–35 kg, Male 40–50 kg
Dall/Thin horn sheep *(Ovis dalli)*	65–140 kg
Goat, Feral *(Capra hircus)*	20–80 kg
Goral *(Naemorhedus griseus)*	35–45 kg
Ibex *(Capra ibex, Capra nubiana, Capra pyrenica)*	40–120 kg
Japanese serow *(Capricornus crispus)*	30–130 kg
Markhor *(Capra falconeri)*	Female 30–40 kg, Male 80–110 kg

(Continued)

Species	Weight [20]
Muskox *(Ovibos moshatus)*	180–400 kg
Rocky mountain goat *(Oreamnos americanus)*	Female 45–70 kg, Male 70–100 kg
Tahr *(Hemitragus, Arabitragus, Nilgiritragus)*	Female 45–70 kg, Male 50–125 kg
Takin *(Budorcas taxicolor)*	Female 150–250 kg, Male 200–400 kg
Urial *(Ovis orientalis arkal)*	Female 40–50 kg, Male 60–100 kg

References

1 Fajt, V.R. and Pugh, D.G. (2002). Commonly used drugs in sheep and goats: suggested dosages. In: *Sheep and Goat Medicine* (ed. D.G. Pugh), 435–444. Philadelphia, PA: Saunders.

2 Gull, J.M. Muntener, C.R., and Hatt, J.M. (2012). Long-acting antibiotics in zoo animals: What do we know? *Proceedings of American Association of Zoo veterinarians*. 82–85.

3 Rivera-Garcia, S., Angelos, J.A., Rowe, J.D. et al. (2014). Pharmacokinetics of Ceftiofur crystalline-free acid following subcutaneous administration of a single dose to sheep. *American Journal of Veterinary Research* 75 (3): 290–295.

4 Bermingham, E.C. and Papich, M.G. (2002). Pharmacokinetics after intravenous and oral administration of Enrofloxacin in sheep. *American Journal of Veterinary Research* 63 (7): 1012–1017.

5 Balcomb, C.C., Angelos, J.A., Chigerwe, M. et al. (2018). Comparative pharmacokinetics of two Florfenicol formulations following intramuscular and subcutaneous administration to sheep. *American Journal of Veterinary Research* 79 (1): 107–114.

6 Escudero, E., Carceles, C.M., and Serrano, J.M. (1994). Pharmacokinetics of Oxytetracycline in goats: modifications induced by a long-acting formula. *The Veterinary Record* 135 (23): 548–552.

7 Jernigan, A.D., St. Jean, G.D., Rings, D.M. et al. (1991). Pharmacokinetics of rifampin in adult sheep. *Veterinary Research* 52 (10): 1626–1629.

8 Romanet, J., Smith, G.W., Leavens, T.L. et al. (2012). Pharmacokinetics and tissue elimination of Tulathromycin following subcutaneous administration in meat goats. *American Journal of Veterinary Research* 73 (10): 1634–1640.

9 Grøndahl, C. (2018). Musk ox sedation and anesthesia. In: *Fowler's Zoo and Wild Animal Medicine Current Therapy*, vol. 9 (ed. R.E. Miller, N. Lamberski and P.P. Calle), 636–640. St. Louis, MO: Elsevier.

10 Stock, M.L., Coetzee, J.F., Kukanich, B. et al. (2013). Pharmacokinetics of intravenously and orally administered meloxicam in sheep. *American Journal of Veterinary Research* 74 (5): 779–783.

11 Casas-Diaz, E., Marco, I., Lopez-Olvera, J.R. et al. (2012). Effect of acepromazine and haloperidol in male Iberian ibex (*Capra pyrenaica*) captured by box-trap. *Journal of Wildlife Diseases* 48 (3): 763–767.

12 Kreeger, T.J. and Arnemo, J.M. (2012). *Handbook of Wildlife Chemical Immobilization*. China: Kreeger.

13 Caulkett, N. and Walzer, C. (2014). Wild sheep and goats. In: *Zoo Animal and Wildlife Immobilization and Anesthesia*, 2e (ed. G. West, D. Heard and N. Caulkett), 857–862. Ames, IA: Wiley Blackwell.

14 Morris, P.J., Bicknese, E., Janssen, D. et al. (2000). Chemical immobilization of Takin (*Budorcas taxicolor*) at the San Diego Zoo. *Annual Proceedings of the International Association of Aquatic Animal Medicine.*
15 Simon, B.T., Scallan, E.M., Odette, O. et al. (2017). Pharmacokinetics and pharmacodynamics of midazolam following intravenous and intramuscular administration to sheep. *American Journal of Veterinary Research* 78 (5): 539–549.
16 Mutlow, A., Isaza, R., Carpenter, J.W. et al. (2004). Pharmacokinetics of carfentanil and naltrexone in domestic goats (*Capra capra*). *Journal of Zoo and Wildlife Medicine* 35 (4): 489–496.
17 Shaw, M.L., Carpenter, J.W., and Galland, J.C. (1993). Comparison of Opiod Antagonists in reversing the immobilization of carfentanil citrate in the domestic goat. *Annual Proceedings of the American Association of Zoo Veterinarians*. 261–264.
18 Foreyt, W.J. (2009). Experimental infection of Bighorn sheep with liver flukes (*Fasciola hepatica*). *Journal of Wildlife Diseases* 45 (4): 1217–1220.
19 Mavangira, V., Cornish, J.M., and Angelos, J.A. (2010). Effect of ammonium chloride supplementation on urine pH and urinary fractional excretion of electrolytes in goats. *Journal of the American Veterinary Medical Association* 237 (11): 1299–1304.
20 Weber, M.A. (2015). Sheep, goats, and goat-like animals. In: *Zoo and Wild Animal Medicine* (ed. R.E. Miller and M. Fowler), 645–649. St. Louis, MO: Elsevier Saunders.

Index

Zoo and Wild Mammal Formulary, First Edition. Alicia Hahn.

d

e

f